Nurse Practitioner's Quick Reference to Clinical Facts

Nurse Practitioner's Quick Reference to Clinical Facts

LIPPINCOTT WILLIAMS & WILKINS
A Wolters Kluwer Company

Philadelphia • Baltimore • New York • London
Buenos Aires • Hong Kong • Sydney • Tokyo

STAFF

Executive Publisher
Judith A. Schilling McCann, RN, MSN

Editorial Director
H. Nancy Holmes

Clinical Director
Joan M. Robinson, RN, MSN

Senior Art Director
Arlene Putterman

Editorial Project Manager
William Welsh

Clinical Project Manager
Mary Perrong, RN, CRNP, MSN,
APRN,BC, CPAN

Editors
Teresa P. Sussman,
Elizabeth Jacqueline Mills

Clinical Editors
Jana L. Sciarra, RN, CRNP, MSN;
Roseanne Hanlon Rafter, RN, MSN, CS

Copy Editors
Kimberly Bilotta (supervisor),
Tom DeZego, Heather Ditch,
Judith Orioli, Carolyn Petersen,
Kelly Taylor, Pamela Wingrod

Designers
ON-TRAK graphics, inc.
(project manager)

Digital Composition Services
Diane Paluba (manager),
Joyce Rossi Biletz, Donna S. Morris

Manufacturing
Patricia K. Dorshaw (director),
Beth J. Welsh

Editorial Assistants
Megan L. Aldinger,
Tara L. Carter-Bell, Linda K. Ruhf

Librarian
Wani Z. Larsen

Indexer
Barbara Hodgson

The clinical treatments described and recommended in this publication are based on research and consultation with nursing, medical, and legal authorities. To the best of our knowledge, these procedures reflect currently accepted practice. Nevertheless, they can't be considered absolute and universal recommendations. For individual applications, all recommendations must be considered in light of the patient's clinical condition and, before administration of new or infrequently used drugs, in light of the latest package insert information. The authors and publisher disclaim any responsibility for any adverse effects resulting from the suggested procedures, from any undetected errors, or from the reader's misunderstanding of the text.

NPQR – D N O S A J J M
06 05 04   10 9 8 7 6 5 4 3 2 1

**Library of Congress
Cataloging-in-Publication Data**

Nurse practitioner's quick reference to clinical facts.
p. ; cm.
Includes bibliographical references and index.
1. Nurse practitioners—Handbooks, manuals, etc. 2. Nursing—Handbooks, manuals, etc. I. Lippincott Williams & Wilkins.
[DNLM: 1. Nursing Process—Handbooks. WY 49 N97294 2005]
RT82.8.N867 2005
610.73—dc22
ISBN 1-58255-336-X (alk. paper)
2004000379

Contents

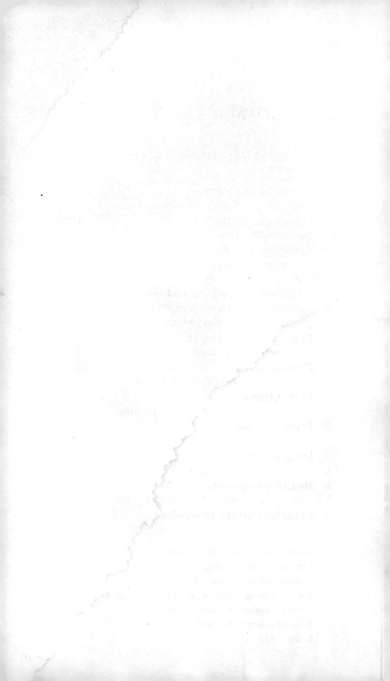

Contributors and consultants

Natalie Burkhalter, RN, MSN, CNS-MS, FNP-BC, ACNP-BC
Associate Professor
Texas A&M International University
Laredo

Cynthia L. Frozena, RN, MSN, CHPN
Medical Writer
Enzymatic Therapy
Green Bay, Wisc.

Linda Fuhrman, RN, MS, ANP
Nurse Practitioner
San Francisco Veterans
  Administration

Catherine Grant, MSN, CRNP
Instructor
Carlow College
Pittsburgh

James J. Greco, MSN, ARNP-BC
Instructor
University of Florida
Gainesville

Janice D. Hausauer, RN, MS, FNP
Adjunct Assistant Professor
Montana State University College of
  Nursing
Bozeman

Shelley Yerger Huffstutler, RN, DSN, CFNP, GNP
Associate Professor of Nursing
Director, Primary Care Nurse
  Practitioner Program
University of Virginia School of
  Nursing
Charlottesville

Sharon L.G. Lee, NP-C, MS, BSN, CCRN
Clinical Educator — Emergency
  Services
Bryan LGH Medical Center
Lincoln, Nebr.

Donna Scemons, RN, MSN, CNS, FNP-C
Family Nurse Practitioner
Healthcare Systems, Inc.
Panorama City, Calif.

Foreword

As nurse practitioners (NPs), we're advancing our scope of care faster than ever before. In the United States alone, more than 100,000 of us are actively bridging gaps in the health care system. From rural clinics to specialized teams in highly regarded medical centers, we've created a niche for ourselves as contributors to high-quality, outcome-oriented care. Every day, we gain more of the public's trust.

Our success is based on our sound clinical decision-making skills and our unique approach to individual and family care. Our ability to assess, treat, and think critically about our patients' presenting signs, symptoms, and conditions is grounded in our solid educational background, which emphasizes history-taking and physical assessment, laboratory testing, and treatment decisions. Recognizing the importance of this background, we've increased the rigor of our professional education requirements to build and maintain our diagnostic acumen as we've grown in numbers. Because of this, finding clinical texts that are substantial enough — and diverse enough — to meet our special needs hasn't always been easy.

Thankfully, *Nurse Practitioner's Quick Reference to Clinical Facts* is an excellent contribution to our growing repertory of ready-reference titles. Its breadth and depth of content is impressive. It doesn't matter if you work in primary care, acute care, long-term care, or any other practice setting — *Nurse Practitioner's Quick Reference to Clinical Facts* is an indispensible clinical companion.

Chapter 1 covers everything you need to know to conduct a thorough patient assessment. It begins by leading you through normal findings for auscultation, inspection, palpation, and percussion of every body system and then provides highly detailed flowcharts that explore some of the most common chief complaints encountered in clinical practice. Beginning with a symptom, each flowchart quickly and easily guides you to an accurate differential diagnosis.

It doesn't get any easier than this.

Chapter 2 on laboratory testing is particularly useful, especially because of the ever-increasing number of diagnostic tests we have to choose from. It covers the most commonly administered diagnostic tests, complete with a test overview, and its purpose, normal findings and reference values, and abnormal findings and their implications. Each of the procedures is described in a clear, concise manner. Students and experienced NPs will find this chapter a great asset in today's explosion of health care technology.

Chapter 3 reviews X-ray interpretation by providing illustrations of some of the most common X-rays results you'll see. If you have any questions about what lung cancer, a pleural effusion, arthritis, or a small-bowel obstruction looks like on film, then this is the chapter for you.

Chapter 4 covers ECG interpretation. No matter how proficient you are in this vital skill, accurate interpretation can sometimes be difficult. This chapter allows you to quickly reference many different ECG waveforms and rhythm strips to help you rapidly identify even the most complicated arrhythmias.

Chapter 5 discusses the wide array of dermatologic disorders that you might encounter in clinical practice. Each entry alerts you to the condition's contagiousness and its causes, clinical presentation, differential diagnosis, management, possible complications, and any applicable patient teaching instructions to provide a complete condition overview.

Chapter 6 on disease management is one of the book's highlights. Not only does it cover everything from acute coronary syndromes to urinary tract infections, each entry provides enough detail to competently manage these diverse diseases and disorders and get your patient on the road to recovery.

Chapter 7 covers emergency care, an important topic for NPs, yet one that's usually overlooked in clinical textbooks. The chapter contains a comprehensive yet succinct discussion of common emergency problems faced by NPs, including corneal abrasions, concussions, and anaphylaxis.

Chapter 8 reviews precautions, which have increased in importance because of the specter of bioterrorism and the recent outbreaks of deadly communicable diseases such as severe acute respiratory syndrome. Remember, safety is always a priority.

Chapter 9 provides step-by-step breakdowns of some of our most commonly performed procedures, such as soft-tissue aspiration, fracture immobilization, and wart removal. After reviewing this chapter, you'll perform these procedures with the utmost of confidence.

Chapter 10 addresses drug hazards and, specifically, how to best manage drug overdoses. With so many drugs in today's marketplace, the importance of knowing the signs and symptoms of overdose and interaction and how to immediately respond can't be overstated. This is a chapter that no NP should be without.

Chapter 11 discusses ways that you can improve your patients' overall health by promoting preventative care over the life span. The chapter provides guidelines for maternal-neonatal, infant and child, adolescent, and adult health, and goes in-depth on such topics as nutrition, exercise, and injury prevention.

Chapter 12, the book's final chapter, tackles the emerging field of complementary therapies. As more and more patients are taking charge of their own health care by pursuing complementary therapies — with or without their health care provider's advice — it's essential that you know the right questions to ask your patients. Your ability to identify alternative therapies that conflict with conventional practices is absolutely vital.

Throughout the text, *Nurse Practitioner's Quick Reference to Clinical Facts* emphasizes key points in many different ways that make this book truly a quick reference for busy NPs. Charts, tables, and illustrations filled with insightful information abound and make answer retrieval quick and easy. Eye-catching icons call your attention to some of the most vital clinical information. *Red flag* highlights special alerts and precautions you need to consider when caring for your patients. *Life span* discusses differences in care among different age-groups, while *Cultural key* discusses differences in care among different ethnic groups. *Clinical pearl* provides best-practice tips and other valuable pearls of information. Appendices include charts on crisis values of laboratory tests, laboratory value changes in elderly patients, potential agents of bioterrorism, and the Food and Drug Administration's list of toxic herbs.

Nurse Practitioner's Quick Reference to Clinical Facts is an indispensable quick resource, a complete guide that you'll use on a daily basis. It will help you to improve your skills and increase your confidence. As an NP and educator of NPs for more than 20 years, I highly recommend it as a clinical reference and as an adjunct to basic textbooks for NP students.

Eileen M. Sullivan-Marx, PhD, CRNP, FAAN
Associate Professor
Associate Dean for Practice & Community Affairs
Shearer Endowed Term Chair for Healthy Community Practices
University of Pennsylvania, School of Nursing
Philadelphia

1
Assessment findings
Arriving at a differential diagnosis

Review of normal findings

To distinguish between health and disease, you must be able to recognize normal assessment findings. Begin by completing a health history that includes the patient's past and present health information and a physical examination of each body system. (See *Obtaining a health history*.) When performing the physical examination, use the following head-to-toe assessment of normal findings as a reference. It's designed to help you quickly zero in on physical abnormalities and evaluate your patient's overall condition.

GENERAL SURVEY

▶ Alert and oriented; responds appropriately
▶ Well-groomed and well-nourished
▶ Vital signs, height, and weight within normal range for age-group

SKIN
Inspection

▶ Color varying from pink to dark brown, depending on ethnic background
▶ Texture smooth and intact
▶ No pallor, jaundice, cyanosis, bruising, erythema, rashes, or lesions
▶ Nail bed color varying from pink to brown depending on skin color
▶ Angle of nail base 160 degrees or less
▶ Normal hair texture and distribution

Palpation

▶ Smooth, warm, dry skin
▶ Turgor good (skin quickly returns to original shape when gently squeezed)

HEAD AND NECK
Inspection

▶ Symmetrical, lesion-free skull
▶ Symmetrical facial structures with no cyanosis or vascular lesions
▶ Unrestricted range of motion in the neck
▶ Ability to shrug the shoulders, a sign of an adequately functioning cranial nerve XI (spinal accessory nerve)
▶ No bulging of the thyroid

Palpation

▶ No lumps or tenderness on the head
▶ Symmetrical strength in the facial muscles, a sign of adequately functioning cranial nerves V and VII (trigeminal and facial nerves)
▶ Symmetrical sensation when stroked with a wisp of cotton on each cheek
▶ Mobile, soft lymph nodes less than $1/2''$ (1.3 cm) with no tenderness
▶ Symmetrical pulses in the carotid arteries
▶ Palpable, symmetrical, lesion-free thyroid and absence of thyroid tenderness
▶ Midline location of the trachea and absence of tracheal tenderness
▶ No crepitus, tenderness, or lesions in the cervical spine
▶ Symmetrical muscle strength in the neck

Auscultation

▶ No bruits heard over carotid arteries or over the thyroid gland

EYES
Inspection

▶ No edema, scaling, or lesions on the eyelids
▶ Eyelids completely covering the corneas when closed

OBTAINING A HEALTH HISTORY

Use a health history to gather subjective data about your patient and explore his previous and current health problems. The information you obtain combined with the results of physical examination and diagnostic testing will assist you in making an accurate patient diagnosis.

Start the history by asking the patient about his general physical and emotional health, and then ask him questions about the specific body systems.

Make the patient comfortable

Before asking your first question, make sure you establish a good rapport with the patient. The following tips may help:
▶ Choose a quiet, private, well-lit interview setting away from distractions.
▶ Introduce yourself, then ask the patient to sit down. Make sure he's comfortably seated.
▶ Explain to the patient that the purpose of the health history and assessment is to identify his problem and provide information for planning care.
▶ Speak slowly and clearly. Avoid the use of medical terms and jargon.
▶ Listen attentively and use reassuring gestures to encourage the patient to talk.
▶ Watch for nonverbal cues that indicate the patient is uncomfortable or unsure about how to answer a question. Make sure that he understands each question.

Ask specific questions

Asking the right question is a critical part of any interview. To obtain a complete health history, gather information from each of the following categories, in sequence:
▶ Biographic data: name, address, phone number, date of birth, birthplace, sex, marital status, ethnic origin, occupation
▶ Source of history: patient, family member, friend
▶ Chief complaint: a brief statement by the patient describing the reason for seeking care
▶ History of present illness: a chronological description about the present illness from the time of symptom onset
▶ Current medications: prescribed and over-the-counter medications, herbal remedies, and supplements
▶ Past medical history: childhood illnesses, accidents, injuries, hospitalizations, surgeries, blood transfusions, serious or chronic illnesses, obstetric history in females, immunizations, and allergies (drug, food, environmental, and latex)
▶ Family history: health status or cause of death of immediate relatives
▶ Psychosocial history: how the patient feels about himself, his place in society, relationships with others, and coping strategies; also involves feelings of safety, which may refer to physical, psychological, emotional, or sexual abuse issues
▶ Activities of daily living: diet and elimination patterns; exercise and sleeping patterns; work and leisure activities; alcohol, tobacco, or illicit drug use; religious observances; and use of safety measures, such as seat belts, bike helmets, and sunblock
▶ Health maintenance: date of last examination or office visit with family physician, dentist, and optometrist; also, screening procedures and immunizations.

(continued)

▶ Eyelid color same as surrounding skin color
▶ Palpebral fissures of equal height
▶ Margin of upper lid falling between the superior pupil margin and the superior limbus

OBTAINING A HEALTH HISTORY *(continued)*

Review of systems
The last part of the health history is a systematic review of each body system to make sure that important symptoms weren't missed. The order of the review of systems is head-to-toe.
▸ General health
▸ Skin and hair
▸ Head
▸ Eyes, ears, and nose
▸ Mouth and throat
▸ Neck
▸ Respiratory system
▸ Cardiovascular system
▸ Breasts
▸ Gastrointestinal system
▸ Urinary system
▸ Reproductive system
▸ Musculoskeletal system
▸ Neurologic system
▸ Endocrine system
▸ Hematologic system
▸ Emotional status

▸ Symmetrical, lesion-free upper eyelids that don't lag or droop when the patient opens his eyes
▸ Evenly distributed eyelashes that curve outward
▸ Globe of eye neither protruding from nor sunken into the orbit
▸ Eyebrows with equal size, color, and distribution
▸ Clear conjunctiva with visible small blood vessels and no signs of drainage
▸ White sclera visible through the conjunctiva
▸ Symmetrical irises of the same color
▸ Transparent anterior chamber that contains no visible material when a penlight is shone into the side of the eye
▸ Transparent, smooth, and bright cornea with no visible irregularities or lesions
▸ Closing of the lids of both eyes when each cornea is stroked with a wisp of cotton, a test of cranial nerve V (trigeminal nerve)
▸ Round, equal-sized pupils that react normally to light and accommodation
▸ Constriction of both pupils when a light is shone on one eye
▸ Lacrimal structures free of exudate, swelling, and excessive tearing
▸ Proper eye alignment
▸ Parallel eye movement in each of the six cardinal fields of gaze
▸ Positive red reflex, sharp disc margins, vessels present all quadrants without arteriovenous crossing deflects, and no hemorrhage or exudates (ophthalmoscopic examination)

Palpation

▸ Absence of eyelid swelling and tenderness
▸ Globes equally firm without feeling overly hard or spongy
▸ Lacrimal sacs don't regurgitate fluid

EARS
Inspection

▸ Bilaterally symmetrical, proportionately sized auricles that have a vertical measurement between $1\frac{1}{2}''$ and $4''$ (4 and 10 cm)
▸ Lip of ear crossing eye-occiput line (an imaginary line extending from the lateral aspect of the eye to the occipital protuberance)
▸ Long axis of ear perpendicular to (or no more than 10 degrees from perpendicular to) the eye-occiput line

- Color match between the ears and facial skin
- No signs of inflammation, lesions, or nodules
- No cracking, thickening, scaling, or lesions behind the ear when the auricle is bent forward
- No visible discharge from auditory canal
- Patent external meatus
- Skin color on the mastoid process that matches the skin color of the surrounding areas
- No redness or swelling
- Pearl-gray tympanic membrane; bright light reflex; landmarks intact; and no perforation, scarring, inflammation, or drainage (otoscopic examination)

Palpation

- No masses or tenderness on the auricle
- No tenderness on the auricle or tragus during manipulation
- Either small, nonpalpable lymph nodes on the auricle or discrete, mobile lymph nodes with no signs of tenderness
- Well-defined, bony edges on the mastoid process with no signs of tenderness

NOSE, MOUTH, AND THROAT

Inspection

- Symmetrical, lesion-free nose with little or no deviation of the septum or discharge
- Little or no nasal flaring
- Nonedematous frontal and maxillary sinuses
- Ability to identify familiar odors
- Pinkish red nasal mucosa with no visible lesions and no purulent drainage
- No evidence of foreign bodies or dried blood in the nose
- Pink lips with no dryness, cracking, lesions, or cyanosis

- Symmetrical facial structures
- Ability to purse the lips and puff out the cheeks, sign of an adequately functioning cranial nerve VII (facial nerve)
- Ability to easily open and close the mouth
- Light pink, moist oral mucosa with no ulcers or lesions
- Visible salivary ducts with no inflammation
- White hard palate
- Pink soft palate
- Pink gums with no tartar, inflammation, or hemorrhage
- All teeth intact with no signs of occlusion, caries, or breakage
- Pink tongue with no swelling, coating, ulcers, or lesions
- Tongue that moves easily and without tremor, sign of a properly functioning cranial nerve XII (hypoglossal nerve)
- No swelling or inflammation on anterior and posterior arches
- No lesions or inflammation on posterior pharynx
- Lesion-free tonsils that are the right size for the patient's age
- Uvula that moves when the patient says "ah" and a gag reflex when a tongue blade touches the posterior pharynx, signs of properly functioning cranial nerves IX (glossopharyngeal) and X (vagus)

Palpation

- No structural deviation, tenderness, or swelling in the external nose
- No tenderness or edema on the frontal and maxillary sinuses
- Lips free from pain and induration
- No lesions, unusual color, tenderness, or swelling on the posterior and lateral surfaces of the tongue
- No tenderness, nodules, or swelling on the floor of the mouth

THORAX AND LUNGS
Inspection
▶ Side-to-side symmetrical chest configuration
▶ Anteroposterior diameter less than the transverse diameter, with a 1:2 to 5:7 ratio in an adult
▶ Normal chest shape with no deformities, such as a barrel chest, kyphosis, retraction, sternal protrusion, and depressed sternum
▶ Costal angle less than 90 degrees with the ribs joining the spine at a 45-degree angle
▶ Quiet, unlabored respirations with no use of accessory neck, shoulder, or abdominal muscles; no intercostal, substernal, or supraclavicular retractions
▶ Symmetrically expanding chest wall during respiration
▶ Normal adult respiratory rate of 16 to 20 breaths/minute; some variation expected, depending on the patient's age
▶ Regular respiratory rhythm with expiration taking about twice as long as inspiration (Men and children breathe diaphragmatically, whereas women breathe thoracically.)
▶ Skin color that matches the rest of the body's complexion

Palpation
▶ Warm, dry skin
▶ No tender spots or bulges in the chest

Percussion
▶ Resonant percussion sounds over the lungs

Auscultation
▶ Loud, high-pitched breath sounds over the trachea
▶ Intense, medium-pitched bronchovesicular breath sounds over the mainstem bronchi, between the scapulae, and below the clavicles
▶ Soft, breezy, low-pitched vesicular breath sounds over most of the peripheral lung fields

HEART
Inspection
▶ No visible pulsations, except at the point of maximal impulse (PMI)
▶ No lifts (heaves) or retractions in the four valve areas of the chest wall

Palpation
▶ No detectable vibrations or thrills
▶ No lifts
▶ No pulsations, except at the PMI and epigastric area (At the PMI, a tapping pulse that's less than ½" [1.3 cm] in diameter [localized] may be felt at the start of systole. In the epigastric area, pulsation from the abdominal aorta may be palpable.)

Auscultation
▶ The first heart sound (S_1), which is the "lub" sound best heard with the diaphragm of the stethoscope over the mitral area when the patient is in a left lateral position (It sounds longer, lower, and louder there than a second heart sound [S_2]. S_1 splitting may be audible in the tricuspid area.)
▶ S_2 sound, which is the "dub" sound heard best with the diaphragm of the stethoscope in the aortic area while the patient sits and leans over (It sounds shorter, sharper, higher, and louder there than S_1 sounds. Normal S_2 splitting may be audible in the pulmonic area on inspiration.)
▶ The third heart sound (S_3), which is normal in children and slender, young adults with no cardiovascular disease (It usually disappears between ages 25 to 35. In an older adult, it may signify heart failure. S_3 may be best heard over the mitral area with the patient in a

supine position and exhaling. It sounds short, dull, soft, and low.)
▶ Murmurs, which may be functional in children and young adults but are abnormal in older adults (Innocent murmurs are soft and short and vary with respirations and patient position. They occur in early systole and are best heard in pulmonic or mitral positions with the patient in a supine position.)

BREASTS AND AXILLAE
Inspection

▶ Breast skin smooth and same color as rest of the skin
▶ Slightly asymmetrical breasts (left breast usually slightly larger)
▶ No edema, erythema, dimpling, or nipple discharge

Palpation

▶ No nodules or unusual tenderness
▶ Firm inframammary ridge at breast's lower edge
▶ Round, elastic nipples
▶ Soft, small, nontender axillary nodes

ABDOMEN
Inspection

▶ Skin free from vascular lesions, jaundice, surgical scars, and rashes
▶ Faint venous patterns (except in thin patients)
▶ Flat, round, or scaphoid abdominal contour
▶ Symmetrical abdomen
▶ Umbilicus positioned midway between the xiphoid process and the symphysis pubis with a flat or concave hemisphere
▶ No variations in the color of the patient's skin
▶ No apparent bulges
▶ Abdominal movement apparent with respiration
▶ Pink or silver-white striae from pregnancy or weight loss

Auscultation

▶ High-pitched, gurgling bowel sounds heard every 5 to 15 seconds through the diaphragm of the stethoscope
▶ Vascular sounds heard through the bell of the stethoscope
▶ Venous hum over the inferior vena cava
▶ No bruits, murmurs, friction rubs, or other venous hums

Percussion

▶ Tympany predominantly over hollow organs, including the stomach, intestines, bladder, abdominal aorta, and gallbladder
▶ Dullness over solid masses, including the liver, spleen, pancreas, kidneys, uterus, and full bladder

Palpation

▶ No tenderness or masses
▶ Abdominal musculature free from tenderness and rigidity
▶ No guarding, rebound tenderness, distention, or ascites
▶ Unpalpable liver except in children (If palpable, liver edge is regular, sharp, and nontender and is felt no more than ¾" [1.9 cm] below the right costal margin.)
▶ Unpalpable spleen
▶ Unpalpable kidneys except in thin patients or those with a flaccid abdominal wall (Right kidney is felt more commonly than left.)

EXTREMITIES
Inspection

▶ No gross deformities
▶ Symmetrical body parts
▶ Good body alignment
▶ No involuntary movements
▶ Smooth gait
▶ Active range of motion (ROM) in all muscles and joints
▶ No pain with active ROM
▶ No visible swelling or inflammation of joints or muscles

▶ Equal bilateral limb length and symmetrical muscle mass
▶ No peripheral edema

Palpation

▶ Normal shape with no swelling or tenderness
▶ Equal bilateral muscle tone, texture, and strength
▶ No involuntary contractions or twitching
▶ Equally strong bilateral pulses

NEUROLOGIC SYSTEM
Inspection

▶ Appropriate mental status, behavior, and thought processes
▶ Coherent speech
▶ Intact memory (remote and recent)
▶ Intact cranial nerves I to XII
▶ Smooth gait
▶ No involuntary movements
▶ Negative for Romberg's sign; no pronator drift
▶ Intact deep tendon reflexes
▶ Intact light touch, pinprick, position vibration, and stereognosis sensations

Palpation

▶ Symmetrical facial muscle strength
▶ Adequate muscle tone and strength

GENITOURINARY SYSTEM
Inspection

▶ No lesions, discoloration, or swelling on the skin over the kidneys and bladder areas
▶ No urethral discharge or ulcerations
▶ Pubic area free from lesions and parasites
In females
▶ Labia majora moist and free from lesions
▶ Normal vaginal discharge
▶ Smooth, round cervix
In males
▶ Slightly wrinkled penis, with color ranging from pink to dark brown, depending on the patient's skin color
▶ Pink, smooth urethral meatus
▶ Scrotum free from swelling and edema, but some sebaceous cysts

Percussion

▶ No costovertebral angle tenderness
▶ Tympany heard over the empty bladder

Palpation

▶ Unpalpable kidneys, except in very thin and elderly patients
▶ Unpalpable bladder
In females
▶ Soft labia, without swelling, hardness, or tenderness
▶ Unpalpable Bartholin's glands
▶ No nodularity, tenderness or bulging of vaginal wall
▶ Smooth, firm cervix that protrudes $1/4''$ to $1 1/4''$ (0.5 to 3 cm) into the vagina; freely movable in all directions
In males
▶ Firm penis with smooth, movable skin
▶ Equally sized, firm, smooth, rubbery testicles that move freely in the scrotal sac
▶ Smooth, discrete, nontender epididymis that's free from swelling and induration
▶ No inguinal or femoral hernias
▶ Smooth, rubbery prostate gland that's about the size of a walnut; doesn't protrude into the rectal lumen

Auscultation

▶ No bruits heard over the renal arteries

Exploring some of the most common chief complaints

A patient's chief complaint is the starting point for almost every initial assessment. To evaluate the complaint thoroughly, you'll need to ask the right health history questions, conduct a physical examination based on the history data you collect, and analyze possible causes of the problem.

The following flowcharts examine 16 complaints frequently encountered in clinical practice. Beginning with a common symptom, each flowchart quickly and easily guides the practitioner to an accurate differential diagnosis. Common medical abbreviations have been used throughout to make the charts easier to read. (See *Flowchart abbreviations*.)

FLOWCHART ABBREVIATIONS

ABC	airway, breathing, and circulation	I.V.	intravenous
ABG	arterial blood gas	JVD	jugular venous distention
ACE	angiotensin-converting enzyme	KUB	kidneys, ureters, and bladder (X-ray)
AFB	acid-fast bacilli	L	left, liter
BP	blood pressure	LFT	liver function tests
BUN	blood urea nitrogen	LLQ	left lower quadrant
C	centigrade; Celsius	LOC	level of consciousness
CBC	complete blood count	LUQ	left upper quadrant
CEA	carcinoembryonic antigen	MI	myocardial infarction
CNS	central nervous system	MRA	magnetic resonance angiography
COPD	chronic obstructive pulmonary disease	MRI	magnetic resonance imaging
CT	computed tomography	NGT	nasogastric tube
CXR	chest X-ray	NPO	nothing by mouth
DX	diagnosis	NSAID	nonsteroidal anti-inflammatory drug
ECG	electrocardiogram	PCI	percutaneous coronary intervention
EMG	electromyogram		
ESR	erythrocyte sedimentation rate	PE	physical examination
F	Fahrenheit	PFT	pulmonary function tests
F/U	follow-up	PRBC	packed red blood cells
Hb	hemoglobin	ROM	range of motion
HCG	human chorionic gonadotropin	SLE	systemic lupus erythematosus
HEENT	head, eyes, ears, nose, and throat	SOB	shortness of breath
		Tc	technetium
HLA	human leukocyte antigen	TEE	transesophageal echocardiogram
HOB	head of bed		
HPI	history of present illness	TMJ	temporomandibular joint
ICP	intracranial pressure	TX	treatment
IU	international unit	UA	urinalysis
		V̇/Q̇	ventilation-perfusion ratio

ABDOMINAL PAIN, ACUTE

HPI

Focused PE: Abdomen, rectum

Abdominal aortic aneurysm
Signs and symptoms
▸ Pulsating periumbilical mass
▸ Systolic bruit over the aorta
▸ Constant upper abdominal pain or lower back pain

LIFE-THREATENING SIGNS AND SYMPTOMS (may signify rupture)
▸ Severe abdominal and back pain
▸ Mottled skin below the waist
▸ Absent femoral and pedal pulses
▸ Lower BP in the legs than in the arms
▸ Abdominal rigidity
▸ Signs of shock

DX: Imaging studies (ultrasonography, CT scan, MRI, angiography)
TX: BP control, reduction of atherosclerotic risk factors, surgery
F/U: BP monitoring as indicated, serial ultrasounds, return visit 1 week after discharge (if surgery is performed)

Diverticulitis (acute)
Signs and symptoms
▸ LLQ pain
▸ Abdominal rigidity and guarding
▸ High-grade fever
▸ Chills
▸ Signs of shock

DX: Labs (CBC, UA, chemistry panel), imaging studies (abdominal upright X-ray, CT scan, ultrasonography)
TX: Low-residue diet, antibiotics, surgery
F/U: Barium enema after acute episode subsides, return visit 1 week after discharge (if surgery is performed)

Ectopic pregnancy
Signs and symptoms
▸ Lower abdominal pain that's sharp, dull, or cramping
▸ Vaginal bleeding
▸ Nausea and vomiting
▸ Urinary frequency
▸ Tender adnexal mass
▸ History of amenorrhea in past 1 to 2 months

LIFE-THREATENING SIGNS AND SYMPTOMS (may signify rupture)
▸ Sharp lower abdominal pain that radiates to the shoulders and neck and becomes extreme with cervical or adnexal palpation
▸ Signs of shock

DX: Labs (urine pregnancy test, serum HCG, CBC), imaging studies (vaginal and abdominal ultrasonography, CT scan, MRI, intravaginal color Doppler flow imaging)
TX: Surgery
F/U: Serial HCG levels (until 0 IU/ L), follow-up imaging if retained placenta is suspected

Renal calculi
Signs and symptoms
▸ Severe abdominal or back pain
▸ Severe colicky pain that travels from the costovertebral angle to the flank, suprapubic region, and external genitalia
▸ Pain that may be excruciating or dull and constant
▸ Pain-induced agitation
▸ Nausea and vomiting
▸ Abdominal distention
▸ Fever and chills
▸ Urinary frequency with hematuria and dysuria

DX: Labs (CBC, BUN, creatine, UA), imaging studies (abdominal X-ray, I.V. urography, spiral CT scan, ultrasound)
TX: Pain relief, increased fluid intake, percutaneous chemolysis, systemic chemolysis, endourologic stone extraction, extracorporeal shock wave lithotripsy
F/U: Urologic referral, if chronic or obstruction; weekly creatinine level until stable; continued urine straining until stone has passed and then stone analysis, if able

Abdominal pain usually results from a GI disorder, but it can also be caused by a reproductive, genitourinary, musculoskeletal, or vascular disorder; drug use; or ingestion of toxins. At times, this symptom signals life-threatening complications.

Appendicitis
Signs and symptoms
▶ Dull discomfort in the epigastric or umbilical region
▶ Anorexia
▶ Nausea and vomiting
▶ Localized pain at McBurney's point
▶ Abdominal rigidity
▶ Rebound tenderness
▶ Positive Rovsing's, psoas, obturator, and cough signs
DX: Labs (CBC, UA, amylase), imaging studies (KUB, CT scan, ultrasound)
TX: Surgery, antibiotics
F/U: Return visits at 2 and 6 weeks after discharge

...if ruptured, may lead to...

Pancreatitis
Signs and symptoms
▶ Fulminating, continuous upper abdominal pain that may radiate to the flanks and back
▶ Nausea and vomiting
▶ Fever
▶ Pallor
▶ Tachycardia
▶ Abdominal rigidity
▶ Rebound tenderness
▶ Hypoactive bowel sounds
▶ Positive Turner's and Cullen's signs (indicate hemorrhagic pancreatitis)
▶ Jaundice
DX: Labs (amylase, lipase, CBC, bilirubin, glucose, electrolytes, LFT), imaging studies (KUB, CT scan, ultrasound)
TX: NPO, bed rest, medication (analgesics, antibiotics), I.V. fluids, electrolyte replacement, and NG tube for severe vomiting and ileus
F/U: Monitoring of amylase levels until normal; if they remain elevated, repeat imaging studies

Peritonitis
Signs and symptoms
▶ Sudden, severe pain that worsens with movement
▶ Vomiting (may be projectile)
▶ Constipation
▶ High-grade fever
▶ Decreased bowel sounds
▶ Rebound tenderness
▶ Abdominal rigidity and guarding
▶ Signs of shock
DX: Labs (peritoneal fluid culture, CBC), imaging studies (abdominal X-ray, CT scan, abdominal sonography)
TX: Bowel decompression, antibiotics, surgery for underlying condition
F/U: Return visit 1 week after discharge, then as needed

Additional differential diagnoses: abdominal cancer • abdominal trauma • acute cholecystitis • acute cholelithiasis • acute hepatitis • adrenal crisis • cholangitis • diabetic ketoacidosis • gastroenteritis • heart failure • hepatic abscess • hepatic amebiasis • hernia (inguinal or ventral) • herpes zoster • intestinal obstruction • intestinal perforation • Meckel's diverticulitis • mesenteric artery ischemia • MI • perforated ulcer • pneumonia • pyelonephritis • retroperitoneal bleed • ruptured ovarian cyst • ruptured spleen • sickle cell crisis • SLE

Other causes: insect toxins

ANXIETY

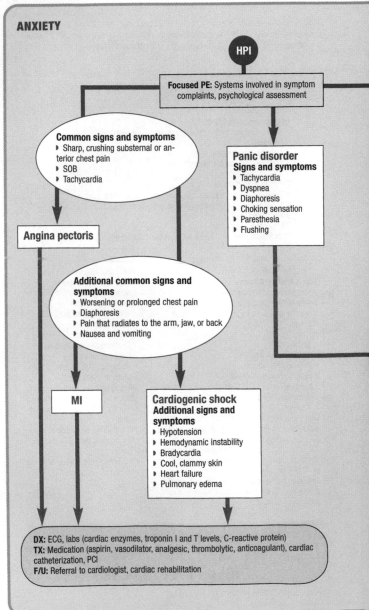

HPI

Focused PE: Systems involved in symptom complaints, psychological assessment

Common signs and symptoms
▸ Sharp, crushing substernal or anterior chest pain
▸ SOB
▸ Tachycardia

Panic disorder
Signs and symptoms
▸ Tachycardia
▸ Dyspnea
▸ Diaphoresis
▸ Choking sensation
▸ Paresthesia
▸ Flushing

Angina pectoris

Additional common signs and symptoms
▸ Worsening or prolonged chest pain
▸ Diaphoresis
▸ Pain that radiates to the arm, jaw, or back
▸ Nausea and vomiting

MI

Cardiogenic shock
Additional signs and symptoms
▸ Hypotension
▸ Hemodynamic instability
▸ Bradycardia
▸ Cool, clammy skin
▸ Heart failure
▸ Pulmonary edema

DX: ECG, labs (cardiac enzymes, troponin I and T levels, C-reactive protein)
TX: Medication (aspirin, vasodilator, analgesic, thrombolytic, anticoagulant), cardiac catheterization, PCI
F/U: Referral to cardiologist, cardiac rehabilitation

A subjective reaction to a real or imagined threat, anxiety is a nonspecific feeling of uneasiness or dread. It may be mild, moderate, or severe. Mild anxiety may cause slight physical or psychological discomfort. Severe anxiety may be incapacitating or even life-threatening.

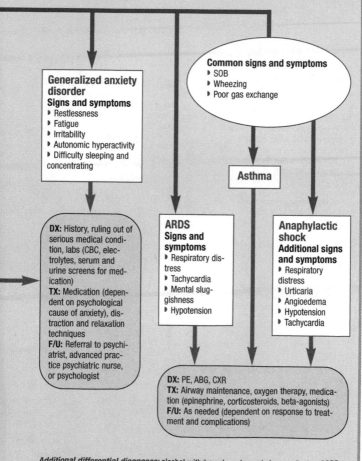

Generalized anxiety disorder
Signs and symptoms
▶ Restlessness
▶ Fatigue
▶ Irritability
▶ Autonomic hyperactivity
▶ Difficulty sleeping and concentrating

Common signs and symptoms
▶ SOB
▶ Wheezing
▶ Poor gas exchange

Asthma

DX: History, ruling out of serious medical condition, labs (CBC, electrolytes, serum and urine screens for medication)
TX: Medication (dependent on psychological cause of anxiety), distraction and relaxation techniques
F/U: Referral to psychiatrist, advanced practice psychiatric nurse, or psychologist

ARDS
Signs and symptoms
▶ Respiratory distress
▶ Tachycardia
▶ Mental sluggishness
▶ Hypotension

Anaphylactic shock
Additional signs and symptoms
▶ Respiratory distress
▶ Urticaria
▶ Angioedema
▶ Hypotension
▶ Tachycardia

DX: PE, ABG, CXR
TX: Airway maintenance, oxygen therapy, medication (epinephrine, corticosteroids, beta-agonists)
F/U: As needed (dependent on response to treatment and complications)

Additional differential diagnoses: alcohol withdrawal • autonomic hyperreflexia • COPD • depression • hyperthyroidism • hyperventilation syndrome • hypoglycemia • mitral valve prolapse • obsessive-compulsive disorder • pheochromocytoma • phobias • pneumonia • pneumothorax • postconcussion syndrome • posttraumatic stress disorder • pulmonary embolism • rabies • somatoform disorder

Other causes: antidepressants • CNS stimulants • sympathomimetics

BACK PAIN

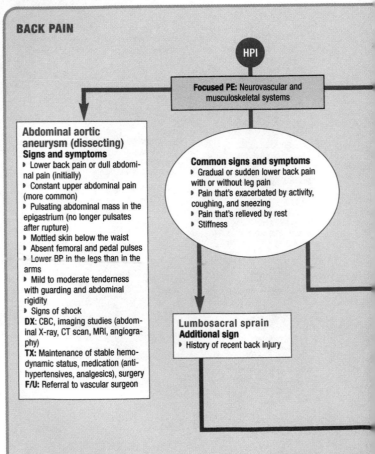

HPI

Focused PE: Neurovascular and musculoskeletal systems

Abdominal aortic aneurysm (dissecting)
Signs and symptoms
▶ Lower back pain or dull abdominal pain (initially)
▶ Constant upper abdominal pain (more common)
▶ Pulsating abdominal mass in the epigastrium (no longer pulsates after rupture)
▶ Mottled skin below the waist
▶ Absent femoral and pedal pulses
▶ Lower BP in the legs than in the arms
▶ Mild to moderate tenderness with guarding and abdominal rigidity
▶ Signs of shock
DX: CBC, imaging studies (abdominal X-ray, CT scan, MRI, angiography)
TX: Maintenance of stable hemodynamic status, medication (antihypertensives, analgesics), surgery
F/U: Referral to vascular surgeon

Common signs and symptoms
▶ Gradual or sudden lower back pain with or without leg pain
▶ Pain that's exacerbated by activity, coughing, and sneezing
▶ Pain that's relieved by rest
▶ Stiffness

Lumbosacral sprain
Additional sign
▶ History of recent back injury

Back pain may herald a spondylogenic, genitourinary, GI, cardiovascular, or neoplastic disorder. Postural imbalance associated with pregnancy may also cause back pain. The onset, location, and distribution of pain and its response to activity and rest provide important clues about the causative disorder.

Ankylosing spondylitis
Signs and symptoms
▶ Sacroiliac pain that travels up the spine and is aggravated by lateral pressure on the pelvis
▶ Pain that's most severe in the morning or after inactivity
▶ Pain that's unrelieved by rest
▶ Local tenderness
▶ Fatigue
▶ Fever
▶ Anorexia
▶ Weight loss
▶ Iritis (occasional)
DX: Labs (histocompatibility antigens, HLA-B27, ESR, CBC), imaging studies (spinal and pelvic X-rays)
TX: NSAIDs, physical therapy, surgery (for severe joint damage and pain)
F/U: Return visit in 6 to 12 months for evaluation of posture and ROM

Intervertebral disk disorder
Additional signs and symptoms
▶ Positive sciatic scratch test
▶ Positive cross straight-leg raising sign
▶ Paresthesia

DX: Imaging studies (spinal X-ray, CT scan, MRI, myelogram), EMG, nerve conduction velocity test
TX: Bed rest, medication (analgesics, NSAIDs, muscle relaxants), surgery (for disk disorder), physical therapy
F/U: Reevaluation 10 days after treatment, then again in 2 months; referral to neurosurgeon

Additional differential diagnoses: acute cauda equina • appendicitis • cholecystitis • chordoma • endometriosis • metastatic tumors • myeloma • pancreatitis (acute) • perforated ulcer • prostate cancer • pyelonephritis (acute) • Reiter's syndrome • renal calculi • sacroiliac strain • spinal neoplasm (benign) • spinal stenosis • spondylolisthesis • transverse process fracture • vertebral compression fracture • vertebral osteomyelitis • vertebral osteoporosis

Other causes: neurologic tests, such as lumbar puncture and myelography

CHEST PAIN, CARDIAC

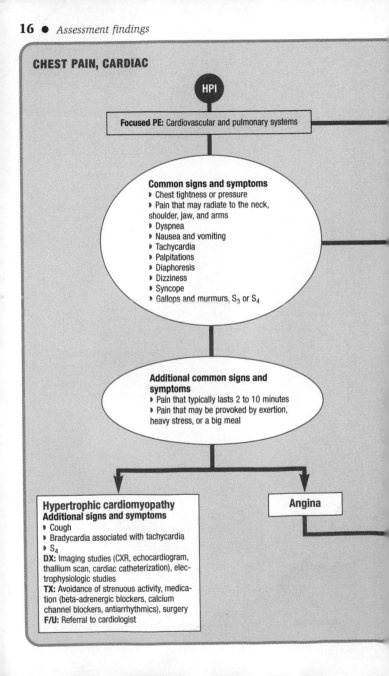

HPI

Focused PE: Cardiovascular and pulmonary systems

Common signs and symptoms
▶ Chest tightness or pressure
▶ Pain that may radiate to the neck, shoulder, jaw, and arms
▶ Dyspnea
▶ Nausea and vomiting
▶ Tachycardia
▶ Palpitations
▶ Diaphoresis
▶ Dizziness
▶ Syncope
▶ Gallops and murmurs, S_3 or S_4

Additional common signs and symptoms
▶ Pain that typically lasts 2 to 10 minutes
▶ Pain that may be provoked by exertion, heavy stress, or a big meal

Hypertrophic cardiomyopathy
Additional signs and symptoms
▶ Cough
▶ Bradycardia associated with tachycardia
▶ S_4
DX: Imaging studies (CXR, echocardiogram, thallium scan, cardiac catheterization), electrophysiologic studies
TX: Avoidance of strenuous activity, medication (beta-adrenergic blockers, calcium channel blockers, antiarrhythmics), surgery
F/U: Referral to cardiologist

Angina

Chest pain usually results from a disorder affecting the thoracic or abdominal organs. An important indicator of several acute and life-threatening cardiopulmonary and GI disorders, chest pain can also result from a musculoskeletal or hematologic disorder, anxiety, or drug therapy.

Pericarditis
Signs and symptoms
▶ Sharp or stabbing precordial or retrosternal pain
▶ Pain that's aggravated by movement, inspiration, or lying supine
▶ Pericardial friction rub
▶ Low-grade fever
▶ Dyspnea
▶ Cough
▶ Dysphagia
DX: Imaging studies (echocardiogram, CT scan, MRI), ECG
TX: Medication (NSAIDs; if bacterial, antibiotics)
F/U: Return visit 2 weeks after treatment

MI
Additional signs and symptoms
▶ Feeling of impending doom
▶ Pain that may escalate to crushing
▶ Hypotension or hypertension
▶ Pallor
▶ Clammy skin

DX: Labs (serial cardiac enzymes, troponin, myoglobin, electrolytes, coagulation studies), imaging studies (echocardiogram, CXR, Tc-99m sestamibi scan, ECG, cardiac catheterization)
TX: Maintenance of ABCs; medication (dependent on severity of myocardial involvement and medical history—antithrombic agents, vasodilators, analgesics, beta-adrenergic agents, thrombolytics, anticoagulants, platelet aggregation inhibitors, anxiolytics, antiarrhythmics); low-fat, low-sodium diet; PCI; surgery
F/U: Referral to cardiologist

Additional differential diagnoses: aortic aneurysm (dissecting) • costochondritis • mediastinitis

Other causes: beta-adrenergic blockers (abrupt withdrawal can cause rebound angina in patients with coronary heart disease) • Chinese restaurant syndrome • cocaine use

CHEST PAIN, PULMONARY

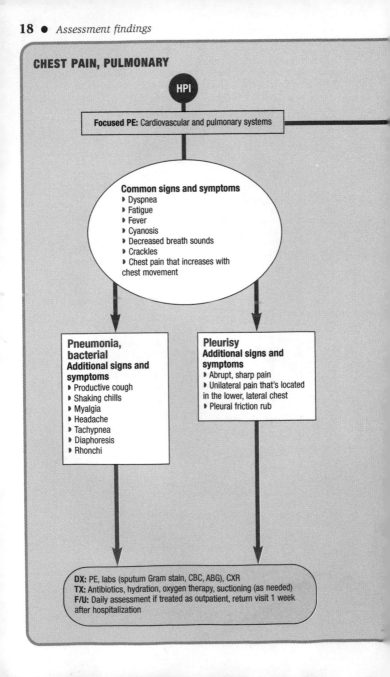

HPI

Focused PE: Cardiovascular and pulmonary systems

Common signs and symptoms
▶ Dyspnea
▶ Fatigue
▶ Fever
▶ Cyanosis
▶ Decreased breath sounds
▶ Crackles
▶ Chest pain that increases with chest movement

Pneumonia, bacterial
Additional signs and symptoms
▶ Productive cough
▶ Shaking chills
▶ Myalgia
▶ Headache
▶ Tachypnea
▶ Diaphoresis
▶ Rhonchi

Pleurisy
Additional signs and symptoms
▶ Abrupt, sharp pain
▶ Unilateral pain that's located in the lower, lateral chest
▶ Pleural friction rub

DX: PE, labs (sputum Gram stain, CBC, ABG), CXR
TX: Antibiotics, hydration, oxygen therapy, suctioning (as needed)
F/U: Daily assessment if treated as outpatient, return visit 1 week after hospitalization

Chest pain usually results from a disorder affecting the thoracic or abdominal organs. An important indicator of several acute and life-threatening cardiopulmonary and GI disorders, chest pain can also result from a musculoskeletal or hematologic disorder, anxiety, or drug therapy.

Common signs and symptoms
- Acute central cyanosis
- Sharp chest pain that's exacerbated with movement
- SOB
- Anxiety
- Tachycardia

Pneumothorax
Additional signs and symptoms
- Asymmetrical chest wall expansion
- Rapid, shallow respirations
- Pallor
- Jugular vein distention
- Absence of breath sounds over the affected lobe

DX: PE, ABG, CXR

TX: Chest tube and oxygen therapy

F/U: Referral to thoracic specialist, return visit 1 week after hospitalization

Pulmonary embolism
Additional signs and symptoms
- Syncope
- Jugular vein distention
- Pulsus paradoxus
- Low-grade fever
- Cough (with blood-tinged sputum)

DX: ABG, imaging studies (CXR, V̇/Q̇ scan, arteriogram, spiral chest CT)

TX: Oxygen therapy, medication (thrombolytic, anticoagulants)

F/U: Referral to pulmonologist, return visit 1 week after hospitalization

Additional differential diagnoses: blastomycosis • bronchitis • interstitial lung disease • lung abscess • lung cancer • pulmonary actinomycosis • pulmonary hypertension • tuberculosis

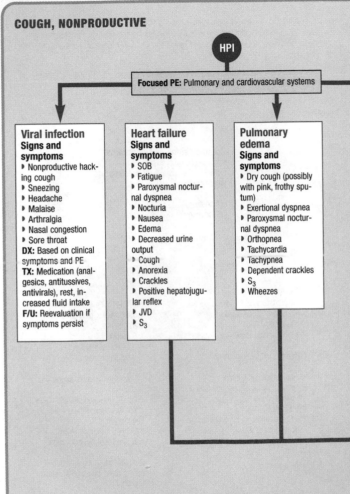

COUGH, NONPRODUCTIVE

HPI

Focused PE: Pulmonary and cardiovascular systems

Viral infection
Signs and symptoms
▶ Nonproductive hacking cough
▶ Sneezing
▶ Headache
▶ Malaise
▶ Arthralgia
▶ Nasal congestion
▶ Sore throat
DX: Based on clinical symptoms and PE
TX: Medication (analgesics, antitussives, antivirals), rest, increased fluid intake
F/U: Reevaluation if symptoms persist

Heart failure
Signs and symptoms
▶ SOB
▶ Fatigue
▶ Paroxysmal nocturnal dyspnea
▶ Nocturia
▶ Nausea
▶ Edema
▶ Decreased urine output
▶ Cough
▶ Anorexia
▶ Crackles
▶ Positive hepatojugular reflex
▶ JVD
▶ S_3

Pulmonary edema
Signs and symptoms
▶ Dry cough (possibly with pink, frothy sputum)
▶ Exertional dyspnea
▶ Paroxysmal nocturnal dyspnea
▶ Orthopnea
▶ Tachycardia
▶ Tachypnea
▶ Dependent crackles
▶ S_3
▶ Wheezes

A nonproductive cough is a noisy, forceful expulsion of air from the lungs that doesn't yield any sputum or blood. It may occur in paroxysms and can worsen by becoming more frequent. An acute cough has a sudden onset and may be self-limiting; a cough that persists beyond 3 months is considered chronic and, in many cases, results from cigarette smoking.

Interstitial lung disease
Signs and symptoms
▶ Progressive dyspnea
▶ Cyanosis
▶ Clubbing
▶ Fine crackles
▶ Fatigue
▶ Variable chest pain
▶ Weight loss
DX: CBC, CXR, PFT, lung biopsy
TX: Removal of source of problem, if known (for example, occupational chemical exposure); supportive therapy; medication (corticosteroids, cytotoxic drugs); single-lung transplantation
F/U: As needed (dependent on the severity of the disease); referral to pulmonologist

GERD
Signs and symptoms
▶ Irritative nonproductive cough
▶ Heartburn
▶ Dysphagia
DX: Barium esophagography, esophageal pH monitoring, upper endoscopy
TX: Lifestyle modification, medication (antacids, histamine-2 receptor antagonists; promotility agents, proton pump inhibitors), surgery
F/U: Referral to a gastroenterologist

DX: ABG, imaging studies (CXR, echocardiography), ECG, pulmonary artery catheterization
TX: Airway maintenance, ventilation and oxygenation; medication (diuretics, ACE inhibitors, inotropic agents, morphine, vasodilation); low-sodium diet
F/U: Referral to cardiologist

Additional differential diagnosis: airway occlusion (partial) • aortic aneurysm (thoracic) • asthma • atelectasis • bronchogenic carcinoma • Hantavirus pulmonary syndrome • laryngeal tumor • laryngitis • legionnaires' disease • pleural effusion • sarcoidosis • sinusitis (chronic)

Other causes: bronchoscopy • inhalants • intermittent positive-pressure breathing • PFTs • tracheal suctioning

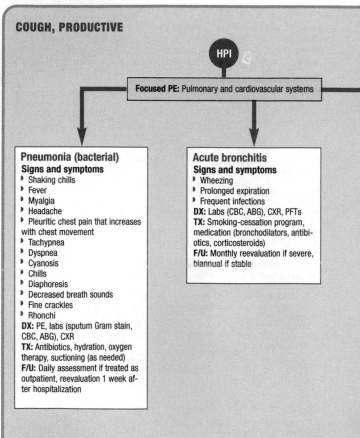

COUGH, PRODUCTIVE

HPI

Focused PE: Pulmonary and cardiovascular systems

Pneumonia (bacterial)
Signs and symptoms
▸ Shaking chills
▸ Fever
▸ Myalgia
▸ Headache
▸ Pleuritic chest pain that increases with chest movement
▸ Tachypnea
▸ Dyspnea
▸ Cyanosis
▸ Chills
▸ Diaphoresis
▸ Decreased breath sounds
▸ Fine crackles
▸ Rhonchi
DX: PE, labs (sputum Gram stain, CBC, ABG), CXR
TX: Antibiotics, hydration, oxygen therapy, suctioning (as needed)
F/U: Daily assessment if treated as outpatient, reevaluation 1 week after hospitalization

Acute bronchitis
Signs and symptoms
▸ Wheezing
▸ Prolonged expiration
▸ Frequent infections
DX: Labs (CBC, ABG), CXR, PFTs
TX: Smoking-cessation program, medication (bronchodilators, antibiotics, corticosteroids)
F/U: Monthly reevaluation if severe, biannual if stable

A productive cough is a sudden, forceful, noisy expulsion of air that contains sputum, blood, or both. The sputum's color, consistency, and odor provide important clues about the patient's condition. Productive coughing can occur as a single cough, or as paroxysmal coughing and can be voluntarily induced, although it's usually a reflexive response to stimulation of the airway mucosa.

Pulmonary tuberculosis
Signs and symptoms
▶ Mild to severe productive cough
▶ Hemoptysis
▶ Malaise
▶ Dyspnea
▶ Pleuritic chest pain
▶ Night sweats
▶ Weight loss
▶ Chest dullness on percussion
DX: Tuberculin skin test, sputum for AFB, CXR, bronchoscopy, open lung biopsy
TX: Medication (antitubercular drugs, specific drugs for resistant strains)
F/U: Referral to pulmonologist

Lung cancer
Signs and symptoms
▶ Chronic cough that produces small amounts of purulent, blood-streaked sputum (bronchogenic carcinoma)
▶ Cough that produces large amounts of frothy sputum (bronchoalveolar carcinoma)
▶ Dyspnea
▶ Anorexia
▶ Fatigue
▶ Weight loss
▶ Chest pain
▶ Fever
▶ Wheezing
DX: Imaging studies (CXR, CT scan, MRI), bronchoscopy, needle biopsy, open lung biopsy
TX: Varies (dependent on the type and stage of the cancer), medication (chemotherapy, analgesia), radiation therapy, surgery
F/U: Referral to oncologist and surgeon

Additional differential diagnoses: actinomycosis • aspiration pneumonitis • asthma (acute) • bronchiectasis • chemical pneumonitis • nocardiosis • psittacosis • pulmonary edema • silicosis

Other causes: bronchoscopy • drugs (expectorants) • respiratory treatments • PFTs

DIARRHEA

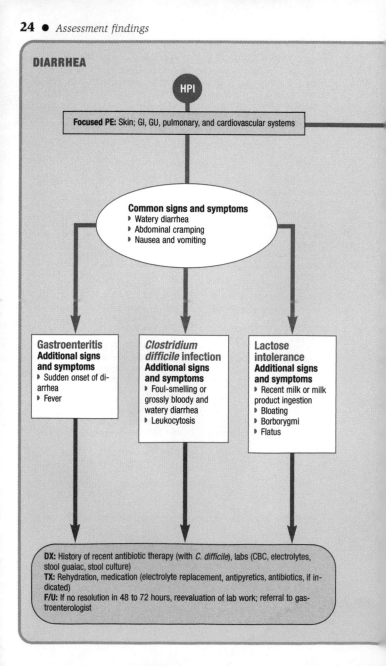

HPI

Focused PE: Skin; GI, GU, pulmonary, and cardiovascular systems

Common signs and symptoms
▶ Watery diarrhea
▶ Abdominal cramping
▶ Nausea and vomiting

Gastroenteritis
Additional signs and symptoms
▶ Sudden onset of diarrhea
▶ Fever

***Clostridium difficile* infection**
Additional signs and symptoms
▶ Foul-smelling or grossly bloody and watery diarrhea
▶ Leukocytosis

Lactose intolerance
Additional signs and symptoms
▶ Recent milk or milk product ingestion
▶ Bloating
▶ Borborygmi
▶ Flatus

DX: History of recent antibiotic therapy (with *C. difficile*), labs (CBC, electrolytes, stool guaiac, stool culture)
TX: Rehydration, medication (electrolyte replacement, antipyretics, antibiotics, if indicated)
F/U: If no resolution in 48 to 72 hours, reevaluation of lab work; referral to gastroenterologist

Diarrhea is an abnormal frequency and liquidity of stools compared with the patient's normal bowel habits. Acute diarrhea may result from acute infection, food sensitivities, stress, fecal impaction, or the effects of certain drugs. Chronic diarrhea may result from food allergies, chronic infection, obstructive or inflammatory bowel disease, malabsorption syndrome, an endocrine disorder, or GI surgery.

Common signs and symptoms
- Increased intestinal motility
- Abdominal pain
- Abdominal tenderness and guarding
- Possible distention

Crohn's disease
Additional signs and symptoms
- Nausea and vomiting
- Fever and chills
- Weakness
- Anorexia and weight loss

DX: Imaging studies (CT scan, barium enema), colonoscopy

TX: Medication (analgesics, electrolyte replacement, mesalamine, corticosteroids), surgery

F/U: Referral to gastroenterologist

Large-bowel cancer
Additional signs and symptoms
- Bloody diarrhea
- Weakness and fatigue
- Anorexia
- Nausea and vomiting

DX: Labs (CBC, CEA, fecal occult blood), imaging studies (barium enema, CT scan, transrectal ultrasound), colonoscopy with biopsy if indicated

TX: Medication (analgesics, chemotherapy), surgery

F/U: Referrals to oncologist and surgeon; after surgery, CEA, LFT, and fecal occult blood test every 3 months for 2 years; annual colonoscopy

Additional differential diagnoses: acute appendicitis • carcinoid syndrome • irritable bowel syndrome • ischemic bowel disease • lead poisoning • malabsorption syndrome • pseudomembranous enterocolitis • rotavirus gastroenteritis • thyrotoxicosis

Other causes: antibiotics (ampicillin, cephalosporins, tetracyclines, clindamycin) • colchicine • dantrolene • digoxin and quinidine (in high doses) • ethacrynic acid • gastrectomy • gastroenterostomy • guanethidine • herbal medicines (ginkgo biloba, ginseng, licorice) • high-dose radiation therapy • lactulose • laxative abuse • magnesium-containing antacids • mefenamic acid • methotrexate • metyrosine • pyloroplasty

DIZZINESS

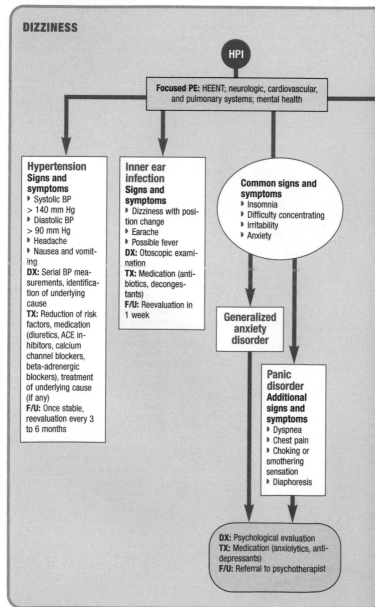

HPI

Focused PE: HEENT; neurologic, cardiovascular, and pulmonary systems; mental health

**Hypertension
Signs and
symptoms**
▶ Systolic BP
> 140 mm Hg
▶ Diastolic BP
> 90 mm Hg
▶ Headache
▶ Nausea and vomiting
DX: Serial BP measurements, identification of underlying cause
TX: Reduction of risk factors, medication (diuretics, ACE inhibitors, calcium channel blockers, beta-adrenergic blockers), treatment of underlying cause (if any)
F/U: Once stable, reevaluation every 3 to 6 months

**Inner ear
infection
Signs and
symptoms**
▶ Dizziness with position change
▶ Earache
▶ Possible fever
DX: Otoscopic examination
TX: Medication (antibiotics, decongestants)
F/U: Reevaluation in 1 week

**Common signs and
symptoms**
▶ Insomnia
▶ Difficulty concentrating
▶ Irritability
▶ Anxiety

**Generalized
anxiety
disorder**

**Panic
disorder
Additional
signs and
symptoms**
▶ Dyspnea
▶ Chest pain
▶ Choking or smothering sensation
▶ Diaphoresis

DX: Psychological evaluation
TX: Medication (anxiolytics, antidepressants)
F/U: Referral to psychotherapist

Dizziness is a sensation of imbalance or faintness sometimes associated with giddiness, weakness, confusion, and blurred or double vision. It typically results from inadequate blood flow and oxygen supply to the cerebrum and spinal cord. It may occur with anxiety, a respiratory or cardiovascular disorder, and postconcussion syndrome. It's a key symptom of certain serious disorders, such as hypertension and vertebrobasilar artery insufficiency.

Cardiac arrhythmias
Signs and symptoms
▶ Palpitations
▶ Tachycardia
▶ Irregular, rapid, or thready pulse
▶ Possible hypotension
DX: Electrolytes, ECG, cardiac monitoring, electrophysiologic study
TX: Antiarrhythmics, electrolyte correction, cardioversion
F/U: Referral to cardiologist

TIA
Signs and symptoms (last fewer than 24 hours)
▶ Unilateral or bilateral diplopia
▶ Visual field deficits
▶ Ptosis
▶ Tinnitus
▶ Dysarthria
▶ Dysphagia
▶ Decreased LOC
▶ Numbness, tingling, weakness on one side of the face, arm, or leg
▶ Unsteady gait and coordination
DX: PE, imaging studies (CT scan, carotid ultrasound, angiography, TEE, MRI, MRA, echocardiogram)
TX: Medication (aspirin, platelet aggregation inhibitors), reduction of risk factors
F/U: Reevaluation every 3 months for 1 year, then annually

Additional differential diagnoses: carotid sinus hypersensitivity • emphysema • hyperventilation syndrome • orthostatic hypotension • postconcussion syndrome

Other causes: antianxiety drugs • antihistamines • antihypertensives • CNS depressants • decongestants • narcotics • St. John's wort • vasodilators

EARACHE

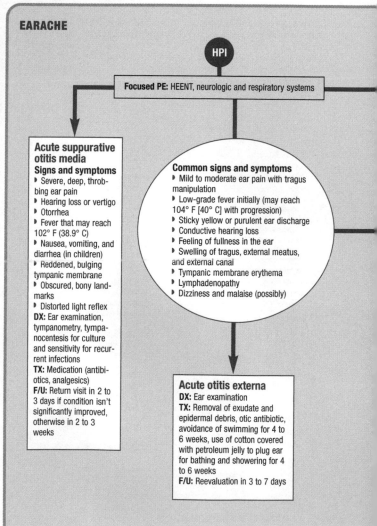

HPI

Focused PE: HEENT, neurologic and respiratory systems

Acute suppurative otitis media
Signs and symptoms
▶ Severe, deep, throbbing ear pain
▶ Hearing loss or vertigo
▶ Otorrhea
▶ Fever that may reach 102° F (38.9° C)
▶ Nausea, vomiting, and diarrhea (in children)
▶ Reddened, bulging tympanic membrane
▶ Obscured, bony landmarks
▶ Distorted light reflex
DX: Ear examination, tympanometry, tympanocentesis for culture and sensitivity for recurrent infections
TX: Medication (antibiotics, analgesics)
F/U: Return visit in 2 to 3 days if condition isn't significantly improved, otherwise in 2 to 3 weeks

Common signs and symptoms
▶ Mild to moderate ear pain with tragus manipulation
▶ Low-grade fever initially (may reach 104° F [40° C] with progression)
▶ Sticky yellow or purulent ear discharge
▶ Conductive hearing loss
▶ Feeling of fullness in the ear
▶ Swelling of tragus, external meatus, and external canal
▶ Tympanic membrane erythema
▶ Lymphadenopathy
▶ Dizziness and malaise (possibly)

Acute otitis externa
DX: Ear examination
TX: Removal of exudate and epidermal debris, otic antibiotic, avoidance of swimming for 4 to 6 weeks, use of cotton covered with petroleum jelly to plug ear for bathing and showering for 4 to 6 weeks
F/U: Reevaluation in 3 to 7 days

Earaches usually result from disorders of the external and middle ear associated with infection, obstruction, or trauma. Their severity ranges from a feeling of fullness or blockage to deep, boring pain; at times, they may be difficult to localize precisely. This common symptom may be intermittent or continuous and may develop suddenly or gradually.

Ménière's disease
Signs and symptoms
▶ Ear fullness
▶ Tinnitus
▶ Severe vertigo
▶ Sensorineural hearing loss
DX: Audiometry, electronystagmography
TX: Salt and fluid restriction, avoidance of nicotine, moderate caffeine and alcohol, medication (diuretics, antiemetic, antivertigo agents), hearing amplification, vestibular exercises
F/U: Reevaluation every 3 months, referral to otolaryngologist (if treatment is ineffective)

Malignant otitis externa
Additional signs and symptoms
▶ Intense itching
▶ Deep-seated nocturnal pain
▶ Parotid gland swelling
▶ Trismus
▶ Swollen external canal with exposed cartilage and temporal bone
▶ Cranial nerve palsy (possibly)
DX: Ear drainage culture
TX: I.V. antibiotics, surgical debridement
F/U: Referral to otolaryngologist

Additional differential diagnoses: abscess (extradural) • barotrauma (acute) • cerumen impaction • chondrodermatitis nodularis chronica helicis • ear canal obstruction by insect • frostbite • furunculosis • herpes zoster oticus (Ramsay Hunt syndrome) • keratosis obturans • mastoiditis (acute) • middle ear tumor • myringitis bullosa • otitis media • perichondritis • petrositis • TMJ infection

EYE PAIN

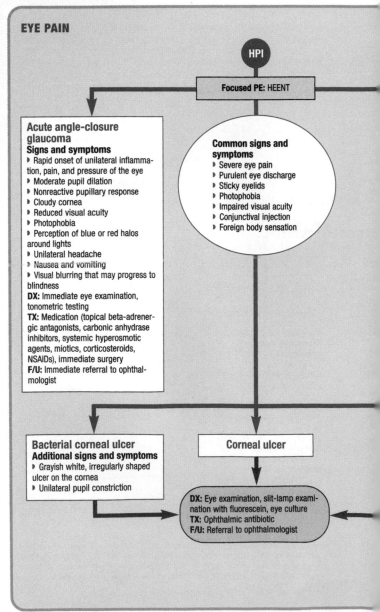

HPI

Focused PE: HEENT

Acute angle-closure glaucoma
Signs and symptoms
▶ Rapid onset of unilateral inflammation, pain, and pressure of the eye
▶ Moderate pupil dilation
▶ Nonreactive pupillary response
▶ Cloudy cornea
▶ Reduced visual acuity
▶ Photophobia
▶ Perception of blue or red halos around lights
▶ Unilateral headache
▶ Nausea and vomiting
▶ Visual blurring that may progress to blindness
DX: Immediate eye examination, tonometric testing
TX: Medication (topical beta-adrenergic antagonists, carbonic anhydrase inhibitors, systemic hyperosmotic agents, miotics, corticosteroids, NSAIDs), immediate surgery
F/U: Immediate referral to ophthalmologist

Common signs and symptoms
▶ Severe eye pain
▶ Purulent eye discharge
▶ Sticky eyelids
▶ Photophobia
▶ Impaired visual acuity
▶ Conjunctival injection
▶ Foreign body sensation

Bacterial corneal ulcer
Additional signs and symptoms
▶ Grayish white, irregularly shaped ulcer on the cornea
▶ Unilateral pupil constriction

Corneal ulcer

DX: Eye examination, slit-lamp examination with fluorescein, eye culture
TX: Ophthalmic antibiotic
F/U: Referral to ophthalmologist

Eye pain may be described as a burning, throbbing, aching, or stabbing sensation in or around the eye. It may also be characterized as a foreign-body sensation. This sign varies from mild to severe; its duration and exact location provide clues to the causative disorder.

Hordeolum
Signs and symptoms
▶ Localized eye pain that increases as the stye grows
▶ Eyelid erythema and edema
▶ Tender red nodule
▶ Slightly blurred vision
DX: Eye examination
TX: Warm compresses
F/U: None necessary unless stye persists

Fungal corneal ulcer
Additional signs and symptoms
▶ Eyelid edema and erythema
▶ Dense, cloudy, central ulcer surrounded by progressively clearer rings

Additional differential diagnoses: astigmatism • blepharitis • burns • chalazion • conjunctivitis • corneal abrasion • corneal erosion • dacryoadenitis • dacryocystitis • episcleritis • foreign body • glaucoma • herpes zoster ophthalmicus • hyphema • interstitial keratitis • iritis (acute) • keratoconjunctivitis sicca • lacrimal gland tumor • migraine headache • optic neuritis • orbital cellulitis • pemphigus • scleritis • sclerokeratitis • trachoma • uveitis

Other causes: contact lenses • ocular surgery

PALPITATIONS

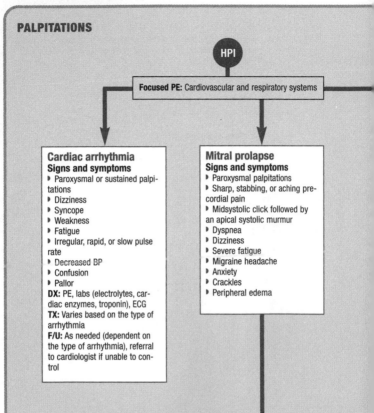

HPI

Focused PE: Cardiovascular and respiratory systems

Cardiac arrhythmia
Signs and symptoms
▶ Paroxysmal or sustained palpitations
▶ Dizziness
▶ Syncope
▶ Weakness
▶ Fatigue
▶ Irregular, rapid, or slow pulse rate
▶ Decreased BP
▶ Confusion
▶ Pallor
DX: PE, labs (electrolytes, cardiac enzymes, troponin), ECG
TX: Varies based on the type of arrhythmia
F/U: As needed (dependent on the type of arrhythmia), referral to cardiologist if unable to control

Mitral prolapse
Signs and symptoms
▶ Paroxysmal palpitations
▶ Sharp, stabbing, or aching precordial pain
▶ Midsystolic click followed by an apical systolic murmur
▶ Dyspnea
▶ Dizziness
▶ Severe fatigue
▶ Migraine headache
▶ Anxiety
▶ Crackles
▶ Peripheral edema

DX: PE, imaging studies (echocardiogram, Doppler ultrasound), cardiac catheterization
TX: None needed (possibly), medication (digoxin, vasodilators, antiarrhythmics, anticoagulants, analgesics), surgery (if symptoms are severe)
F/U: As needed (dependent on the severity of signs and symptoms)

Palpitations are a conscious awareness of one's heartbeat. They're usually felt over the precordium or in the throat or neck and may be regular or irregular, fast or slow, paroxysmal or sustained. Although usually insignificant, palpitations may result from a cardiac or metabolic disorder or from the effects of certain drugs.

Mitral stenosis
Signs and symptoms
▶ Sustained palpitations
▶ Dyspnea and fatigue on exertion
▶ Loud S_1 or opening snap and rumbling diastolic murmur at the apex
▶ Atrial gallop
▶ Orthopnea
▶ Chest discomfort
▶ Paroxysmal nocturnal dyspnea
▶ Hemoptysis
▶ Signs of right-sided heart failure
▶ Arrhythmias

Anxiety attack (acute)
Signs and symptoms
▶ Diaphoresis
▶ Facial flushing
▶ Trembling
▶ Impending sense of doom
▶ SOB
DX: Tests to rule out underlying illness or substance abuse
TX: Antianxiety agents, psychotherapy if recurrent
F/U: As needed (dependent on the recurrence of attacks), referral to psychologist

Additional differential diagnoses: anemia • hypertension • hypocalcemia • hypoglycemia • pheochromocytoma • thyrotoxicosis

Other causes: drugs that precipitate cardiac arrhythmias or increase cardiac output (cardiac glycosides, sympathomimetics, cocaine, ganglionic blockers, atropine) • herbal drugs, such as ginseng and ephedra

PYROSIS

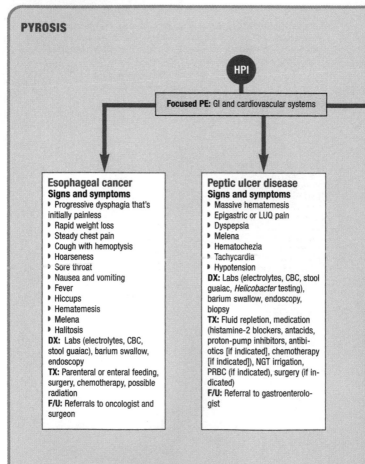

HPI

Focused PE: GI and cardiovascular systems

Esophageal cancer
Signs and symptoms
▶ Progressive dysphagia that's initially painless
▶ Rapid weight loss
▶ Steady chest pain
▶ Cough with hemoptysis
▶ Hoarseness
▶ Sore throat
▶ Nausea and vomiting
▶ Fever
▶ Hiccups
▶ Hematemesis
▶ Melena
▶ Halitosis
DX: Labs (electrolytes, CBC, stool guaiac), barium swallow, endoscopy
TX: Parenteral or enteral feeding, surgery, chemotherapy, possible radiation
F/U: Referrals to oncologist and surgeon

Peptic ulcer disease
Signs and symptoms
▶ Massive hematemesis
▶ Epigastric or LUQ pain
▶ Dyspepsia
▶ Melena
▶ Hematochezia
▶ Tachycardia
▶ Hypotension
DX: Labs (electrolytes, CBC, stool guaiac, *Helicobacter* testing), barium swallow, endoscopy, biopsy
TX: Fluid repletion, medication (histamine-2 blockers, antacids, proton-pump inhibitors, antibiotics [if indicated], chemotherapy [if indicated]), NGT irrigation, PRBC (if indicated), surgery (if indicated)
F/U: Referral to gastroenterologist

Pyrosis is a substernal burning sensation that rises in the chest and may radiate to the neck or throat. It's caused by reflux of gastric contents into the esophagus and is frequently accompanied by regurgitation. Because increased intra-abdominal pressure contributes to reflux, pyrosis commonly occurs with pregnancy, ascites, or obesity. It also accompanies various GI disorders, connective tissue diseases, and the use of certain drugs.

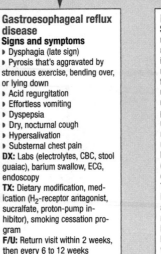

Gastroesophageal reflux disease
Signs and symptoms
▶ Dysphagia (late sign)
▶ Pyrosis that's aggravated by strenuous exercise, bending over, or lying down
▶ Acid regurgitation
▶ Effortless vomiting
▶ Dyspepsia
▶ Dry, nocturnal cough
▶ Hypersalivation
▶ Substernal chest pain
DX: Labs (electrolytes, CBC, stool guaiac), barium swallow, ECG, endoscopy
TX: Dietary modification, medication (H_2-receptor antagonist, sucralfate, proton-pump inhibitor), smoking cessation program
F/U: Return visit within 2 weeks, then every 6 to 12 weeks

Hiatal hernia
Signs and symptoms
▶ Eructation after eating
▶ Pyrosis that worsens when lying down
▶ Regurgitation of sour-tasting fluid
▶ Abdominal distention
▶ Dull, substernal or epigastric pain
▶ Dysphagia
▶ Nausea
▶ Cough
DX: History, imaging studies (barium swallow, CT scan), endoscopy
TX: Diet modification, repositioning (sleeping with HOB elevated and avoiding lying down after meals), medication (antacids, histamine-2 blockers)
F/U: None unless symptoms worsen

Additional differential diagnoses: esophageal diverticula or stenosis • gastritis • obesity • scleroderma

Other causes: acetohexamide • anticholinergic agents • aspirin • drugs with anticholinergic effects • NSAIDs • tolbutamide

VISION LOSS

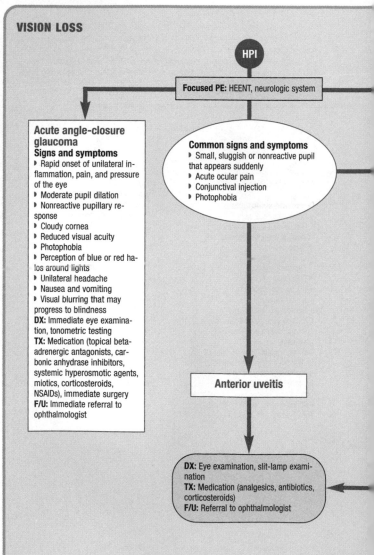

HPI

Focused PE: HEENT, neurologic system

Acute angle-closure glaucoma
Signs and symptoms
▸ Rapid onset of unilateral inflammation, pain, and pressure of the eye
▸ Moderate pupil dilation
▸ Nonreactive pupillary response
▸ Cloudy cornea
▸ Reduced visual acuity
▸ Photophobia
▸ Perception of blue or red halos around lights
▸ Unilateral headache
▸ Nausea and vomiting
▸ Visual blurring that may progress to blindness
DX: Immediate eye examination, tonometric testing
TX: Medication (topical beta-adrenergic antagonists, carbonic anhydrase inhibitors, systemic hyperosmotic agents, miotics, corticosteroids, NSAIDs), immediate surgery
F/U: Immediate referral to ophthalmologist

Common signs and symptoms
▸ Small, sluggish or nonreactive pupil that appears suddenly
▸ Acute ocular pain
▸ Conjunctival injection
▸ Photophobia

Anterior uveitis

DX: Eye examination, slit-lamp examination
TX: Medication (analgesics, antibiotics, corticosteroids)
F/U: Referral to ophthalmologist

Vision loss — the inability to perceive visual stimuli — can be sudden or gradual and temporary or permanent. The deficit can range from a slight impairment of vision to total blindness. It can result from an ocular, neurologic, or systemic disorder or from trauma or a reaction to a certain drug. A sudden vision loss can signal an ocular emergency and require immediate referral to an ophthalmologist.

Retinal detachment
Signs and symptoms
▶ Painless vision loss that may be rapid or may occur over several days
▶ Flashing light sensation
▶ Shower of floaters
▶ Shadow in peripheral vision
▶ Wavy distortion
▶ Decreased visual acuity
DX: Visual field testing, slit-lamp examination, ultrasonography
TX: None in certain cases, surgery
F/U: Referral to ophthalmologist

Posterior uveitis
Additional signs and symptoms
▶ Blurred vision
▶ Decreased visual acuity
▶ Distorted pupil shape
▶ Floaters
▶ Optic nerve edema

Additional differential diagnoses: Alzheimer's disease • amaurosis fugax • cataract • concussion • diabetic retinopathy • endophthalmitis • hereditary corneal dystrophies • herpes zoster • hyphema • keratitis • ocular trauma • optic atrophy • optic neuritis • Paget's disease • papilledema • pituitary tumor • retinal artery occlusion (central) • retinal vein occlusion (central) • senile macular degeneration • Stevens-Johnson syndrome • temporal arteritis • trachoma • vitreous hemorrhage

Other causes: cardiac glycosides • chloroquine therapy • ethambutol • indomethacin • methanol toxicity • phenylbutazone • quinine

VOMITING

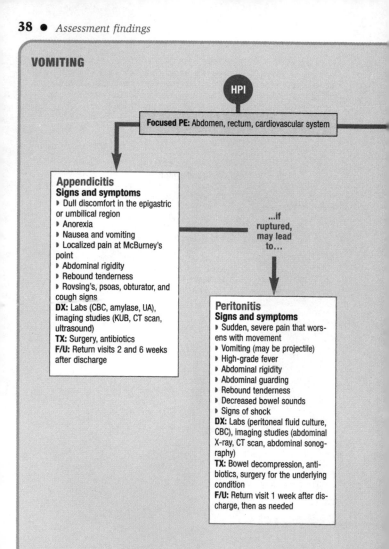

HPI

Focused PE: Abdomen, rectum, cardiovascular system

Appendicitis
Signs and symptoms
▶ Dull discomfort in the epigastric or umbilical region
▶ Anorexia
▶ Nausea and vomiting
▶ Localized pain at McBurney's point
▶ Abdominal rigidity
▶ Rebound tenderness
▶ Rovsing's, psoas, obturator, and cough signs
DX: Labs (CBC, amylase, UA), imaging studies (KUB, CT scan, ultrasound)
TX: Surgery, antibiotics
F/U: Return visits 2 and 6 weeks after discharge

...if ruptured, may lead to...

Peritonitis
Signs and symptoms
▶ Sudden, severe pain that worsens with movement
▶ Vomiting (may be projectile)
▶ High-grade fever
▶ Abdominal rigidity
▶ Abdominal guarding
▶ Rebound tenderness
▶ Decreased bowel sounds
▶ Signs of shock
DX: Labs (peritoneal fluid culture, CBC), imaging studies (abdominal X-ray, CT scan, abdominal sonography)
TX: Bowel decompression, antibiotics, surgery for the underlying condition
F/U: Return visit 1 week after discharge, then as needed

Vomiting is the forceful expulsion of gastric contents through the mouth. Characteristically preceded by nausea, it occurs with fluid and electrolyte imbalances; infections; and metabolic, endocrine, labyrinthine, central nervous system, and cardiac disorders. It can also result from drug therapy, surgery, radiation, pregnancy, stress, anxiety, pain, alcohol intoxication, overeating, or ingestion of distasteful foods or liquids.

Pancreatitis
Signs and symptoms
▶ Vomiting that's usually preceded by nausea (early symptom)
▶ Steady, severe epigastric or LUQ pain that may radiate to the back
▶ Restlessness
▶ Abdominal tenderness and rigidity
▶ Rebound tenderness
▶ Jaundice
▶ Hypoactive bowel sounds
▶ Fever
▶ Tachycardia
▶ Possible Turner's or Cullen's sign
▶ Signs of shock if severe
DX: Labs (amylase, lipase, CBC, bilirubin, glucose, electrolytes, calcium, albumin, LFT), imaging studies (CT scan, abdominal ultrasound)
TX: Symptomatic treatment, initially NPO, I.V. fluids, medication (analgesics, electrolyte replacement), NG tube for severe vomiting or ileus
F/U: Reevaluation of amylase levels until normal; if levels remain elevated, repeated imaging studies

Gastroenteritis
Signs and symptoms
▶ Nausea
▶ Vomiting (commonly of undigested food)
▶ Diarrhea
▶ Abdominal cramping
▶ Fever
▶ Malaise
▶ Hyperactive bowel sounds
▶ Abdominal pain and tenderness (possibly)
DX: History, labs if prolonged (electrolytes, stool culture),
TX: Rest; NPO until 4 hours after vomiting ceases, gradual increase in oral intake
F/U: None needed unless unresponsive to treatment

Additional differential diagnoses: adrenal insufficiency • bulimia • cholecystitis (acute) • cholelithiasis • cirrhosis • ectopic pregnancy • electrolyte imbalances • food poisoning • gastric cancer • gastritis • heart failure • hepatitis • hyperemesis gravidarum • increased ICP • infection • intestinal obstruction • labyrinthitis • mesenteric artery ischemia • mesenteric venous thrombosis • metabolic acidosis • MI • migraine headache • motion sickness • peptic ulcer • preeclampsia • renal and urologic disorders • thyrotoxicosis • ulcerative colitis

Other causes: drugs (such as antineoplastic agents, opiates, ferrous sulfate, levodopa, oral potassium, chloride replacement, estrogens, sulfasalazine, antibiotics, quinidine, anesthetic agents, and overdoses of cardiac glycosides and theophylline) • radiation

WEIGHT LOSS, EXCESSIVE

HPI

Focused PE: All systems

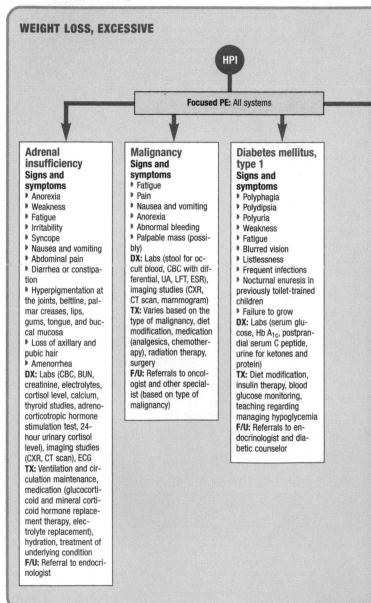

Adrenal insufficiency
Signs and symptoms
▶ Anorexia
▶ Weakness
▶ Fatigue
▶ Irritability
▶ Syncope
▶ Nausea and vomiting
▶ Abdominal pain
▶ Diarrhea or constipation
▶ Hyperpigmentation at the joints, beltline, palmar creases, lips, gums, tongue, and buccal mucosa
▶ Loss of axillary and pubic hair
▶ Amenorrhea
DX: Labs (CBC, BUN, creatinine, electrolytes, cortisol level, calcium, thyroid studies, adrenocorticotropic hormone stimulation test, 24-hour urinary cortisol level), imaging studies (CXR, CT scan), ECG
TX: Ventilation and circulation maintenance, medication (glucocorticoid and mineral corticoid hormone replacement therapy, electrolyte replacement), hydration, treatment of underlying condition
F/U: Referral to endocrinologist

Malignancy
Signs and symptoms
▶ Fatigue
▶ Pain
▶ Nausea and vomiting
▶ Anorexia
▶ Abnormal bleeding
▶ Palpable mass (possibly)
DX: Labs (stool for occult blood, CBC with differential, UA, LFT, ESR), imaging studies (CXR, CT scan, mammogram)
TX: Varies based on the type of malignancy, diet modification, medication (analgesics, chemotherapy), radiation therapy, surgery
F/U: Referrals to oncologist and other specialist (based on type of malignancy)

Diabetes mellitus, type 1
Signs and symptoms
▶ Polyphagia
▶ Polydipsia
▶ Polyuria
▶ Weakness
▶ Fatigue
▶ Blurred vision
▶ Listlessness
▶ Frequent infections
▶ Nocturnal enuresis in previously toilet-trained children
▶ Failure to grow
DX: Labs (serum glucose, Hb A$_{1c}$, postprandial serum C peptide, urine for ketones and protein)
TX: Diet modification, insulin therapy, blood glucose monitoring, teaching regarding managing hypoglycemia
F/U: Referrals to endocrinologist and diabetic counselor

Weight loss can reflect decreased food intake or absorption, increased metabolic requirements, or a combination of the three. Its causes include endocrine, neoplastic, GI, and psychiatric disorders; nutritional deficiencies; infections; and neurologic lesions that cause paralysis and dysphagia. It may also accompany a condition that prevents sufficient food intake or may be the metabolic consequence of poverty, fad diets, excessive exercise, or certain drugs.

Anorexia nervosa
Signs and symptoms
▶ Primary or secondary amenorrhea
▶ Emaciated appearance
▶ Compulsive behavior patterns
▶ Constipation
▶ Loss of scalp hair and lanugo on the face and arms
▶ Skeletal muscle atrophy
▶ Sleep disturbances
DX: Malnourished state, labs (electrolytes, CBC, renal studies, LFT, thyroid levels)
TX: Parenteral nutrition, psychological and nutritional counseling
F/U: Weekly return visits, then monthly visits if weight gain occurs; inpatient therapy if the condition doesn't improve

Thyrotoxicosis
Signs and symptoms
▶ Ptosis
▶ Progressive exophthalmus
▶ Increased tearing
▶ Visual changes
▶ Lid edema
▶ Lid lag
▶ Photophobia
▶ Enlarged thyroid
▶ Nervousness
▶ Heat intolerance
▶ Tremors
▶ Palpitations
▶ Tachycardia
▶ Dyspnea
DX: PE, thyroid function studies, imaging studies (thyroid scan, ultrasound)
TX: Medication (antithyroid therapy, radioiodine, beta$_2$-adrenergic blockers)
F/U: Thyroid function testing 6 weeks after treatment is initiated, then biannually if at euthyroid state

Additional differential diagnoses: Crohn's disease • cryptosporidiosis • depression • esophagitis • gastroenteritis • leukemia • lymphoma • pulmonary tuberculosis • stomatitis • thyrotoxicosis • ulcerative colitis • Whipple's disease

Other causes: amphetamines • chemotherapeutic agents • inappropriate dosages of thyroid preparations • laxative abuse

2

Laboratory tests

Understanding the results in context

ALANINE AMINO-TRANSFERASE

The alanine aminotransferase (ALT) test is used to measure serum levels of ALT, one of two enzymes that catalyze a reversible amino group transfer reaction in the Krebs cycle. ALT, which is necessary for tissue energy production, is found primarily in the liver, with lesser amounts in the kidneys, heart, and skeletal muscles. It's a sensitive indicator of acute hepatocellular disease.

Purpose

▸ To detect and evaluate treatment of acute hepatic disease, especially hepatitis and cirrhosis without jaundice
▸ To distinguish between myocardial and hepatic tissue damage (used with aspartate aminotransferase)
▸ To assess hepatotoxicity of some drugs

Reference values

Serum ALT levels range from 8 to 50 U/L (SI, 0.14 to 0.85 µkat/L).

Abnormal findings

Very high serum ALT levels (up to 50 times normal) suggest viral or severe drug-induced hepatitis or other hepatic disease with extensive necrosis. Moderate to high levels may indicate infectious mononucleosis, chronic hepatitis, intrahepatic cholestasis or cholecystitis, early or improving acute viral hepatitis, or severe hepatic congestion due to heart failure.

Slight to moderate elevations of serum ALT may appear in any condition that produces acute hepatocellular injury, such as active cirrhosis and drug-induced hepatitis. Marginal elevations occasionally occur in acute myocardial infarction, reflecting secondary hepatic congestion or the release of small amounts of ALT from myocardial tissue.

ANTINUCLEAR ANTIBODIES

Antinuclear antibodies (ANA) are antibodies to nuclear antigens that are present in the serum of patients who have connective tissue disorders. In such conditions as systemic lupus erythematosus (SLE), scleroderma, and certain infections, the body's immune system may perceive portions of its own cell nuclei as foreign and may produce antinuclear antibodies (ANAs). Specific ANAs include antibodies to deoxyribonucleic acid (DNA), nucleoprotein, histones, nuclear ribonucleoprotein, and other nuclear constituents.

Because they don't penetrate living cells, ANAs are harmless but sometimes form antigen-antibody complexes that cause tissue damage (as in SLE). Because of multiorgan involvement, test results alone aren't diagnostic. Diagnosis is based primarily on the presence of clinical signs and symptoms; a positive test result helps confirm the diagnosis. (See *Incidence of antinuclear antibodies in various disorders,* page 44.)

Purpose

▸ To help confirm the diagnosis of connective tissue disorders
▸ To monitor the effectiveness of therapy for connective tissue disorders

Normal findings

Test results are reported as positive (with pattern and serum titer noted) or negative.

INCIDENCE OF ANTINUCLEAR ANTIBODIES IN VARIOUS DISORDERS

The chart below indicates the percentage of patients with certain disorders whose serum contains antinuclear antibodies (ANAs). About 40% of elderly people and 5% of the general population also have positive ANA findings.

Disorder	Positive ANA
Systemic lupus erythematosus (SLE)	95% to 100%
Lupoid hepatitis	95% to 100%
Felty's syndrome	95% to 100%
Progressive systemic sclerosis (scleroderma)	75% to 80%
Drug-associated SLE-like syndrome (hydralazine, procainamide, isoniazid)	Approximately 50%
Sjögren's syndrome	40% to 75%
Rheumatoid arthritis	25% to 60%
Healthy family member of SLE patient	Approximately 25%
Chronic discoid lupus erythematosus	15% to 50%
Juvenile arthritis	15% to 30%
Polyarteritis nodosa	15% to 25%
Miscellaneous diseases	10% to 50%
Dermatomyositis, polymyositis	10% to 30%
Rheumatic fever	Approximately 5%

Abnormal findings

Although this test is a sensitive indicator of ANAs, it isn't specific for SLE. Low titers may occur in patients with viral diseases, chronic hepatic disease, collagen vascular disease, and autoimmune diseases and in some healthy adults; the incidence increases with age. The higher the titer, the more specific the test is for SLE (titer often exceeds 1:256).

The pattern of nuclear fluorescence helps identify the type of immune disease present. A peripheral pattern is almost exclusively associated with SLE because it indicates the presence of anti-DNA antibodies; sometimes anti-DNA antibodies are measured by radioimmunoassay if ANA titers are high or a peripheral pattern is observed. A homogeneous, or diffuse, pattern is also associated with SLE as well as with related connective tissue disorders; a nucleolar pattern, with scleroderma; and a speckled, irregular pattern, with mixed connective tissue disorders (for example, SLE and scleroderma).

ARTERIAL BLOOD GAS ANALYSIS

Arterial blood gas (ABG) analysis is used to measure the partial pressures of oxygen (Pao_2) and carbon dioxide ($Paco_2$) and the pH of an arterial sample. Oxygen saturation (Sao_2) and bicarbonate (HCO_3^-) values are also measured. A blood sample for ABG analysis may be drawn by percutaneous arterial puncture or from an arterial line.

Purpose

▶ To evaluate gas exchange in the lungs
▶ To assess integrity of the ventilatory control system
▶ To determine the acid-base level of the blood
▶ To monitor respiratory therapy

Reference values

Normal ABG values fall within the following ranges:
▶ Pao_2: 80 to 100 mm Hg (SI, 10.6 to 13.3 kPa)
▶ $Paco_2$: 35 to 45 mm Hg (SI, 4.7 to 5.3 kPa)
▶ *pH*: 7.35 to 7.45 (SI, 7.35 to 7.45)
▶ Sao_2: 94% to 100% (SI, 0.94 to 1)
▶ HCO_3^-: 22 to 26 mEq/L (SI, 22 to 26 mmol/L).

Abnormal findings

Acid base balance disturbances result from abnormalities in the metabolic or respiratory systems. A pH greater than 7.45 indicates alkalosis; a pH less than 7.35 indicates acidosis. A $Paco_2$ above 45 mm Hg indicates hypoventilation or hypercapnia; below 35 mm Hg, hyperventilation or hypocapnia. The $Paco_2$ value can also signal a respiratory acid-base imbalance. A value above 45 mm Hg points to respiratory acidosis; below 35 mm Hg, respiratory alkalosis. (See *Recognizing acid-base disorders*, page 46.) An HCO_3^- value above 26 mEq/L points to metabolic, or kidney-related, alkalosis; below 22 mEq/L, metabolic acidosis.

When interpreting ABG results, it's important to remember that Pao_2 decreases at altitudes greater than 3,000 feet and that an increase in dead space will result in a decrease in O_2 and an increase in Pao_2 in the alveoli.

✽ **LIFE SPAN** *Pao_2 also decreases with age due to changes in lung compliance.*

Hypoxemia, which is indicated by a Pao_2 of less than 50 mm Hg, results from hypoventilation, diffusion abnormalities, shunting of blood from the alveoli, and ventilation-perfusion defects. Hypoventilation may result from medications that suppress respiratory drive, thoracic trauma, paralysis of the respiratory muscles, or other disorders that create a high resistance to breathing.

ASPARTATE AMINO-TRANSFERASE

Aspartate aminotransferase (AST) is one of two enzymes that catalyze the conversion of the nitrogenous portion of an amino acid to an amino acid residue. It's essential to energy production in the Krebs cycle. AST is found in the cytoplasm and mitochondria of many cells, primarily in the liver, heart, skeletal muscles, kidneys, pancreas, and red blood cells. It's released into serum in proportion to cellular damage.

Purpose

▶ To aid detection and differential diagnosis of acute hepatic disease
▶ To monitor patient progress and prognosis in cardiac and hepatic diseases
▶ To aid diagnosis of myocardial infarction (MI) in correlation with creatine kinase and lactate dehydrogenase levels

Reference values

AST levels range from 8 to 46 U/L (SI, 0.14 to 0.78 µkat/L) in males and from 7 to 34 U/L (SI, 0.12 to 0.58 µkat/L) in females. Normal values for infants are typically higher.

RECOGNIZING ACID-BASE DISORDERS

This chart lists the arterial blood gas (ABG) values, possible causes, and clinical effects associated with acid-base disorders.

Disorders and ABG findings	Possible causes	Signs and symptoms
Respiratory acidosis (excess CO_2 retention)		
▶ pH < 7.35 (SI, < 7.35) ▶ HCO_3^- > 26 mEq/L (SI, > 26 mmol/L) (if compensating) ▶ $Paco_2$ > 45 mm Hg (SI, > 5.3 kPa)	▶ Central nervous system depression from drugs, injury, or disease ▶ Asphyxia or airway obstruction ▶ Hypoventilation due to pulmonary, cardiac, musculoskeletal, or neuromuscular disease	▶ Diaphoresis, headache, tachycardia, confusion, restlessness, apprehension
Respiratory alkalosis (excess CO_2 excretion)		
▶ pH > 7.45 (SI, > 7.45) ▶ HCO_3^- < 22 mEq/L (SI, < 22 mmol/L) (if compensating) ▶ $Paco_2$ < 35 mm Hg (SI, < 4.7 kPa)	▶ Hyperventilation due to anxiety, pain, or improper ventilator settings ▶ Respiratory stimulation caused by drugs, disease, hypoxia, fever, or high room temperature ▶ Gram-negative bacteremia	▶ Rapid, deep breathing; paresthesia; light-headedness; twitching; anxiety; fear
Metabolic acidosis (HCO_3^- loss, acid retention)		
▶ pH < 7.35 (SI, < 7.35) ▶ HCO_3^- < 22 mEq/L (SI, < 22 mmol/L) ▶ $Paco_2$ < 35 mm Hg (SI, < 4.7 kPa) (if compensating)	▶ HCO_3^- depletion due to renal disease, diarrhea, or small-bowel fistulas ▶ Excessive production of organic acids due to hepatic disease, endocrine disorders (including diabetes mellitus), hypoxia, shock, and drug intoxication ▶ Inadequate excretion of acids due to renal disease	▶ Rapid, deep breathing; fruity breath; fatigue; headache; lethargy; drowsiness; nausea; vomiting; coma (if severe)
Metabolic alkalosis (HCO_3^- retention, acid loss)		
▶ pH > 7.45 (SI, > 7.45) ▶ HCO_3^- > 26 mEq/L (SI, > 26 mmol/L) ▶ $Paco_2$ > 45 mm Hg (SI, > 5.3 kPa) (if compensating)	▶ Loss of hydrochloric acid from prolonged vomiting or gastric suctioning ▶ Loss of potassium due to increased renal excretion (as in diuretic therapy) or steroid overdose ▶ Excessive alkali ingestion	▶ Slow, shallow breathing; hypertonic muscles, restlessness; twitching; confusion; irritability; apathy; tetany; seizures; coma (if severe)

Abnormal findings

AST levels fluctuate in response to the extent of cellular necrosis, being transiently and minimally increased early in the disease process and extremely increased during the most acute phase. Depending on when the initial specimen is drawn, AST levels may increase, indicating increasing disease severity and tissue damage, or decrease, indicating disease resolution and tissue repair.

Maximum AST elevations (greater than 20 times normal) may indicate acute viral hepatitis, severe skeletal muscle trauma, extensive surgery, drug-induced hepatic injury, or severe passive liver congestion.

High AST levels (10 to 20 times normal) may indicate severe MI, severe infectious mononucleosis, or alcoholic cirrhosis. High AST levels also occur during the prodromal or resolving stages of conditions that cause maximum AST elevations.

Moderate to high AST levels (5 to 10 times normal) may indicate dermatomyositis, Duchenne's muscular dystrophy, or chronic hepatitis. Moderate to high AST levels also occur during prodromal and resolving stages of diseases that cause high AST elevations.

Low to moderate AST levels (2 to 5 times normal) occur at some time during the preceding conditions or diseases or may indicate hemolytic anemia, metastatic hepatic tumors, acute pancreatitis, pulmonary emboli, delirium tremens, or fatty liver. AST levels rise slightly after the first few days of biliary duct obstruction.

BLOOD UREA NITROGEN

The blood urea nitrogen (BUN) test is used to measure the nitrogen fraction of urea, the chief end product of protein metabolism. Formed in the liver from ammonia and ex-creted by the kidneys, urea constitutes 40% to 50% of the blood's nonprotein nitrogen. The BUN level reflects protein intake and renal excretory capacity but is a less reliable indicator of uremia than the serum creatinine level.

Purpose

▶ To evaluate kidney function and aid diagnosis of renal disease
▶ To aid assessment of hydration

Reference values

BUN values normally range from 8 to 20 mg/dl (SI, 2.9 to 7.5 mmol/L), with slightly higher values in elderly patients.

Abnormal findings

Elevated BUN levels occur in renal disease, reduced renal blood flow (due to dehydration, for example), urinary tract obstruction, and increased protein catabolism (such as burn injuries).

Low BUN levels occur in severe hepatic damage, malnutrition, and overhydration.

CARCINO-EMBRYONIC ANTIGEN

Carcinoembryonic antigen (CEA) is a protein normally found in embryonic entodermal epithelium and fetal GI tissue. Production of CEA stops before birth, but it may begin again later if a neoplasm develops. Because CEA levels are also raised by biliary obstruction, alcoholic hepatitis, chronic heavy smoking, and other conditions, this test can't be used as a general indicator of cancer. However, measurement of enzyme CEA levels by immunoassay is useful for staging and monitoring treatment of certain cancers.

Purpose

▶ To monitor the effectiveness of cancer therapy
▶ To assist in preoperative staging of colorectal cancers, assess adequacy of surgical resection, and test for recurrence of colorectal cancers

Reference values

Normal serum CEA values are less than 5 ng/ml (SI, < 5 mg/L).

Abnormal findings

If CEA levels are higher than normal before surgical resection, chemotherapy, or radiation therapy, their return to normal within 6 weeks suggests successful treatment. However, persistently elevated CEA levels suggest residual or recurrent tumor.

High CEA levels are characteristic in various malignant conditions, particularly endodermally derived neoplasms of the GI organs and the lungs, and in certain nonmalignant conditions, such as benign hepatic disease, hepatic cirrhosis, alcoholic pancreatitis, and inflammatory bowel disease.

Elevated CEA concentrations may also result from nonendodermal carcinomas, such as breast cancer and ovarian cancer.

Chronic smokers may also have elevated CEA levels.

CHOLESTEROL, TOTAL

The quantitative analysis of serum cholesterol measures the circulating levels of free cholesterol and cholesterol esters; it reflects the level of the two forms in which this biochemical compound appears in the body.

Cholesterol, a structural component in cell membranes and plasma lipoproteins, is absorbed from the diet and synthesized in the liver and other body tissues. The body uses cholesterol for numerous functions, including steroid and hormone synthesis (sex hormones as well as adrenal steroids), cell membrane biogenesis, and formation of bile acids. The human body can produce all the cholesterol it requires, although researchers estimate that 20% to 40% is obtained through diet. A diet high in saturated fat raises cholesterol levels by stimulating absorption of lipids, including cholesterol, from the intestine; a diet low in saturated fat lowers cholesterol levels.

Elevated serum cholesterol levels, elevated low-density lipoproteins (LDLs), and decreased high-density lipoproteins (HDLs) may be associated with an increased risk of atherosclerosis-related diseases, especially coronary heart disease. (See *Lipoprotein levels in adults.*)

● **CLINICAL PEARL** *Cholesterol levels shouldn't be measured immediately after a myocardial infarction (MI) because of falsely low readings. In these patients, cholesterol levels should be evaluated 3 months after the MI.*

Purpose

▶ To assess the risk of atherosclerosis and coronary artery disease (CAD)
▶ To evaluate fat metabolism
▶ To aid in monitoring the effects of other disease processes, such as nephrotic syndrome, diabetes mellitus, pancreatitis, hepatic disease, and hypothyroidism and hyperthyroidism
▶ To assess the efficacy of lipid-lowering drug therapy

Reference values

Total cholesterol levels vary with age and sex. Total cholesterol val-

LIPOPROTEIN LEVELS IN ADULTS

Value	Indications
Low-density lipoprotein cholesterol	
< 100 mg/dl (SI, < 2.59 mmol/L)	Optimal
100 to 129 mg/dl (SI, 2.59 to 3.34 mmol/L)	Above optimal
130 to 159 mg/dl (SI, 3.36 to 4.12 mmol/L)	Borderline high
160 to 189 mg/dl (SI, 4.14 to 4.90 mmol/L)	High
≥ 190 mg/dl (SI, ≥ 4.92 mmol/L)	Very high
High-density lipoprotein cholesterol	
< 40 mg/dl (SI, < 1.03 mmol/L)	Low
≥ 60 mg/dl (SI, ≥ 1.55 mmol/L)	Desirable
Total cholesterol	
< 200 mg/dl (SI, < 5.18 mmol/L)	Desirable
200 to 239 mg/dl (SI, 5.18 to 6.19 mmol/L)	Borderline high
≥ 240 mg/dl (SI, ≥ 6.2 mmol/L)	High

Adapted from National Institute of Health, National Heart, Lung, and Blood Institute. *ATP III Guidelines At-A-Glance. Quick Desk Reference.* May 2001. Publication No. 01-3305.

ues for adults and children are as follows:

▶ *Adults:* desirable: < 200 mg/dl (SI, < 5.18 mmol/L); borderline high: 200 to 239 mg/dl (5.18 to 6.19 mmol/L); high: ≥ 240 mg/dl (SI, ≥ 6.2 mmol/L).
▶ *Children and adolescents ages 12 to 18:* desirable: < 170 mg/dl (SI, < 4.39 mmol/L); borderline high: 170 to 199 mg/dl (SI, 4.40 to 5.16 mmol/L); high: ≥ 200 mg/dl (SI, ≥ 5.18 mmol/L).

Abnormal findings

The cholesterol level needs to be evaluated in the context of the entire risk factor analysis for each individual patient. If the level is abnormal, a second cholesterol test should be completed in 1 week to verify the results. Marked fluctuations can occur from day to day. A decision to begin treatment will be based on the number of risk factors and a patient's prior cardiovascular history.

An elevated serum cholesterol level (hypercholesterolemia) may indicate an increased risk for CAD as well as incipient hepatitis, lipid disorders, bile duct blockage, nephrotic syndrome, obstructive jaundice, pancreatitis, and hypothyroidism. Hypercholesterolemia associated with increased intake of fats and cholesterol-rich foods requires dietary changes and, possibly, medication to retard absorption of cholesterol.

A low serum cholesterol level (hypocholesterolemia) is commonly associated with malnutrition, cellular necrosis of the liver, or hyperthyroidism. Abnormal cholesterol levels commonly require further testing to pinpoint the causative disorder, depending on the type of abnormality and the presence of overt signs. Abnormal levels associated with cardiovascular diseases, for example, may require lipoprotein phenotyping.

CLINICAL PEARL *If a genetic lipid disorder is discovered, family members should be screened for cholesterol abnormalities.*

CREATINE KINASE

Creatine kinase (CK) is an enzyme that's present in brain tissue, skeletal muscle, and myocardial muscle. Serum CK can be fractionated to determine the source of CK: CK-BB, brain tissue; CK-MM, skeletal muscle; and CK-MB, myocardial muscle (with small amounts originating from skeletal muscle).

Purpose

▶ To detect and diagnose acute myocardial infarction (MI) and reinfarction (CK-MB is primarily used)
▶ To evaluate possible causes of chest pain and to monitor the severity of myocardial ischemia after cardiac surgery, cardiac catheterization, and cardioversion (CK-MB is primarily used)
▶ To detect musculoskeletal disorders that aren't neurogenic in origin, such as Duchenne muscular dystrophy (total CK is primarily used), rhabdomyolysis, and early dermatomyositis

Reference values

Total CK values determined by ultraviolet or kinetic measurement range from 55 to 170 U/L (SI, 0.94 to 2.89 μkat/L) for men and from 30 to 135 U/L (SI, 0.51 to 2.3 μkat/L) for women. CK levels may be significantly higher in muscular people.

LIFE SPAN *Infants up to age 1 have levels 2 to 4 times higher than those in adults, possibly reflecting birth trauma and striated muscle development.*

Normal ranges for isoenzyme levels are as follows: CK-BB, undetectable; CK-MB, 0 to 5%; CK-MM, 90% to 100%.

Abnormal findings

CK-MM makes up 99% of total CK normally present in serum. Detectable CK-BB isoenzyme may indicate, but doesn't confirm, a diagnosis of brain tissue injury, widespread malignant tumors, severe shock, or renal failure.

CK-MB levels greater than 5% of total CK indicate MI, especially if the lactate dehydrogenase isoenzyme ratio (LD_1/LD_2) is greater than 1 (flipped LD). In acute MI and after cardiac surgery, CK-MB begins to increase within 2 to 4 hours, peaks within 12 to 24 hours, and usually returns to normal within 24 to 48 hours; persistent elevations and increasing levels indicate ongoing myocardial damage. Total CK follows roughly the same pattern but increases slightly later. CK-MB levels may not increase in heart failure or during angina pectoris not accompanied by myocardial cell necrosis. (See *Release of cardiac enzymes and proteins.*)

Serious skeletal muscle injury that occurs in certain muscular dystrophies, polymyositis, and severe myoglobinuria may produce a mild CK-MB increase because a small amount of this isoenzyme is present in some skeletal muscles.

Increasing CK-MM values follow skeletal muscle damage from trauma, such as surgery and I.M. injections, and from diseases, such as dermatomyositis and muscular dystrophy (values may be 50 to 100 times normal). A moderate increase in CK-MM levels develops in patients with hypothyroidism; sharp increases occur with muscle activity caused by agitation, such as during an acute psychotic episode.

RELEASE OF CARDIAC ENZYMES AND PROTEINS

Because they're released by damaged tissue, serum proteins and isoenzymes (catalytic proteins that vary in concentration in specific organs) can help identify the compromised organ and assess the extent of damage. After acute myocardial infarction, cardiac enzymes and proteins rise and fall in a characteristic pattern, as shown in the graph below

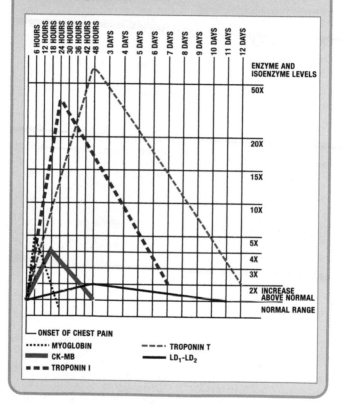

Total CK levels may be increased in patients with severe hypokalemia, carbon monoxide poisoning, malignant hyperthermia, and alcoholic cardiomyopathy. They may also be increased after seizures and, occasionally, in patients who have suffered pulmonary or cerebral infarctions.

CREATININE, SERUM

The serum creatinine test provides a more sensitive measure of renal

damage than blood urea nitrogen levels. Creatinine is a nonprotein end product of creatine metabolism that appears in serum in amounts proportional to the body's muscle mass.

Purpose

▶ To assess glomerular filtration
▶ To screen for renal damage

Reference values

Creatinine concentrations normally range from 0.8 to 1.2 mg/dl (SI, 62 to 115 µmol/L) in males and 0.6 to 0.9 mg/dl (SI, 53 to 97 µmol/L) in females.

Abnormal findings

Elevated serum creatinine levels generally indicate renal disease that has seriously damaged 50% or more of the nephrons. Elevated levels may also be associated with gigantism and acromegaly.

ELECTROLYTES, SERUM

Electrolytes are vital to many bodily functions. They're responsible for depolarization of cell membranes, which enables muscle movement and nerve conduction. They maintain fluid balance by controlling the diffusion of fluids and particles between compartments. Other chemical processes are dependent on electrolytes for energy production or acid-base balance.

Sodium, the major extracellular cation, is the major determinant of extracellular osmolarity. Potassium, the major intracellular cation, is important in maintaining membrane potential in neuromuscular tissue. Chloride, the major extracellular anion, is an important buffer in acid-base balance.

Purpose

▶ To evaluate the serum concentrations of electrolytes

Reference values

Normally, serum sodium levels range from 135 to 145 mEq/L (SI, 135 to 145 mmol/L), serum potassium levels range from 3.5 to 5 mEq/L (SI, 3.5 to 5 mmol/L), and serum chloride levels range from 100 to 108 mEq/L (SI, 100 to 108 mmol/L).

Abnormal values

Abnormally low sodium levels (hyponatremia) may result from dilutional factors, such as excess water intake, inappropriate secretion of antidiuretic hormone, and osmotic dilution secondary to hyperglycemia. Inadequate sodium intake, the loss of sodium into other compartments (such as in ascites and edema), and conditions causing increased sodium loss (such as Addison's disease, diarrhea, vomiting, and renal tubular dysfunction) are other causes.

Abnormally high sodium levels (hypernatremia) usually result from excess sodium intake or inadequate water intake but may also be secondary to excessive sweating, thermal burns, diabetes insipidus, and osmotic diuresis. Disorders that inhibit sodium loss, such as Cushing's syndrome and hyperaldosteronism, are other causes.

Abnormally low potassium levels (hypokalemia) may result from insufficient intake or diuretic therapy but may also be secondary to hyperaldosteronism, Cushing's syndrome, renal tubular acidosis, excessive licorice intake, and loss of potassium through the GI tract. Alkalosis and administration of insulin, glucose, and calcium result in a shift from the intravascular compartment to the intracellular space.

Above-normal serum potassium values (hyperkalemia) are usually the result of renal insufficiency or failure. They may also result from excessive intake of potassium or decreased loss due to Addison's disease, hyperaldosteronism, or aldosterone-inhibiting diuretics. Acidosis, infection, crushing injury to tissues, and malignant hyperthermia may result in the potassium shifting to the intracellular compartment.

Chloride abnormalities usually accompany changes in serum sodium concentrations.

ERYTHROCYTE SEDIMENTATION RATE

The erythrocyte sedimentation rate (ESR) measures the degree of erythrocyte settling in a blood sample during a specified time period. The ESR is a sensitive but nonspecific test that's frequently the earliest indicator of disease when other chemical or physical signs are normal. The ESR commonly increases significantly in widespread inflammatory disorders; elevations may be prolonged in localized inflammation and malignant disease.

Purpose

▶ To monitor inflammatory or malignant disease
▶ To aid detection and diagnosis of occult disease, such as tuberculosis, tissue necrosis, and connective tissue disease

Reference values

The ESR normally ranges from 0 to 10 mm/hour (SI, 0 to 10 mm/h) in children, 0 to 10 mm/hour (SI, 0 to 10 mm/h) in males, and 0 to 20 mm/hour (SI, 0 to 20 mm/h) in females. Rates gradually increase after age 50.

Abnormal findings

The ESR rises in pregnancy, anemia, acute or chronic inflammation, tuberculosis, paraproteinemias (especially multiple myeloma and Waldenström's macroglobulinemia), rheumatic fever, rheumatoid arthritis, and some malignant diseases.

Polycythemia, sickle cell anemia, hyperviscosity, and low plasma fibrinogen or globulin levels tend to decrease the ESR.

ESTROGEN, SERUM

Estrogens (and progesterone) are secreted by the ovaries. They're responsible for the development of secondary female sexual characteristics and for normal menstruation; levels are usually undetectable in children. These hormones are secreted by ovarian follicular cells during the first half of the menstrual cycle and by the corpus luteum during the luteal phase and during pregnancy. In menopause, estrogen secretion drops to a constant, low level.

This radioimmunoassay measures serum levels of estradiol, estrone, and estriol (the only estrogens that appear in serum in measurable amounts) and has diagnostic significance in evaluating female gonadal dysfunction. Tests of hypothalamic-pituitary function may be required to confirm the diagnosis.

Purpose

▶ To determine sexual maturation and fertility
▶ To aid diagnosis of gonadal dysfunction, such as precocious or delayed puberty, menstrual disorders (especially amenorrhea), and infertility
▶ To determine fetal well-being
▶ To aid diagnosis of tumors known to secrete estrogen

Reference values

Normal serum estrogen levels for premenopausal women vary widely during the menstrual cycle, ranging from 26 to 149 pg/ml (SI, 90 to 550 pmol/L). The range for post-menopausal women is 0 to 34 pg/ml (SI, 0 to 125 pmol/L).

Serum estrogen levels in men range from 12 to 34 pg/ml (SI, 40 to 125 pmol/L). In children younger than age 6, the normal level of serum estrogen is 3 to 10 pg/ml (SI, 10 to 36 pmol/L).

Abnormal findings

Decreased estrogen levels may indicate primary hypogonadism, or ovarian failure, as in Turner's syndrome or ovarian agenesis; secondary hypogonadism, as in hypopituitarism; or menopause.

Abnormally high estrogen levels may occur with estrogen-producing tumors, in precocious puberty, and in severe hepatic disease, such as cirrhosis, that prevents clearance of plasma estrogens. High levels may also result from congenital adrenal hyperplasia (increased conversion of androgens to estrogen).

GLUCOSE, FASTING PLASMA

The fasting plasma glucose (or fasting blood sugar) test is used to measure plasma glucose levels after at least an 8-hour fast. This test is commonly used to screen for diabetes mellitus, in which absence or deficiency of insulin allows persistently high glucose levels.

Purpose

▶ To screen for diabetes mellitus
▶ To monitor drug or diet therapy in patients with diabetes mellitus

Reference values

The normal range for fasting plasma glucose varies according to the laboratory procedure. Generally, normal values for an adult after an 8-hour fast are less than 110 mg/dl (SI, < 6.1 mmol/L); for children ages 2 to 18 years after an 8-hour fast, values are 60 to 100 mg/dl (SI, 3.3 to 5.6 mmol/L).

Abnormal findings

Confirmation of diabetes mellitus requires fasting plasma glucose levels of 126 mg/dl (SI, 7 mmol/L) or greater obtained on two or more occasions. In patients with borderline or transient elevated levels, a 2-hour postprandial plasma glucose test or oral glucose tolerance test may be performed to confirm diagnosis.

Increased fasting plasma glucose levels can also result from pancreatitis, recent acute illness (such as myocardial infarction), Cushing's syndrome, acromegaly, and pheochromocytoma. Hyperglycemia may also stem from chronic hepatic disease, nephrotic syndrome, brain tumor, sepsis, or gastrectomy with dumping syndrome and is typical in eclampsia, anoxia, and seizure disorder.

Low plasma glucose levels can result from hyperinsulinism, insulinoma, von Gierke's disease, functional and reactive hypoglycemia, myxedema, adrenal insufficiency, congenital adrenal hyperplasia, hypopituitarism, malabsorption syndrome, and some cases of hepatic insufficiency.

HEMATOCRIT

A hematocrit (HCT) test may be done separately or as part of a complete blood cell count. It measures percentage by volume of packed red blood cells (RBCs) in a whole blood sample; for example, an HCT of 40% indicates that a 100-ml sample of blood contains 40 ml of packed RBCs. Packing is achieved by centrifuging anticoagulated whole blood in a capillary tube so that red cells are tightly packed without hemolysis.

Purpose

▶ To aid diagnosis of polycythemia, anemia, or abnormal states of hydration
▶ To aid calculation of erythrocyte indices

Reference values

HCT is usually measured electronically. The results are 3% lower than manual measurements, which trap plasma in the column of packed RBCs.

Reference values vary, depending on the type of sample, the laboratory performing the test, and the patient's age and sex, as follows:
▶ *Neonates at birth:* 55% to 68% (SI, 0.55 to 0.68)
▶ *Neonates age 1 week:* 47% to 65% (SI, 0.47 to 0.65)
▶ *Neonates age 1 month:* 37% to 49% (SI, 0.37 to 0.49)
▶ *Infants age 3 months:* 30% to 36% (SI, 0.3 to 0.36)
▶ *Infants age 1:* 29% to 41% (SI, 0.29 to 0.41)
▶ *Children age 10:* 36% to 40% (SI, 0.36 to 0.4)
▶ *Adult males:* 42% to 52% (SI, 0.42 to 0.52)
▶ *Adult females:* 36% to 48% (SI, 0.36 to 0.48).

Abnormal findings

Low HCT suggests anemia, hemodilution, or massive blood loss. High HCT indicates polycythemia or hemoconcentration due to blood loss and dehydration.

HEMOGLOBIN

The hemoglobin (Hb) test, which is usually performed as a part of a complete blood cell count, is used to measure the amount of Hb found in a deciliter (100 ml) of whole blood. Hb concentration correlates closely with the red blood cell (RBC) count and affects the Hb-RBC ratio (mean corpuscular hemoglobin [MCH] and mean corpuscular hemoglobin concentration [MCHC]).

Purpose

▶ To measure the severity of anemia or polycythemia and to monitor response to therapy
▶ To obtain data for calculating MCH and MCHC

Reference values

Hb concentration varies depending on the type of sample drawn and the patient's age and sex:
▶ *Neonates at birth:* 17 to 22 g/dl (SI, 170 to 220 g/L)
▶ *Neonates age 1 week:* 15 to 20 g/dl (SI, 150 to 200 g/L)
▶ *Neonates age 1 month:* 11 to 15 g/dl (SI, 110 to 150 g/L)
▶ *Children:* 11 to 13 g/dl (SI, 110 to 130 g/L)
▶ *Adult males:* 14 to 17.4 g/dl (SI, 140 to 174 g/L)
▶ *Males after middle age:* 12.4 to 14.9 g/dl (SI, 124 to 149 g/L)
▶ *Adult females:* 12 to 16 g/dl (SI, 120 to 160 g/L)
▶ *Females after middle age:* 11.7 to 13.8 g/dl (SI, 117 to 138 g/L)

Those who are more physically active or who live in high altitudes may have higher values.

Abnormal findings

Low Hb concentration may indicate anemia, recent hemorrhage, or fluid retention, causing hemodilution.

Elevated Hb suggests hemoconcentration from polycythemia or dehydration.

HEMOGLOBIN, GLYCOSYLATED

The glycosylated hemoglobin test (or hemoglobin A_{1c} [HbA_{1c}] test) reflects the average plasma glucose level over the preceding 2- to 3-month period. The process in which glucose binds to the hemoglobin molecule (glycohemoglobin) is called glycosylation. When the glucose concentration is increased because of an insulin deficiency, glycosylation is irreversible. Because the average lifespan of a red blood cell is 120 days, the average plasma glucose can be calculated by measuring the HbA_{1c}.

Purpose

▶ To assess control of diabetes mellitus by assessing the average plasma glucose level over the previous 2 to 3 months

Reference values

HbA_{1c} values are reported as a percentage of the total hemoglobin level within an erythrocyte. HbA_{1c} normally constitutes 4% to 6% (SI, 0.04 to 0.06) of the total hemoglobin.

Abnormal findings

In diabetes, the patient has good control of blood glucose concentrations when the HbA_{1c} value is less than 6% (SI, < 0.06).

Hemoglobinopathies (hemoglobin C, D, and S) will cause false low values due to the shortened life span of the RBC in these conditions. Patients with acute or chronic blood loss secondary to hemorrhage may also have false-low values. The presence of hemoglobin F may result in falsely elevated values.

HEPATITIS TESTS

This panel of tests confirms a diagnosis of hepatitis and identifies the causative type. (See *Hepatitis panel.*)

HUMAN CHORIONIC GONADOTROPIN, SERUM

Human chorionic gonadotropin (hCG) is a glycoprotein hormone produced by developing embryonic tissue and the placenta. If conception occurs, a specific assay for hCG, commonly called the beta-subunit assay, may detect this hormone in the blood 9 days after ovulation. This interval coincides with the implantation of the fertilized ovum into the uterine wall. The hormone is present in blood and also in urine whenever there's living chorionic or placental tissue.

Purpose

▶ To detect pregnancy
▶ To determine adequacy of hormonal production in high-risk pregnancies (for example, habitual abortion)
▶ To aid diagnosis of trophoblastic tumors, such as hydatidiform moles and choriocarcinoma, and tumors that ectopically secrete hCG
▶ To monitor treatment for induction of ovulation and conception

Reference values

Normally, hCG levels are less than 4 IU/L. During pregnancy, however, hCG levels increase as the pregnancy progresses. They'll peak between 30,000 and 100,000 IU/L at 60 to 80 days after the last menstrual period. After 120 days, the levels decline and remain between 5,000 and 10,000 IU/L for the rest of the pregnancy.

HEPATITIS PANEL

These tests are performed on patients with symptoms of hepatitis. Positive results not only confirm a hepatitis diagnosis but differentiate the type and status of the infection as well.

Test	Purpose	Implication of positive result
Anti-HAV (antibody to hepatitis A virus [HAV] antigen; also called *HAV-Ab*)	▶ To rule out HAV infection ▶ To determine immune status to HAV	▶ Indicates need for supportive care and education ▶ Can test for anti-HAV immunoglobulin (Ig) M and anti-HAV IgG ▶ Presence of IgG: indicates unlikely cause of current symptoms and immunity to HAV
Anti-HBc (IgG and IgM) (antibody to hepatitis B virus [HBV] core antigen)	▶ To differentiate acute from chronic HBV infection	▶ Is occasionally falsely positive ▶ Must be interpreted in context of other tests ▶ Indicates HBV infection as this marker doesn't appear after vaccination ▶ If primarily anti-HBc IgM result: reveals acute hepatitis B (infected usually less than 6 months) and needs follow-up ▶ If primarily anti-HBc IgG result: reveals chronic hepatitis B and needs follow-up
Anti-HBeAg (antibody to hepatitis Be antigen)	▶ To select patients for interferon therapy ▶ To select patients for liver transplantation	▶ If anti-HBeAg is present: indicates favorable prognosis because body has mounted a defensive attack against HBV ▶ Usually appears 8 to 16 weeks after exposure to HBV antigen; indicates an immune response has occurred
Anti-HbsAg (antibody to hepatitis B surface antigen; also called *anti-HBs*)	▶ To check immune status to HBV	▶ Indicates immune response to HBV due to HBV infection, HBV immunoglobulin, or HBV vaccination ▶ In acute infection, detectable after HbsAg disappears

(continued)

HEPATITIS PANEL *(continued)*

Test	Purpose	Implication of positive result
Anti-HCV (antibody to hepatitis C virus [HCV]) enzyme-linked immunosorbent assay (ELISA)	▶ To aid differential diagnosis of HCV ▶ To screen blood donors (ELISA-1 and ELISA-2: inexpensive, simple to perform, high sensitivity [ELISA-2 more sensitive])	▶ Does *not* indicate immunity ▶ Appears 2 to 6 months after acute HCV infection, but may take up to 1 year ▶ In the presence of elevated LFTs: diagnostic for hepatitis C and needs follow-up ▶ Low specificity compared to RNA testing*
Anti-HDV (antibody to hepatitis D virus [HDV])	▶ To detect antibodies to HDV ribonucleic acid (RNA) by polymerase chain reaction (HDV is a defective RNA virus that replicates efficiently only in the presence of HbsAg.)	▶ If positive for HDV: indicates poor prognosis ▶ 50% of patients with fulminant HBV also have HDV
HbeAg (hepatitis Be antigen)	▶ To measure viral replication	▶ High levels: very infectious patient
HbsAg (also called hepatitis-associated antigen and Australia antigen)	▶ To screen blood donors and high-risk populations ▶ As part of prenatal testing ▶ To establish differential diagnosis of viral hepatitis	▶ Needs follow-up ▶ Elevation for more than 6 months indicative of chronic hepatitis B infection
HBV deoxyribonucleic acid	▶ To measure viral presence (not antibodies) ▶ To confirm HBV if HBV screen is positive result but liver function tests (LFTs) are normal	▶ Confirms HBV status and requires careful follow-up care
HCV RNA (also called *enzyme immunoassay 2 [EIA-2], HCV RNA RT-PCR [reverse transcriptase-polymerase chain reaction]*)	▶ To measure viral presence (not antibodies) ▶ To confirm hepatitis C virus (HCV) status (gold standard because it's the most sensitive, but it's expensive and requires technical skill) ▶ To confirm HCV if HCV screen is positive but LFTs are normal	▶ Confirms HCV status and requires careful follow-up care

*A second-generation recombinant immunoblot assay (also called RIBA) is a commonly used supplemental assay, particularly in patients with normal alanine aminotransferase levels. The reactivity of antibodies toward each antigen band is reported as 1+ to 4+. If two or more bands react with an intensity of at least 1+, the result is indeterminate; however, the bands c22-3 and c33c are strongly associated with HCV RNA and even an indeterminate result that includes one of them may indicate positive HCV infection.

Abnormal findings

Elevated hCG beta-subunit levels indicate pregnancy; significantly higher concentrations are present in a multiple pregnancy. Increased levels may also suggest hydatidiform mole, trophoblastic neoplasms of the placenta, and nontrophoblastic carcinomas that secrete hCG (including gastric, pancreatic, and ovarian adenocarcinomas). Low hCG beta-subunit levels can occur in ectopic pregnancy or pregnancy of less than 9 days. Beta-subunit levels can't differentiate between pregnancy and tumor recurrence because they're high in both conditions.

HUMAN IMMUNO-DEFICIENCY VIRUS

These tests detect antibodies, antigens, or ribonucleic acid caused by human immunodeficiency virus (HIV) in serum. HIV is the virus that causes acquired immunodeficiency syndrome (AIDS). Transmission occurs by direct exposure of a person's blood to body fluids containing the virus. The virus may be transmitted from one person to another through exchange of contaminated blood and blood products, during sexual intercourse with an infected partner, when I.V. drugs are shared, and from an infected mother to her child during pregnancy or breast-feeding.

Initial identification of HIV is usually achieved through enzyme-linked immunosorbent assay. Positive findings are confirmed by Western blot test and immuno-fluorescence. (See *HIV testing,* pages 60 and 61.)

Purpose

▸ To screen for HIV in high-risk patients
▸ To screen donated blood for HIV

Normal findings

Test results are normally negative. However, HIV-1 or HIV-2 antibodies may fall to undetectable levels in the final stages of AIDS. A positive result, indicating the presence of antibodies, necessitates further investigation.

⬤⬤⬤ RED FLAG *Immunocompro-*
⬤⬤⬤ *mised patients may not produce these antibodies.*

Abnormal findings

The test detects exposure to HIV-1 or HIV-2 1 to 6 months after infection occurs; antibody to p24 is commonly the first HIV-1 antibody detectable. However, the test doesn't identify patients who have been exposed to the virus but haven't yet made antibodies. Most patients with AIDS have antibodies to HIV. A positive test for the HIV antibody can't determine whether a patient harbors actively replicating virus or when the patient will manifest signs and symptoms of AIDS.

Many apparently healthy people have been exposed to HIV and have circulating antibodies. The test results for such people aren't false-positives.

INTERNATIONAL NORMALIZED RATIO

The International Normalized Ratio (INR) system is viewed as the best means of standardizing measurement of prothrombin time to monitor oral anticoagulant therapy. It isn't used as a screening test for coagulopathies.

Purpose

▸ To evaluate effectiveness of oral anticoagulant therapy

(Text continues on page 62.)

HIV TESTING

Test type	Specimen (mode of collection)	Test complexity*
Standard human immunodeficiency virus (HIV) test	Serum or plasma (phlebotomy)	High
Rapid test	Serum, plasma, whole blood (phlebotomy, fingerstick)	Moderate§
Home sample collection test++	Dried blood spot (fingerstick)	High
Oral fluid test	Oral mucosal transudate (oral fluid collection device)	High
Urine-based test	Urine (Urine cup)	High

KEY

* Complexity of specimen collection and testing as categorized by the Clinical Laboratory Improvement Amendments (CLIA). (Schochetman, G., and George, J.R., eds. *AIDS Testing: A Comprehensive Guide to Technical, Medical, Social, Legal, and Management Issues,* 2nd ed. New York: Springer-Verlag, 1994).

+ All licensed enzyme immunoassays (EIAs) detect HIV-1 but not all detect HIV-2. EIAs that can detect HIV-1 and HIV-2 are required for blood donor screening and are recommended for diagnostic screening only where HIV-2 infection is likely. No licensed confirmatory test exists for HIV-2. Although current tests detect most HIV-1 group O infections, few detect all such infections.

§ The one rapid test licensed by FDA, Abbott Murex Single Use Diagnostic System (SUDS) HIV-1 test (Abbott Laboratories, Inc., Abbott Park, Illinois) is classified as a moderate-complexity test and requires on-site laboratory testing capability. Future rapid tests could be classified by CLIA as "waived" and not require on-site laboratory testing capability, depending on the expertise required to perform this test correctly.

Screening; confirmatory	Strains detected+	Provision of results
Enzyme immunoassay (EIA); Western blot or immunofluorescence assay (IFA)	HIV-1 and HIV-2	*HIV negative* Test result at return visit (typically a few days to 1 to 2 weeks) *HIV positive* Confirmed result at return visit
Rapid EIA; Western blot/IFA¶	HIV-1	*HIV negative* Test result at time of testing (typically 10 to 60 minutes) *HIV positive* Preliminary positive test result at time of testing;** confirmed result at return visit
EIA; Western blot/IFA	HIV-1	*HIV negative* Test result when patient calls (typically 3 to 7 days) *HIV positive* Confirmed result when patient calls
EIA; oral mucosal transudate Western blot	HIV-1	*HIV negative* Test result at return visit (typically 1 to 2 weeks) *HIV positive* Confirmed result at return visit
EIA; urine Western blot	HIV-1	*HIV negative* Test result at return visit (typically 1 to 2 weeks) *HIV positive* Test result at return visit; further confirmation by blood sample recommended because of lower specificity of urine Western blot compared with serum-based Western blot/IFA

¶ Future rapid tests might be able to be confirmed with a second rapid test to provide an immediate test result with high sensitivity, specificity, and predictive value comparable with EIA/Western blot (Stetler, H.C., et al. "Field Evaluation of Rapid HIV Serologic Tests for Screening and Confirming HIV-1 infection in Honduras," *AIDS* 1997;11:369-75).

** Information on providing "preliminary" positive test results from a single rapid test is available elsewhere (CDC. Update: HIV Counseling and Testing using Rapid Tests — United States, 1995. *MMWR* 1998;47:211-15).

++ Home sample collection is different from home-use testing. FDA has approved home sample collection but not home-use HIV test kits (Kassler, W.J. "Advances in HIV Testing Technology and Their Potential Impact on Prevention," *AIDS Educ Prev* 1997;9[suppl B]:27-40).

Source: Centers for Disease Control and Prevention. "Revised Guidelines for HIV Counseling, Testing, and Referral," *Morbidity and Mortality Weekly Report* 50(RR-19):1-58, November 2001.

Reference values

Normal INR for patients receiving warfarin therapy is 2.0 to 3.0. For those with prosthetic heart valves, an INR of 2.5 to 3.5 is suggested. Verify the patient's maintenance range with the cardiologist.

Abnormal findings

An increased INR may indicate disseminated intravascular coagulation, cirrhosis, hepatitis, vitamin K deficiency, or salicylate intoxication or may be due to massive blood transfusion.

LYME DISEASE SEROLOGY

Lyme disease is a multisystem disorder characterized by dermatologic, neurologic, cardiac, and rheumatic manifestations in various stages. Epidemiologic and serologic studies implicate a common tick-borne spirochete, *Borrelia burgdorferi*, as the cause. Serologic tests for Lyme disease, both indirect immunofluorescent and enzyme-linked immunosorbent assays, measure antibody response to this spirochete and indicate current infection or past exposure. Serologic tests are able to identify 50% of patients with early-stage Lyme disease and all patients with later complications of carditis, neuritis, and arthritis, as well as patients in remission.

Purpose

▶ To confirm a diagnosis of Lyme disease

Normal findings

Normal serum values are nonreactive.

Abnormal findings

A positive Lyme disease serology can help confirm diagnosis, but it isn't definitive because the tests aren't able to detect infection until a sufficient amount of antibodies are produced, which may take as long as 2 to 4 months after the tick bite. Other treponemal diseases and high rheumatoid factor titers can cause false-positive results. More than 15% of patients with Lyme disease fail to develop antibodies.

MYOGLOBIN

The myoglobin test detects the presence of myoglobin—a red pigment found in the cytoplasm of cardiac and skeletal muscle cells—in the blood. Myoglobin functions as an oxygen-binding muscle protein. It's released into the bloodstream in patients with ischemia, trauma, or inflammation of the muscle.

Purpose

▶ To estimate damage to skeletal or cardiac muscle tissue (as a nonspecific test)
▶ To predict flare-ups of polymyositis
▶ To determine specifically whether myocardial infarction (MI) has occurred

Reference values

Normal myoglobin values are 0 to 0.09 µg/ml (SI, 5 to 70 µ/L).

Abnormal findings

Besides an MI, increased myoglobin levels may occur with acute alcohol intoxication, dermatomyositis, hypothermia (with prolonged shivering), muscular dystrophy, polymyositis, rhabdomyolysis, severe burn injuries, trauma, severe renal failure, and systemic lupus erythematosus.

PARTIAL THROMBOPLASTIN TIME

The partial thromboplastin time (PTT) is used to evaluate all the clotting factors of the intrinsic pathway except platelets by measuring the time required for formation of a fibrin clot after the addition of calcium and phospholipid emulsion to a plasma sample. An activator, such as kaolin, is used to shorten clotting time.

Purpose

▶ To aid preoperative screening for bleeding tendencies
▶ To screen for congenital coagulation deficiencies of the clotting factors
▶ To monitor heparin therapy

Reference values

Normally, a fibrin clot forms 21 to 35 seconds (SI, 21 to 35 s) after addition of reagents. For a patient on anticoagulant therapy, ask the attending physician to specify the reference values for the therapy being delivered.

Abnormal findings

Prolonged PTT may indicate a deficiency of certain plasma clotting factors, the presence of heparin, or the presence of fibrin split products, fibrinolysins, or circulating anticoagulants that act as antibodies to specific clotting factors.

PLATELET COUNT

Platelets, or thrombocytes, are the smallest formed elements in blood. They promote coagulation and the formation of a hemostatic plug in vascular injury. The platelet count test is one of the most important screening tests of platelet function because it assesses bleeding disorders associated with disease processes such as malignancies and liver disease. Accurate counts are vital.

Purpose

▶ To evaluate platelet production
▶ To assess effects of chemotherapy or radiation therapy on platelet production
▶ To diagnose and monitor severe thrombocytosis or thrombocytopenia
▶ To confirm a visual estimate of platelet number and morphology from a stained blood film

Reference values

Normal platelet counts range from 140,000 to 400,000/µl (SI, 140 to 400 x 10^9/L) in adults and from 150,000 to 450,000/µl (SI, 150 to 450 x 10^9/L) in children.

Abnormal findings

A decreased platelet count (thrombocytopenia) can result from aplastic or hypoplastic bone marrow; infiltrative bone marrow disease such as leukemia, or disseminated infection; megakaryocytic hypoplasia; ineffective thrombopoiesis due to folic acid or vitamin B_{12} deficiency; pooling of platelets in an enlarged spleen; increased platelet destruction due to drugs or immune disorders; disseminated intravascular coagulation; Bernard-Soulier syndrome; or mechanical injury to platelets.

An increased platelet count (thrombocytosis) can result from hemorrhage, infectious disorders, iron deficiency anemia, recent surgery, pregnancy, splenectomy, or inflammatory disorders. In such cases, the platelet count returns to normal after the patient recovers from the primary disorder. However, the count remains elevated in primary thrombocythemia, myelofibro-

sis with myeloid metaplasia, polycythemia vera, and chronic myel-
ogenous leukemia.

When the platelet count is abnormal, diagnosis usually requires further studies, such as complete
blood cell count, bone marrow
biopsy, direct antiglobulin test (direct Coombs' test), and serum protein electrophoresis.

PROSTATE-SPECIFIC ANTIGEN

Prostate-specific antigen (PSA) is a
glucoprotein that's produced by the
prostatic ductal epithelium. It's
present in the serum in normal,
benign hyperplastic, and malignant
prostatic tissue as well as in metastatic prostatic carcinoma. Serum
PSA levels are used to monitor the
spread or recurrence of prostate
cancer and to evaluate the patient's
response to treatment. PSA is intended for screening of prostatic
disorders but isn't specific for
prostate cancer.

Purpose

▶ To screen for prostate disorders
▶ To monitor the course of prostate
cancer and aid evaluation of treatment

Reference values

Normal serum values are as fol-
lows:
▶ *Ages 40 to 50:* 2 to 2.8 ng/ml (SI,
2 to 2.8 µg/L)
▶ *Ages 51 to 60:* 2.9 to 3.8 ng/ml
(SI, 2.9 to 3.8 µg/L)
▶ *Ages 61 to 70:* 4 to 5.3 ng/ml (SI,
4 to 5.3 µg/L)
▶ *Ages 71 and older:* 5.6 to 7.2 ng/
ml (SI, 5.6 to 7.2 µg/L).

Abnormal findings

About 80% of patients with prostate cancer have pretreatment PSA
values greater than 4 ng/ml. However, PSA results alone don't confirm a diagnosis of prostate cancer.
About 20% of patients with benign
prostatic hyperplasia also have levels greater than 4 ng/ml. Further
assessment and testing, including
tissue biopsy, are needed to confirm
cancer.

PROTHROMBIN TIME

Prothrombin time (PT) measures
the time required for a fibrin clot to
form in a citrated plasma sample after addition of calcium ions and tissue thromboplastin (factor III).

Purpose

▶ To provide an overall evaluation
of extrinsic coagulation factors V,
VII, and X and of prothrombin and
fibrinogen
▶ To monitor response to oral anticoagulant therapy

Reference values

Normally, PTs range from 10 to 13
seconds (SI, 10 to 13 s). Times vary,
however, depending on the source
of tissue thromboplastin and the
type of sensing devices used to
measure clot formation. In a patient
receiving oral anticoagulants, PT is
usually maintained between 2 and
2.5 times the normal control value.

Abnormal findings

Prolonged PT may indicate deficiencies in fibrinogen; prothrombin; factor V, VII, or X (specific assays can
pinpoint such deficiencies); or vitamin K as well as hepatic disease. It
may also result from ongoing oral
anticoagulant therapy. Prolonged PT
that exceeds 2½ times the control is
commonly associated with abnormal bleeding.

RED BLOOD CELL COUNT

The red blood cell (RBC) count, also called an *erythrocyte count,* is part of a complete blood cell count. It's used to detect the number of RBCs in a microliter (µl), or cubic millimeter (mm³), of whole blood.

Purpose

▶ To provide data for calculating mean corpuscular volume and mean corpuscular hemoglobin, which reveal RBC size and hemoglobin content
▶ To support other hematologic tests for diagnosing anemia or polycythemia

Reference values

Normal RBC values vary, depending on the type of sample and on the patient's age and sex, as follows:
▶ *Adult males:* 4.5 to 5.5 million RBCs/µl (SI, 4.5 to 5.5 × 10^{12}/L) of venous blood
▶ *Adult females:* 4 to 5 million RBCs/µl (SI, 4 to 5 × 10^{12}/L) of venous blood
▶ *Children:* 4.6 to 4.8 million RBCs/µl (SI, 4.6 to 4.8 × 10^{12}/L) of venous blood
▶ *Full-term neonates:* 4.4 to 5.8 million RBCs/µl (SI, 4.4 to 5.8 × 10^{12}/L) of capillary blood at birth, decreasing to 3 to 3.8 million RBCs/µl (SI, 3 to 3.8 × 10^{12}/L) at age 2 months and increasing slowly thereafter.

Normal values may exceed these levels in patients living at high altitudes or those who are very active.

Abnormal findings

An elevated RBC count may indicate absolute or relative polycythemia. A depressed count may indicate anemia, fluid overload, or hemorrhage beyond 24 hours. Further tests, such as stained cell examination, hematocrit, hemoglobin, red cell indices, and white cell studies, are needed to confirm the diagnosis.

RED CELL INDICES

Using the results of the red blood cell (RBC) count, hematocrit, and total hemoglobin (Hb) tests, red cell indices (erythrocyte indices) provide important information about the size, Hb concentration, and Hb weight of an average RBC.

Purpose

▶ To aid diagnosis and classification of anemias

Reference values

The indices tested include mean corpuscular volume (MCV), mean corpuscular Hb (MCH), and mean corpuscular Hb concentration (MCHC).

MCV, the ratio of hematocrit (packed cell volume) to the RBC count, expresses the average size of the erythrocytes and indicates whether they're undersized (microcytic), oversized (macrocytic), or normal (normocytic). MCH, the Hb-RBC ratio, gives the weight of Hb in an average red cell. MCHC, the ratio of Hb weight to hematocrit, defines the concentration of Hb in 100 ml of packed RBCs. It helps to distinguish normally colored (normochromic) RBCs from paler (hypochromic) RBCs.

The range of normal red cell indices is as follows:
▶ *MCV:* 84 to 99 µm³
▶ *MCH:* 26 to 32 pg/cell
▶ *MCHC:* 30 to 36 g/dl.

Abnormal findings

Low MCV and MCHC indicate microcytic, hypochromic anemias caused by iron deficiency anemia, pyridoxine-responsive anemia, or thalassemia. A high MCV suggests macrocytic anemias caused by megaloblastic anemias, folic acid or vitamin B_{12} deficiency, inherited disorders of deoxyribonucleic acid synthesis, or reticulocytosis. Because MCV reflects the average volume of many cells, a value within the normal range can encompass RBCs of varying size, from microcytic to macrocytic.

THYROID-STIMULATING HORMONE

Thyroid-stimulating hormone (TSH), or thyrotropin, promotes increases in the size, number, and activity of thyroid cells and stimulates the release of triiodothyronine and thyroxine. These hormones affect total body metabolism and are essential for normal growth and development.

This test measures serum TSH levels by radioimmunoassay. It can detect primary hypothyroidism and determine whether the hypothyroidism results from thyroid gland failure or from pituitary or hypothalamic dysfunction. Normal serum TSH levels rule out primary hypothyroidism. This test may not distinguish between low-normal and subnormal levels, especially in secondary hypothyroidism.

Purpose

▶ To confirm or rule out primary hypothyroidism and distinguish it from secondary hypothyroidism
▶ To monitor drug therapy in patients with primary hypothyroidism

Reference levels

Normal TSH values range from 0.3 to 5 mU/ml (SI, 0.3 to 5 mU/L).

Abnormal findings

TSH levels may be slightly elevated in euthyroid patients with thyroid cancer. Extremely high levels suggest primary hypothyroidism or, possibly, endemic goiter.

Low or undetectable TSH levels may be normal but occasionally indicate secondary hypothyroidism (with inadequate secretion of TSH or thyrotropin-releasing hormone), hyperthyroidism (Graves' disease), and thyroiditis; both disorders are marked by hypersecretion of thyroid hormones, which suppresses TSH release.

THYROXINE

Thyroxine (T_4) is an amine secreted by the thyroid gland in response to thyroid-stimulating hormone (TSH) and, indirectly, thyrotropin-releasing hormone. The rate of secretion is normally regulated by a complex system of negative and positive feedback mechanisms.

Only a fraction of T_4 (about 0.05%) circulates freely in the blood; the rest binds strongly to plasma proteins, primarily thyroxine-binding globulin (TBG). This minute fraction is responsible for the clinical effects of thyroid hormone. TBG binds so tenaciously that T_4 survives in the plasma for a relatively long time, with a half-life of about 6 days. This immunoassay should be interpreted in conjunction with the TBG level or as part of a free thyroxine index.

Purpose

▶ To evaluate thyroid function
▶ To aid diagnosis of hyperthyroidism and hypothyroidism
▶ To monitor response to antithyroid medication in hyperthyroidism or to thyroid replacement therapy in hypothyroidism

Reference values

Normally, total T_4 levels range from 5 to 13.5 µg/dl (SI, 64.3 to 173.7 nmol/L).

Abnormal findings

Abnormally elevated T_4 levels are consistent with primary and secondary hyperthyroidism, including excessive T_4 (levothyroxine) replacement therapy (factitious or iatrogenic hyperthyroidism). Subnormal levels suggest primary or secondary hypothyroidism or may be due to T_4 suppression by normal, elevated, or replacement levels of triiodothyronine (T_3). In doubtful cases of hypothyroidism, TSH measurement may be indicated.

Normal T_4 levels don't guarantee euthyroidism; for example, normal readings occur in T_3 thyrotoxicosis. Overt signs of hyperthyroidism require further testing.

THYROXINE AND TRIIODO-THYRONINE (FREE)

These tests, often done simultaneously, measure serum levels of free thyroxine (FT_4) and free triiodothyronine (FT_3), the minute portions of T_4 and T_3 not bound to thyroxine-binding globulin (TBG) and other serum proteins. These unbound hormones are responsible for the thyroid's effects on cellular metabolism. Measurement of free hormone levels is the best indicator of thyroid function.

Because of disagreement as to whether FT_4 or FT_3 is the better indicator, laboratories commonly measure both. The disadvantages of these tests include a cumbersome and difficult laboratory method, inaccessibility, and cost. This test may be useful in the 5% of patients in whom the standard T_3 or T_4 tests fail to produce diagnostic results.

Purpose

▶ To measure the metabolically active form of the thyroid hormones
▶ To aid diagnosis of hyperthyroidism and hypothyroidism when TBG levels are abnormal

Reference values

Normal range for FT_4 is 0.9 to 2.3 ng/dl (SI, 10 to 30 pmol/L); for FT_3, 260 to 480 pg/dl (SI, 4 to 7.4 pmol/L). Values vary, depending on the laboratory.

Abnormal findings

Elevated FT_4 and FT_3 levels indicate hyperthyroidism, unless peripheral resistance to thyroid hormone is present. T_3 thyrotoxicosis, a distinct form of hyperthyroidism, yields high FT_3 levels with normal or low FT_4 values. Low FT_4 levels usually indicate hypothyroidism, except in patients receiving replacement therapy with T_3. Patients receiving thyroid therapy may have varying levels of FT_4 and FT_3, depending on the preparation used and the time of sample blood collection.

TRIGLYCERIDES

Serum triglyceride analysis provides quantitative analysis of triglycerides — the main storage form of lipids — that constitute about 95% of fatty tissue. Although not diagnostic itself, the triglyceride test permits early identification of hyperlipidemia and the risk of coronary artery disease (CAD).

Purpose

▶ To screen for hyperlipidemia or pancreatitis

▶ To help identify nephrotic syndrome and poorly controlled diabetes mellitus
▶ To determine the risk of CAD
▶ To calculate low-density lipoprotein cholesterol level using the Freidewald equation

Reference values

Reference values for triglyceride levels are as follows:
▶ *Normal:* < 150 mg/dl (SI, < 1.70 mmol/L)
▶ *Borderline high:* 150 to 199 mg/dl (SI, 1.70 to 2.25 mmol/L)
▶ *High:* 200 to 499 mg/dl (SI, 2.26 to 5.64 mmol/L)
▶ *Very high:* ≥ 500 mg/dl (SI, ≥ 5.65 mmol/L).

Abnormal findings

Increased or decreased serum triglyceride levels suggest a clinical abnormality; additional tests are required for a definitive diagnosis.

A mild to moderate increase in serum triglyceride levels indicates biliary obstruction, diabetes mellitus, nephrotic syndrome, endocrinopathy, or overconsumption of alcohol. Markedly increased levels without an identifiable cause reflect congenital hyperlipoproteinemia and necessitate lipoprotein phenotyping to confirm the diagnosis. Decreased serum triglyceride levels are rare and occur mainly in patients with malnutrition or abetalipoproteinemia.

TRIIODO-THYRONINE

This highly specific radioimmunoassay measures total (bound and free) serum content of triiodothyronine (T_3) to investigate clinical indications of thyroid dysfunction. Like thyroxine (T_4) secretion, T_3 secretion occurs in response to thyroid-stimulating hormone (TSH) and, secondarily, thyrotropin-releasing hormone.

Although T_3 is present in the bloodstream in minute quantities and is metabolically active for only a short time, its impact on body metabolism dominates that of T_4. Another significant difference between the two major thyroid hormones is that T_3 binds less firmly to thyroxine-binding globulin. Consequently, T_3 persists in the bloodstream for a short time; half disappears in about 1 day, whereas half of T_4 disappears in 6 days.

Purpose

▶ To aid diagnosis of T_3 thyrotoxicosis
▶ To aid diagnosis of hypothyroidism and hyperthyroidism
▶ To monitor clinical response to thyroid replacement therapy in hypothyroidism

Reference values

Normal serum T_3 levels range from 80 to 200 ng/dl (SI, 1.2 to 3 nmol/L).

Abnormal findings

Serum T_3 and serum T_4 levels usually rise and fall in tandem. However, in T_3 thyrotoxicosis, T_3 levels rise while total and free T_4 levels remain normal. T_3 thyrotoxicosis occurs in patients with Graves' disease, toxic adenoma, or toxic nodular goiter. T_3 levels also surpass T_4 levels in patients receiving thyroid replacement therapy containing more T_3 than T_4. In iodine-deficient areas, the thyroid may produce larger amounts of the more cellularly active T_3 than of T_4 in an effort to maintain the euthyroid state.

Generally, T_3 levels appear to be a more accurate diagnostic indicator of hyperthyroidism. Although both

T_3 and T_4 levels are increased in about 90% of patients with hyperthyroidism, there's a disproportionate increase in T_3. In some patients with hypothyroidism, T_3 levels may fall within the normal range and not be diagnostically significant.

A rise in serum T_3 levels normally occurs during pregnancy. Low T_3 levels may appear in euthyroid patients with systemic illness (especially hepatic or renal disease), during severe acute illness, and after trauma or major surgery; in such patients, TSH levels are within normal limits. Low serum T_3 levels are found in some euthyroid patients with malnutrition.

TROPONIN-I AND TROPONIN-T

Troponin (cardiac troponin-I [cTn I]) is the contractile regulatory protein of striated muscle (slow-twitch and fast-twitch skeletal muscle and cardiac muscle). Cardiac muscle produces specific forms of troponin: cTn I and cardiac troponin-T (cTn T). They're released into the circulation after cellular necrosis.

Purpose

▶ To rule out myocardial infarction on initial presentation, especially when the patient didn't seek care immediately after onset of symptoms; highest sensitivity occurs after 10 hours

Reference values

Laboratories may give varying results, with some calling a result abnormal if it shows any detectable levels and others giving a range for abnormal levels.

Normally, cTn I levels are less than 0.4 µg/ml, and cTn T levels are less than 0.1 µg/ml. cTn I levels below 0.4 µg/ml aren't suggestive of cardiac injury, and levels of 0.5 to 1.9 µg/ml are indeterminate for cardiac injury. cTn I levels greater than 2.0 µg/ml suggest cardiac injury. Results of a qualitative cTn T rapid immunoassay that are greater than 0.2 µg/ml are considered positive for cardiac injury. When quantitative serum assays for cTn T are done, the upper limit for normal is 0.1 µg/ml. As long as tissue injury continues, the troponin levels will remain high.

Abnormal findings

Troponin levels rise rapidly and are detectable within 1 hour of myocardial cell injury. cTn I levels aren't detectable in people without cardiac injury.

WHITE BLOOD CELL COUNT

A white blood cell (WBC) count, also called a *leukocyte count,* is part of a complete blood cell count. It indicates the number of white cells in a microliter (µl, or cubic millimeter) of whole blood.

WBC counts can vary by as much as 2,000 cells/µl (SI, 2 x 10^9/L) on any given day, due to strenuous exercise, stress, or digestion. The WBC count may increase or decrease significantly with certain diseases but is diagnostically useful only when the patient's WBC differential and clinical status are considered.

Purpose

▶ To determine infection or inflammation
▶ To determine the need for further tests, such as the WBC differential or bone marrow biopsy
▶ To monitor response to chemotherapy or radiation therapy

Reference values

The WBC count ranges from 4,000 to 10,000/µl (SI, 4 to 10 x 10^9/L).

Abnormal findings

An elevated WBC count (leukocytosis) often signals infection, such as an abscess, meningitis, appendicitis, or tonsillitis. A high count may also result from leukemia or from tissue necrosis due to burns, a myocardial infarction, or gangrene.

A low WBC count (leukopenia) indicates bone marrow depression that may result from viral infections or from toxic reactions, such as those after treatment with an antineoplastic, ingestion of mercury or other heavy metals, or exposure to benzene or arsenicals. Leukopenia characteristically accompanies influenza, typhoid fever, measles, infectious hepatitis, mononucleosis, and rubella.

WHITE BLOOD CELL DIFFERENTIAL

The white blood cell (WBC) differential is used to evaluate the distribution and morphology of WBCs, providing more specific information about a patient's immune system than the WBC count alone.

WBCs are classified as one of five major types of leukocytes—neutrophils, eosinophils, basophils, lymphocytes, and monocytes. The differential count is the percentage of each type of WBC in the blood. The total number of each type of WBC is obtained by multiplying the percentage of each type by the total WBC count.

INTERPRETING WBC DIFFERENTIAL VALUES

The differential count measures the types of white blood cells (WBCs) as a percentage of the total WBC count (the relative value). The absolute value is obtained by multiplying the relative value of each cell type by the total WBC count. Both the relative and absolute values must be considered to obtain an accurate diagnosis.

For example, consider a patient whose WBC count is 6,000/µl (SI, 6 × 10^9/L) and whose differential shows 30% (SI, 0.3) neutrophils and 70% (SI, 0.7) lymphocytes. His relative lymphocyte count seems to be quite high (lymphocytosis), but when this figure is multiplied by his WBC count (6,000 × 70% = 4,200 lymphocytes/µl) (SI, [6 × 10^9/L] × 9.79 = 4.2 × 10^9/L lymphocytes), it's well within the normal range.

However, this patient's neutrophil count (30%) (SI, 0.3) is low; when this figure is multiplied by the WBC count (6,000 × 30% = 1,800 neutrophils/ml) (SI, [6 × 10^9/L] × 0.30 = 1.8 × 10^9/L neutrophils), the result is a low absolute number, which may mean depressed bone marrow.

The normal percentages of WBC type in adults are:
Neutrophils: 54% to 75% (SI, 0.54 to 0.75)
Eosinophils: 1% to 4% (SI, 0.01 to 0.04)
Basophils: 0% to 1% (SI, 0 to 0.01)
Monocytes: 2% to 8% (SI, 0.02 to 0.08)
Lymphocytes: 25% to 40% (SI, 0.25 to 0.40).

High levels of these leukocytes are associated with various allergic diseases and reactions to parasites. An eosinophil count is sometimes ordered as a follow-up test when an elevated or depressed eosinophil level is reported.

Purpose

▶ To evaluate the body's capacity to resist and overcome infection
▶ To detect and identify various types of leukemia
▶ To determine the stage and severity of an infection
▶ To detect allergic reactions and parasitic infections and to assess their severity (eosinophil count)
▶ To distinguish viral from bacterial infections

Reference values

For normal values for the five types of WBCs classified in the differential for adults and children, see *Interpreting WBC differential values*.

For an accurate diagnosis, differential test results must always be interpreted in relation to the total WBC count.

Abnormal findings

Abnormal differential patterns provide evidence for a wide range of disease states and other conditions.

3
Common X-rays
Deciphering the images

Understanding an X-ray

When a radiologist assesses X-ray film, it's usually to find an answer to a particular problem or question. Examples include whether a chest tube or central line is positioned correctly, where there's fluid in the lungs, and whether the bowel loops are distended.

Comparing an X-ray film with previous films is helpful, particularly when assessing a progression of a clinical situation, such as pneumonia or pneumothorax. The patient's position when the film is taken should be noted because distance from the X-ray source can change the apparent size of structures. For instance, the heart may appear enlarged in an anterioposterior projection rather than in a posteroanterior projection because it was closer to the X-ray tube (and farther from the film) when exposed.

A decubitus film may be a better projection for assessing fluid levels in the abdomen because the fluid is in a dependent position. Likewise, the quality and diagnostic usefulness of a portable film taken in a semi-upright position versus a full upright position are compromised because of fluid collecting in layers posteriorly and because the lungs aren't fully expanded. Typically, the physician will order the X-ray to be done at the bedside or in the radiology department. Although it may be more convenient not to transport the patient, posteroanterior and lateral films taking in the radiology department ensure higher quality and greater diagnostic accuracy.

Differences in film quality, sharpness of detail, patient motion, lightness versus darkness of structures, and patient positioning can affect the diagnostic usefulness of an X-ray and should be monitored.

An X-ray should be considered a tool to aid the clinician in confirming a diagnosis or clinical finding. Wheezes or crackles in the lung bases heard on auscultation may be confirmed by the presence of fluid-filled, dense areas seen on a chest X-ray. However, usually an ordinary X-ray can't give the clinician all the

---

FACTORS IN RADIATION PROTECTION

If you need to be with a patient or in the vicinity when X-rays are being taken, you need to be aware of your own safety as well as your patient's. These three factors affect your protection.

Time
Duration of exposure to the X-rays (Cutting exposure time by 50% cuts the dose by 50%.)

Distance
Distance from the source of the X-rays (Exposure decreases with distance, according to the inverse-square law; doubling the distance cuts exposure by 25%. A distance of 6′ (1.8 m) is generally considered the minimum.)

Shielding
Protects against scatter radiation (Effective barriers include lead aprons, gloves, thyroid shields, leaded or photosensitive glass, walls, and fixed or movable partitions.)

information needed to make a diagnosis. In that case, the clinician may use another imaging modality to view anatomy or to identify a pathological process.

If you're present when X-rays are taken, take safety factors into account. (See *Factors in radiation protection,* page 73.)

X-rays of the torso

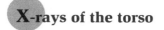

NORMAL CHEST X-RAY

Bony and soft landmarks in this normal chest and upper abdomen X-ray stand out in this posteroanterior view.

Tracheal air shadow
Clavicles
Aortic notch
Ribs
Vertebrae
Lungs
Heart
Breasts
Diaphragm
Costophrenic angles
Liver
Stomach gas
Spleen

FOREIGN OBJECT IN LUNG

The child in the X-rays on this page has inhaled an object that has lodged in the left bronchus. The anteroposterior chest X-ray taken during inspiration seems normal. An X-ray taken during expiration shows the effect of the foreign object. Trapped air has hyperinflated the left lung ➤ The mediastinum has shifted right ➛ and, compared to the inspiratory X-ray, the dark air-filled area on the left has become more lucent.

INSPIRATION

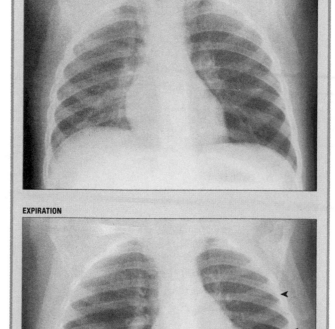

EXPIRATION

LOBAR PNEUMONIA

Typical signs of lobar pneumonia that involve the left lower lobe ⇨ are apparent in this chest X-ray. Borders of the heart shadow and the left hemidiaphragm are hidden (silhouette sign). Visible are mediastinal shift to the left, depressed left hilum, and atelectasis (indicated by the smaller left lung) ➤.

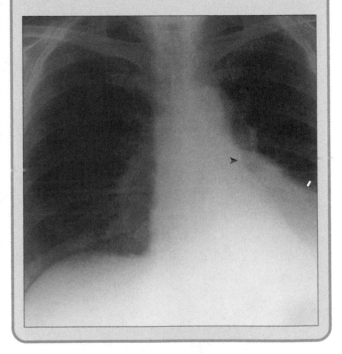

LUNG CANCER

In this chest X-ray, bronchogenic lung cancer shows up as a large mass ➡ with central cavitation ➤ in the right hilar area. Opacity of the right lower lobe indicates atelectasis caused by the tumor.

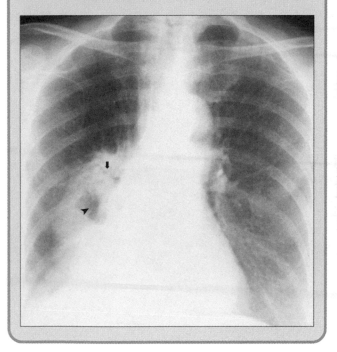

PLEURAL EFFUSION

This posteroanterior chest X-ray of a patient with heart failure reveals pleural effusion. The right costophrenic angle is blunted by pleural fluid and the upper border of the pleural fluid ▷ is concave.

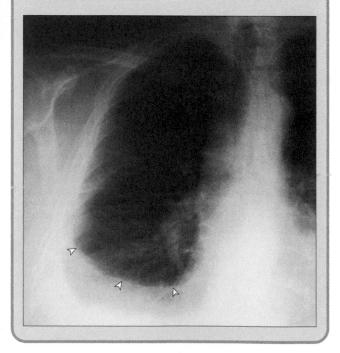

PNEUMOTHORAX WITH SUBCUTANEOUS EMPHYSEMA

This posteroanterior chest X-ray shows a pneumothorax as well as subcutaneous and mediastinal emphysema ⇨. Because the chest tube ⇨ has migrated outside the pleural space, the pneumothorax ▷ is larger than it was originally.

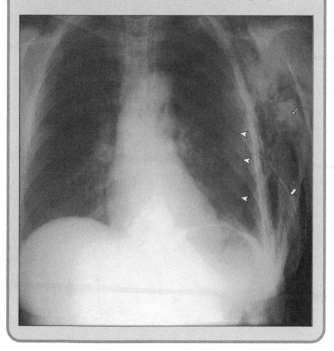

PULMONARY CHANGES WITH ASTHMA

The effects of asthma are apparent in this posteroanterior chest X-ray. The lungs ➤ are hyperinflated, the heart ▷ small, and the diaphragm ⇨ depressed.

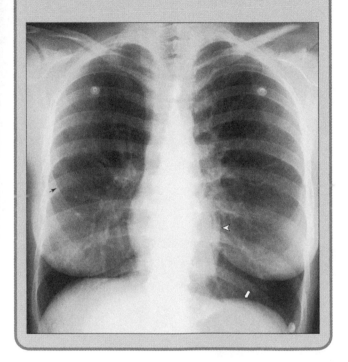

RIB FRACTURES

This anteroposterior chest X-ray of a trauma patient shows lateral fractures of the fifth → and sixth ➡ ribs on the left side. Displacement and associated fractures of the left clavicle ➤ and left scapula ➤ have created separation at the fracture sites.

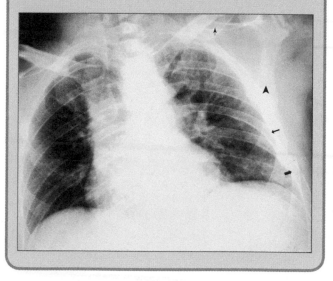

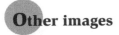ther images

BONE TUMOR

A well-defined, eccentric, bubbly expansible tumor ▷ in the distal femoral diaphysis is clear in this plain X-ray.

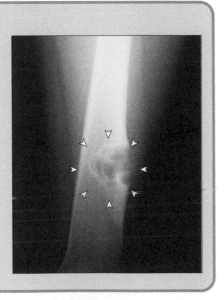

LEG FRACTURES

This anteroposterior X-ray of the left leg and ankle shows the results of trauma. Visible are an oblique, comminuted fracture of the tibia ➤ and lateral displacement of distal parts as well as a comminuted avulsion-type fracture of the medial malleolus ➡.

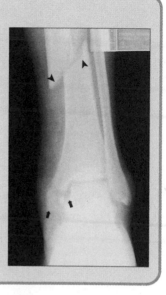

OSTEOARTHRITIS OF THE KNEE

This plain X-ray of a right knee shows narrowing of the medial joint space ➤ and mild osteophyte formation ▷.

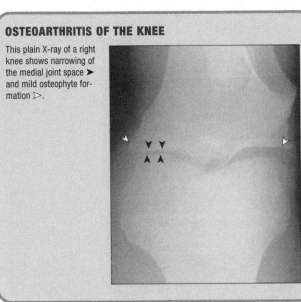

RHEUMATOID ARTHRITIS OF THE HAND

This plain X-ray of the left hand shows classic signs of advanced rheumatoid arthritis. Periarticular soft tissue swelling ⇢ is evident as are many erosions involving the distal ulna, carpals, metacarpals, and phalanges ▷. Joint spaces are narrowed. In addition, periarticular osteoporosis encircles the metacarpal and phalangeal joints ✻.

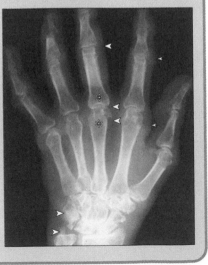

ROTATOR CUFF TEAR AND MENISCAL TEAR

The shoulder shown in this magnetic resonance imaging (MRI) scan (top) clearly has a torn right rotator cuff ▷. In the sagittal MRI image (bottom), an oblique tear ➤ is evident in the posterior horn of the medial meniscus.

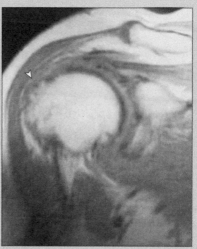

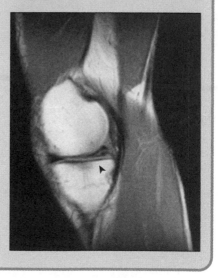

SMALL-BOWEL OBSTRUCTION

In this plain abdominal X-ray, dilated, gas-filled bowel loops ▷ and a lack of colon gas indicate an obstruction of the small bowel.

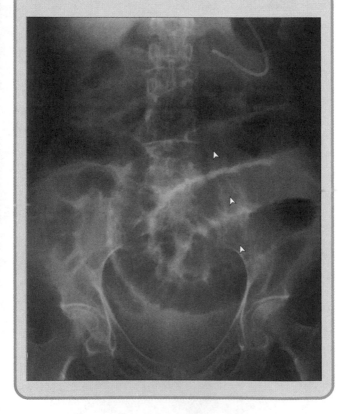

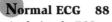

4
ECGs
Interpreting them with ease and accuracy

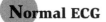

Normal ECG

ANALYZING THE ECG WAVEFORM

An electrocardiogram (ECG) complex represents the electrical events occurring in one cardiac cycle. A complex consists of five waveforms labeled with the letters P, Q, R, S, and T. The letters Q, R, and S are referred to as a unit, the QRS complex. The ECG tracing represents the conduction of electrical impulses from the atria to the ventricles. (See *ECG waveform components*.)

▶ The P wave is the first component of the normal ECG waveform. It represents atrial depolarization.

▶ The PR interval tracks the atrial impulse from the atria through the atrioventricular (AV) node, bundle of His, and the right and left bundle branches. It begins with atrial depolarization and ends with the beginning of ventricular depolarization.

▶ QRS complex follows the P wave and represents ventricular depolarization.

▶ The ST segment represents the end of ventricular depolarization and the beginning of ventricular repolarization. The point that marks the end of the QRS complex and the beginning of the ST segment is known as the J point.

▶ The T wave represents ventricular repolarization.

▶ The QT interval measures the time needed for ventricular depolarization and repolarization.

▶ The U wave probably represents His-Purkinje repolarization. It's uncommon and not routinely measured. The U wave is best seen when the heart rate is slow; it follows the T wave and occurs before the next P wave.

HOW TO READ AN ECG RHYTHM STRIP: AN 8-STEP METHOD

Analyzing a rhythm strip is a skill developed through practice. You can use several methods, as long as you're consistent. (See *The 8-step method of rhythm strip analysis*.)

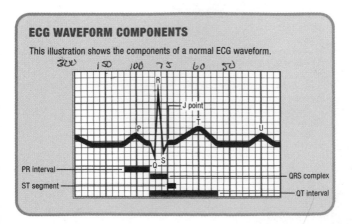

ECG WAVEFORM COMPONENTS

This illustration shows the components of a normal ECG waveform.

THE 8-STEP METHOD OF RHYTHM STRIP ANALYSIS

Rhythm strip analysis requires a sequential and systematic approach. The following eight steps provide a good outline for you to follow.

Step 1: Determine rhythm
To determine the heart's atrial and ventricular rhythms, use either the paper-and-pencil method or the caliper method.

To determine the atrial rhythm, measure the P-P intervals, the intervals between consecutive P waves. These intervals should occur regularly, with only small variations associated with respirations. Then compare the P-P intervals in several cycles. Consistently similar P-P intervals indicate regular atrial rhythm; dissimilar P-P intervals indicate irregular atrial rhythm.

To determine the ventricular rhythm, measure the intervals between two consecutive R waves in the QRS complexes. If an R wave isn't present, use either the Q wave or the S wave of consecutive QRS complexes. The R-R intervals should occur regularly. Then compare R-R intervals in several cycles. As with atrial rhythms, consistently similar intervals mean a regular rhythm; dissimilar intervals point to an irregular rhythm.

After completing your measurements, ask yourself:
▸ Is the rhythm regular or irregular? Consider a rhythm with only slight variations, up to 0.04 second, to be regular.
▸ If the rhythm is irregular, is it slightly irregular or markedly so? Does the irregularity occur in a pattern (a regularly irregular pattern)?

Step 2: Calculate rate
You can use one of three methods to determine atrial and ventricular heart rates from an electrocardiogram (ECG) waveform. Although these methods can provide accurate information, you shouldn't rely solely on them when assessing your patient. Keep in mind that the ECG waveform represents electrical, not mechanical, activity; therefore, although an ECG can show that ventricular depolarization has occurred, it doesn't mean that ventricular contraction has occurred. To determine this, you must assess the patient's pulse.
▸ *Times-ten method.* The simplest, quickest, and most common way to calculate rate is the times-ten method, especially if the rhythm is irregular. ECG paper is marked in increments of 3 seconds, or 15 large boxes. To calculate the atrial rate, obtain a 6-second strip, count the number of P waves on it, and multiply by 10. Ten 6-second strips equal 1 minute. Calculate ventricular rate the same way, using the R waves.
▸ *1,500 method.* If the heart rhythm is regular, use the 1,500 method, so named because 1,500 small squares equal 1 minute. Count the number of small squares between identical points on two consecutive P waves, and then divide 1,500 by that number to get the atrial rate. To obtain the ventricular rate, use the same method with two consecutive R waves.
▸ *Sequence method.* The third method of estimating heart rate is the sequence method, which requires memorizing a sequence of numbers. For atrial rate, find a P wave that peaks on a heavy black line, and assign the following numbers to the next six heavy black lines: 300, 150, 100, 75, 60, and 50. Then find the next P wave peak and estimate the atrial rate, based on the number assigned to the nearest heavy black line. Estimate the ventricular rate the same way, using the R wave.

(continued)

THE 8-STEP METHOD OF RHYTHM STRIP ANALYSIS *(continued)*

Step 3: Evaluate P waves
When examining a rhythm strip for P waves, ask yourself:
▶ Are P waves present?
▶ Do the P waves have a normal configuration?
▶ Do all the P waves have a similar size and shape?
▶ Is there one P wave for every QRS complex?

Step 4: Determine PR interval duration
To measure the PR interval, count the small squares between the start of the P wave and the start of the QRS complex; then multiply the number of squares by 0.04 second. After performing this calculation, ask yourself:
▶ Does the duration of the PR interval fall within normal limits, 0.12 to 0.20 second (or 3 to 5 small squares)?
▶ Is the PR interval constant?

Step 5: Determine QRS complex duration
When determining QRS complex duration, make sure you measure straight across from the end of the PR interval to the end of the S wave, not just to the peak. Remember, the QRS complex has no horizontal components. To calculate duration, count the number of small squares between the beginning and end of the QRS complex and multiply this number by 0.04 second. Then ask yourself:
▶ Does the duration of the QRS complex fall within normal limits, 0.06 to 0.10 second?
▶ Are all QRS complexes the same size and shape? (If not, measure each one and describe them individually.)
▶ Does a QRS complex appear after every P wave?

Step 6: Evaluate T wave
Examine the T waves on the ECG strip. Then ask yourself:
▶ Are T waves present?
▶ Do all of the T waves have a normal shape?
▶ Could a P wave be hidden in a T wave?
▶ Do all T waves have a normal amplitude?
▶ Do the T waves have the same deflection as the QRS complexes?

Step 7: Determine QT interval duration
Count the number of small squares between the beginning of the QRS complex and the end of the T wave, where the T wave returns to the baseline. Multiply this number by 0.04 second. Ask yourself:
▶ Does the duration of the QT interval fall within normal limits, 0.36 to 0.44 second?

Step 8: Evaluate other components
Note the presence of ectopic or aberrantly conducted beats or other abnormalities. Also, check the ST segment for abnormalities, and look for the presence of a U wave.
   Next, interpret your findings by classifying the rhythm strip according to one or all of the following:
▶ site of origin of the rhythm: for example, sinus node, atria, atrioventricular node, or ventricles
▶ rate: normal (60 to 100 beats/minute), bradycardia (less than 60 beats/minute), or tachycardia (greater than 100 beats/minute)
▶ rhythm: normal or abnormal; for example, flutter, fibrillation, heart block, escape rhythm, or other arrhythmias.

NORMAL SINUS RHYTHM

When the heart functions normally, the sinoatrial (SA) node acts as the primary pacemaker, initiating the electrical impulses. The SA node assumes this role because its automatic firing rate exceeds that of the heart's other pacemakers, allowing cells to depolarize spontaneously.

Normal sinus rhythm records an impulse that starts with the sinus node and progresses to the ventricles through a normal conduction pathway — from the sinus node to the atria and atrioventricular (AV) node, through the bundle of His, to the bundle branches, and onto the Purkinje fibers. Normal sinus rhythm is the standard against which all other rhythms are compared; you need to be able to recognize normal sinus rhythm before you can recognize an arrhythmia. (See *Characteristics and interpretation of normal sinus rhythm*.)

Based on an electrical disturbance's location, arrhythmias can be classified as sinus, atrial, junctional, or ventricular arrhythmias or AV blocks. Functional disturbances in the SA node produce sinus arrhythmias. Enhanced automaticity of atrial tissue or reentry may produce atrial arrhythmias, the most common arrhythmias.

Junctional arrhythmias originate in the area around the AV node and bundle of His. These arrhythmias usually result from a suppressed higher pacemaker, blocked impulses at the AV node, or enhanced automaticity or reentry mechanism.

Ventricular arrhythmias originate in ventricular tissue below the bi-

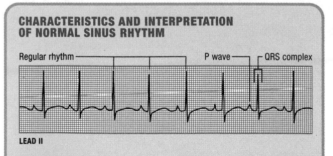

CHARACTERISTICS AND INTERPRETATION OF NORMAL SINUS RHYTHM

Regular rhythm   P wave   QRS complex

LEAD II

Atrial rhythm: regular
Ventricular rhythm: regular
Atrial rate: 60 to 100 beats/minute (80 beats/minute shown)
Ventricular rate: 60 to 100 beats/minute (80 beats/minute shown)
P wave: normally shaped (All P waves have similar size and shape; a P wave precedes each QRS complex.)
PR interval: within normal limits (0.12 to 0.20 second) and constant (0.20-second duration shown)

QRS complex: within normal limits (0.06 to 0.10 second) (All QRS complexes have the same configuration. The duration shown here is 0.12 second.)
T wave: normally shaped; upright and rounded in lead II (Each QRS complex is followed by a T wave.)
QT interval: within normal limits (0.36 to 0.44 second) and constant (0.44-second duration shown)

furcation of the bundle of His. These rhythms may result from reentry or enhanced automaticity or after depolarization.

An AV block results from an abnormal interruption or delay of atrial impulse conduction to the ventricles. It may be partial or total and may occur in the AV node, bundle of His, or Purkinje system.

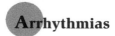

Arrhythmias

SINUS ARRHYTHMIA

In sinus arrhythmia, the heart rate stays within normal limits, but the rhythm is irregular and corresponds to the respiratory cycle and variations in vagal tone. During inspiration, an increased volume of blood returns to the heart, reducing vagal tone and increasing sinus rate. During expiration, venous return decreases, vagal tone increases, and sinus rate slows. (See *Characteristics and interpretation of sinus arrhythmia*.)

Conditions unrelated to respiration may also produce sinus arrhythmia. These conditions include an inferior wall myocardial infarction and digoxin toxicity.

Sinus arrhythmia is easily recognized in elderly, pediatric, and sedated patients. The patient's pulse rate increases with inspiration and decreases with expiration. Usually, the patient is asymptomatic.

Intervention

Treatment isn't necessary, unless the patient is symptomatic or the sinus arrhythmia stems from an un-

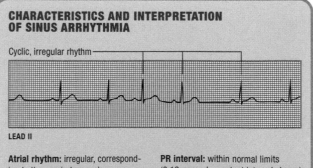

CHARACTERISTICS AND INTERPRETATION OF SINUS ARRHYTHMIA

Cyclic, irregular rhythm

LEAD II

Atrial rhythm: irregular, corresponding to the respiratory cycle
Ventricular rhythm: irregular, corresponding to the respiratory cycle
Atrial rate: within normal limits; varies with respiration (60 beats/minute shown)
Ventricular rate: within normal limits; varies with respiration (60 beats/minute shown)
P wave: normal size and configuration (One P wave precedes each QRS complex.)

PR interval: within normal limits (0.16-second, constant interval shown)
QRS complex: normal duration and configuration (0.06-second duration shown)
T wave: normal size and configuration
QT interval: within normal limits (0.36-second interval shown)
Other: phasic slowing and quickening of the rhythm

derlying cause. If symptoms are associated with symptomatic bradycardia, atropine may be administered.

SINUS BRADYCARDIA

Characterized by a sinus rate of less than 60 beats/minute, sinus bradycardia usually occurs as the normal response to a reduced demand for blood flow. (See *Characteristics and interpretation of sinus bradycardia*.) It's common among athletes, whose well-conditioned hearts can maintain stroke volume with reduced effort. It may also be caused by drugs, such as cardiac glycosides, calcium channel blockers, and beta-adrenergic blockers. Sinus bradycardia may occur after an inferior wall myocardial infarction involving the right coronary artery, which provides the blood supply to the sinoatrial node. The rhythm may develop during sleep and in patients with increased intracranial pressure. It may also result from vagal stimulation caused by vomiting or defecating. Pathological sinus bradycardia may occur with sick sinus syndrome.

The patient with sinus bradycardia is asymptomatic if he's able to compensate for the drop in heart rate by increasing stroke volume. If not, he may have signs and symptoms of decreased cardiac output, such as hypotension, syncope, confusion, and blurred vision. *vagal syncope*

Intervention

If the patient is asymptomatic, treatment isn't necessary. If he has signs and symptoms, treatment aims to identify and correct the underlying cause. The heart rate may be increased with such drugs as atropine. A temporary (transcutaneous or transvenous) or permanent pacemaker may be necessary if the bradycardia persists.

CHARACTERISTICS AND INTERPRETATION OF SINUS BRADYCARDIA

Regular rhythm with rate less than 60 beats/minute

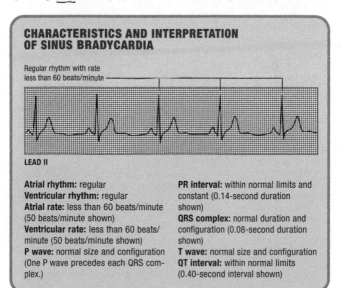

LEAD II

Atrial rhythm: regular
Ventricular rhythm: regular
Atrial rate: less than 60 beats/minute (50 beats/minute shown)
Ventricular rate: less than 60 beats/minute (50 beats/minute shown)
P wave: normal size and configuration (One P wave precedes each QRS complex.)

PR interval: within normal limits and constant (0.14-second duration shown)
QRS complex: normal duration and configuration (0.08-second duration shown)
T wave: normal size and configuration
QT interval: within normal limits (0.40-second interval shown)

SINUS TACHYCARDIA

Sinus tachycardia is an acceleration of firing of the sinoatrial node beyond its normal discharge rate. In an adult, it's characterized by a sinus rate of more than 100 beats/minute. (The rate rarely exceeds 180 beats/minute except during strenuous exercise. The maximum rate achieved with exercise decreases with age.) (See *Characteristics and interpretation of sinus tachycardia*.)

A normal response to cellular demands for increased oxygen delivery and blood flow commonly produces sinus tachycardia. Conditions that cause such a demand include heart failure, shock, anemia, exercise, fever, hypoxia, pain, and stress. Drugs that stimulate the beta receptors in the heart also cause sinus tachycardia. They include aminophylline, epinephrine, dobutamine, and dopamine. Alcohol, caffeine, and nicotine may also produce sinus tachycardia.

An elevated heart rate increases myocardial oxygen demands. If the patient can't meet these demands (for example, because of coronary artery disease), ischemia and further myocardial damage may occur.

Intervention

Treatment focuses on finding the primary cause. If it's high catecholamine levels, a beta-adrenergic blocker may slow the heart rate. After myocardial infarction, persistent

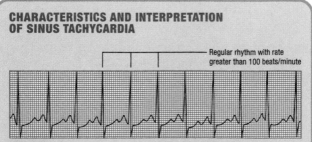

CHARACTERISTICS AND INTERPRETATION OF SINUS TACHYCARDIA

Regular rhythm with rate greater than 100 beats/minute

LEAD II

Atrial rhythm: regular
Ventricular rhythm: regular
Atrial rate: 100 to 160 beats/minute (110 beats/minute shown)
Ventricular rate: 100 to 160 beats/minute (110 beats/minute shown)
P wave: normal size and configuration (One P wave precedes each QRS complex. As the sinus rate reaches about 150 beats/minute, the P wave merges with the preceding T wave and may be difficult to identify. Examine the descending slope of the preceding T wave closely for notches, indicating the presence of the P wave. The P wave shown is normal.)
PR interval: within normal limits and constant (0.16-second duration shown)
QRS complex: normal duration and configuration (0.10-second shown)
T wave: normal size and configuration
QT interval: within normal limits and constant (0.36-second duration shown)
Other: gradual onset and cessation

sinus tachycardia may precede heart failure or cardiogenic shock.

SINUS ARREST

In sinus arrest, the normal sinus rhythm is interrupted by an occasional, prolonged failure of the sinoatrial node to initiate an impulse. Sinus arrest, therefore, is caused by episodes of failure in the automaticity of impulse formation of the SA node. The atria aren't stimulated, and an entire PQRST complex is missing from the electrocardiogram (ECG) strip. Except for the missing complex, or pause, the ECG usually remains normal. (See *Characteristics and interpretation of sinus arrest.*)

During a sinus arrest, the sinus node resets itself so that when the impulse is initiated, the complex following the pause will be out of the cycle and the rate frequently different than the rate before the pause.

Sinus arrest may result from an acute inferior wall myocardial infarction, increased vagal tone, or use of certain drugs, such as cardiac glycosides, calcium channel blockers, and beta-adrenergic blockers. The arrhythmia may also be linked to sick sinus syndrome. The patient has an irregular pulse rate associated with the sinus rhythm pauses. If the pauses are infrequent, the patient is asymptomatic. If they occur frequently and last for several

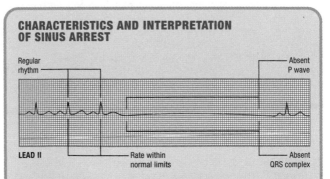

CHARACTERISTICS AND INTERPRETATION OF SINUS ARREST

Atrial rhythm: regular, except for the missing complex

Ventricular rhythm: regular, except for the missing complex

Atrial rate: within normal limits but varies because of pauses (94 beats/minute shown)

Ventricular rate: within normal limits but varies because of pauses (94 beats/minute shown)

P wave: normal size and configuration (One P wave precedes each QRS complex but is absent during a pause.)

PR interval: within normal limits and constant when the P wave is present; not measurable when the P wave is absent (0.20-second duration shown on all complexes surrounding the arrest)

QRS complex: normal duration and configuration; absent during pause (0.08-second duration shown)

T wave: normal size and configuration; absent during pause

QT interval: within normal limits; not measurable during pause (0.40-second, constant interval shown)

seconds, the patient may have signs of decreased cardiac output.

Intervention

For a symptomatic patient, treatment focuses on maintaining cardiac output and discovering the cause of the sinus arrest. If indicated, atropine may be given, or a temporary (transcutaneous or transvenous) or permanent pacemaker may be inserted.

PREMATURE ATRIAL CONTRACTIONS

Premature atrial contractions (PACs) usually result from an irritable focus in the atria that supersedes the sinoatrial node as the pacemaker for one or more beats. (See *Characteristics and interpretation of premature atrial contractions.*) Although PACs commonly occur in normal hearts, they're also associated with coronary and valvular heart disease. In an inferior wall myocardial infarction (MI), PACs may indicate a concomitant right atrial infarct. In an anterior wall MI, PACs are an early sign of left-sided heart failure. They may also warn of a more severe atrial arrhythmia, such as atrial flutter or atrial fibrillation.

Possible causes include digoxin toxicity, hyperthyroidism, elevated catecholamine levels, acute respiratory failure, and chronic obstructive pulmonary disease. Alcohol, caf-

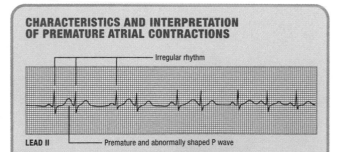

CHARACTERISTICS AND INTERPRETATION OF PREMATURE ATRIAL CONTRACTIONS

— Irregular rhythm

LEAD II — Premature and abnormally shaped P wave

Atrial rhythm: irregular (Incomplete compensatory pause follows premature arterial contraction [PAC]. Underlying rhythm may be regular.)
Ventricular rhythm: irregular (Incomplete compensatory pause follows PAC. Underlying rhythm may be regular.)
Atrial rate: varies with underlying rhythm (90 beats/minute shown)
Ventricular rate: varies with underlying rhythm (90 beats/minute shown)
P wave: premature and abnormally shaped; possibly lost in previous T wave (Varying configurations indicate multiform PACs.)

PR interval: usually normal but may be shortened or slightly prolonged, depending on the origin of ectopic focus (0.16-second, constant interval shown)
QRS complex: usually normal duration and configuration (0.08-second, constant duration shown)
T wave: usually normal configuration; may be distorted if the P wave is hidden in the previous T wave
QT interval: usually normal (0.36-second, constant interval shown)
Other: may occur in bigeminy or couplets

feine, or tobacco use can also trigger PACs. Patients who eliminate or control those factors can usually correct the arrhythmia.

Intervention

Symptomatic patients may be treated with beta-adrenergic blockers or calcium channel blockers.

ATRIAL TACHYCARDIA

Atrial tachycardia is a supraventricular tachycardia, which means that the impulse originates above the ventricles; in this rhythm the impulse originates in the atria. The rapid atrial rate shortens diastole,

resulting in a loss of atrial kick, reduced cardiac output, reduced coronary perfusion, and ischemic myocardial changes.

Although atrial tachycardia can occur in healthy patients, it's usually associated with high catecholamine levels, digoxin toxicity, myocardial infarction, cardiomyopathy, hyperthyroidism, hypertension, and valvular heart disease. Three types of atrial tachycardia exist: atrial tachycardia with block, multifocal atrial tachycardia (MAT), and paroxysmal atrial tachycardia (PAT). (See *Characteristics and interpretation of atrial tachycardia.*)

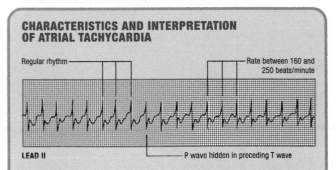

CHARACTERISTICS AND INTERPRETATION OF ATRIAL TACHYCARDIA

Regular rhythm ——— Rate between 160 and 250 beats/minute

LEAD II ——— P wave hidden in preceding T wave

Atrial rhythm: regular
Ventricular rhythm: regular
Atrial rate: three or more successive ectopic atrial beats at a rate of 160 to 250 beats/minute (210 beats/minute shown)
Ventricular rate: varies with atrioventricular conduction ratio (210 beats/minute shown)
P wave: 1:1 ratio with QRS complex, though often indiscernible because of rapid rate; may be hidden in previous ST segment or T wave
PR interval: may be unmeasurable if P wave can't be distinguished from preceding T wave (If P wave is pres-

ent, PR interval is short when conduction through the AV node is 1:1. On this strip, the PR interval isn't discernible.)
QRS complex: usually normal unless aberrant intraventricular conduction is present (0.10-second duration shown)
T wave: may be normal or inverted if ischemia is present (inverted T waves shown)
QT interval: usually normal but may be shorter because of rapid rate (0.20-second interval shown)
Other: appearance of ST-segment and T-wave changes if tachyarrhythmia persists longer than 30 minutes

Intervention

If the patient has atrial tachycardia or PAT and is symptomatic, prepare for immediate cardioversion. If the patient is stable, the physician may perform carotid sinus massage (if no bruits are present) or order drug therapy, such as adenosine (Adenocard), a calcium channel blocker, a beta-adrenergic blocker, or digoxin (Lanoxin). If each preceding treatment is ineffective in rhythm conversion, then consider procainamide or amiodarone. If these measures fail, cardioversion may be necessary.

ATRIAL FLUTTER

Characterized by an atrial rate of 300 beats/minute or more, atrial flutter results from multiple reentry circuits within the atrial tissue. On the electrocardiogram, the P waves lose their normal appearance due to rapid atrial rate and blend together in a saw tooth configuration called *flutter waves.* These waves are the hallmark of atrial flutter. (See *Characteristics and interpretation of atrial flutter.*)

Causes of atrial flutter include conditions that enlarge atrial tissue and elevate atrial pressures. Atrial flutter is associated with myocardial infarction, increased catecholamine levels, hyperthyroidism, and digoxin toxicity. A ventricular rate of 300 beats/minute suggests the presence of an anomalous pathway.

If the patient's pulse rate is normal, he usually has no symptoms. If his pulse rate is high, he'll probably have signs and symptoms of decreased cardiac output, such as hypotension and syncope.

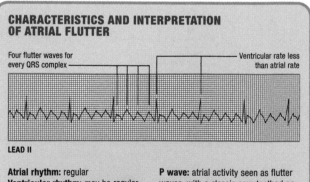

CHARACTERISTICS AND INTERPRETATION OF ATRIAL FLUTTER

Four flutter waves for every QRS complex

Ventricular rate less than atrial rate

LEAD II

Atrial rhythm: regular
Ventricular rhythm: may be regular or irregular, depending on the conduction ratio (regular rhythm shown)
Atrial rate: 300 to 350 beats/minute (300 beats/minute shown)
Ventricular rate: variable (70 beats/minute shown)

P wave: atrial activity seen as flutter waves, with a classic saw-toothed appearance
PR interval: not measurable
QRS complex: usually normal but can be distorted by the underlying flutter waves (0.10-second, normal duration shown)
T wave: unidentifiable
QT interval: not measurable

Intervention

If the patient is symptomatic, prepare for immediate cardioversion. The focus of treatment for stable patients with atrial flutter includes controlling the rate and converting the rhythm. Specific interventions depend on the patient's cardiac function, whether preexcitation syndromes are involved, and the duration (less than or greater than 48 hours) of the arrhythmia. For example, in atrial flutter with normal cardiac function and duration of rhythm less than 48 hours, cardioversion may be considered; for duration greater than 48 hours, avoid nonemergent cardioversion unless the patient has been adequately anticoagulated.

Drugs that may be ordered to control the rate include amiodarone, ibutilide, procainamide, calcium channel blockers, and beta-adrenergic blockers.

ATRIAL FIBRILLATION

Defined as chaotic, asynchronous electrical activity in the atrial tissue, atrial fibrillation results from impulses in many reentry pathways. These multiple and multidirectional impulses cause the atria to quiver instead of contracting regularly. (See *Characteristics and interpretation of atrial fibrillation*)

With this arrhythmia, blood may pool in the left atrial appendage and form thrombi that can be ejected into the systemic circulation. An associated rapid ventricular rate can decrease cardiac output.

Possible causes include valvular disorders, hypertension, coronary

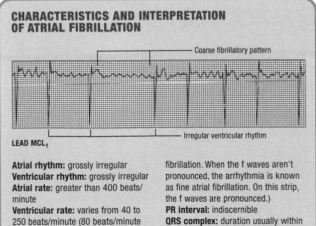

CHARACTERISTICS AND INTERPRETATION OF ATRIAL FIBRILLATION

Coarse fibrillatory pattern

LEAD MCL₁

Irregular ventricular rhythm

Atrial rhythm: grossly irregular
Ventricular rhythm: grossly irregular
Atrial rate: greater than 400 beats/minute
Ventricular rate: varies from 40 to 250 beats/minute (80 beats/minute shown)
P wave: absent; appearance of erratic baseline fibrillatory waves (f waves) (When the f waves are pronounced, the arrhythmia is called coarse atrial

fibrillation. When the f waves aren't pronounced, the arrhythmia is known as fine atrial fibrillation. On this strip, the f waves are pronounced.)
PR interval: indiscernible
QRS complex: duration usually within normal limits, with aberrant intraventricular conduction (0.08-second duration shown)
T wave: indiscernible
QT interval: not measurable

artery disease, myocardial infarction, chronic lung disease, ischemia, thyroid disorders, and Wolff-Parkinson-White syndrome. The disorder may also result from high adrenergic tone secondary to physical exertion, sepsis or alcohol withdrawal, and the use of such drugs as aminophylline (theophyl-line ethylenediamine) and cardiac glycosides.

Intervention

If the patient is symptomatic, synchronized cardioversion should be used immediately. Vagal stimulation may be used to slow the ventricular response, but it won't convert the arrhythmia. Drugs that may be ordered to slow atrioventricular conduction include calcium channel blockers and beta-adrenergic blockers. Digoxin may be ordered if the patient is stable. After the rate

slows, if conversion to a normal sinus rhythm hasn't occurred, amiodarone (Cordarone), procainamide (Pronestyl), flecainide, or sotalol may be ordered. If atrial fibrillation is of several days' duration, anticoagulant therapy is recommended before pharmacologic or electrical conversion. If atrial fibrillation is of recent onset, ibutilide (Corvert) may be used to convert the rhythm.

JUNCTIONAL RHYTHM

Junctional rhythm, also referred to as *junctional escape rhythm*, occurs in the atrioventricular junctional tissue, producing retrograde depolarization of the atrial tissue and antegrade depolarization of the ventricular tissue. It results from conditions that depress sinoatrial node function, such as an inferior wall

---

CHARACTERISTICS AND INTERPRETATION OF JUNCTIONAL RHYTHM

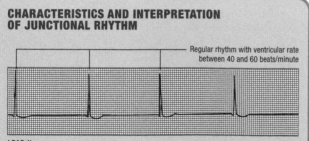

Regular rhythm with ventricular rate between 40 and 60 beats/minute

LEAD II

Atrial rhythm: regular
Ventricular rhythm: regular
Atrial rate: if discernible, 40 to 60 beats/minute (On this strip, the rate isn't discernible.)
Ventricular rate: 40 to 60 beats/minute (40 beats/minute shown)
P wave: usually inverted; may precede, follow, or fall within the QRS complex; may be absent (On this strip, the P wave is absent.)

PR interval: less than 0.12 second and constant if the P wave precedes the QRS complex; otherwise, not measurable (not measurable on this strip)
QRS complex: duration normal; configuration usually normal (0.08-second duration shown)
T wave: usually normal configuration
QT interval: usually normal (0.32-second duration shown)

myocardial infarction (MI), digoxin toxicity, and vagal stimulation. The arrhythmia may also stem from an increased automaticity of the junctional tissue, which can be brought about by digoxin toxicity or ischemia associated with an inferior wall MI. (See *Characteristics and interpretation of junctional rhythm.*)

Junctional rhythm is a regular rhythm with a ventricular rate of 40 to 60 beats/minute. A junctional rhythm with a ventricular rate of 60 to 100 beats/minute is known as an accelerated junctional rhythm. If the ventricular rate exceeds 100 beats/minute, the arrhythmia is called *junctional tachycardia.*

Intervention

Treatment aims to identify and manage the arrhythmia's primary cause. If the patient is symptomatic, treatment may include atropine to increase the sinus or junctional rate. Alternately, the physician may insert a pacemaker or use transcutaneous pacing to maintain an effective heart rate.

ACCELERATED JUNCTIONAL RHYTHM

An accelerated junctional rhythm is an arrhythmia that originates in the atrioventricular (AV) junction and is usually caused by enhanced automaticity of the AV junctional tissue. It's called "accelerated" because it occurs at a rate of 60 to 100 beats/minute, exceeding the inherent junctional rate of 40 to 60 beats/minute. (See *Characteristics and interpretation of accelerated junctional rhythm.*)

Digoxin toxicity is a common cause of accelerated junctional rhythm. Other causes include electrolyte disturbances, valvular heart

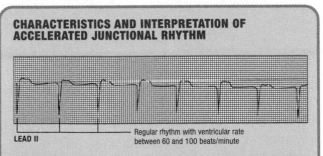

CHARACTERISTICS AND INTERPRETATION OF ACCELERATED JUNCTIONAL RHYTHM

LEAD II — Regular rhythm with ventricular rate between 60 and 100 beats/minute

Atrial rhythm: regular
Ventricular rhythm: regular
Atrial rate: if discernible, 60 to 100 beats/minute (On this strip, the rate isn't discernible.)
Ventricular rate: 60 to 100 beats/minute (75 beats/minute shown)
P wave: usually inverted; may precede, follow, or fall within the QRS complex; may be absent (On this strip, the P wave is absent.)

PR interval: less than 0.12 second and constant if the P wave precedes the QRS complex; otherwise, not measurable (not measurable on this strip)
QRS complex: duration normal; configuration usually normal (0.10-second duration shown)
T wave: usually normal configuration
QT interval: usually normal (0.32-second duration shown)

disease, heart failure, and inferior or posterior myocardial infarction.

Patients are generally asymptomatic because the rate corresponds to the normal inherent firing rate of the sinoatrial node. The patient may become symptomatic if atrial depolarization occurs after or simultaneously with ventricular depolarization, which results in a loss of atrial kick.

Intervention

Treatment aims to identify and manage the arrhythmia's primary cause. Assessing the patient for signs and symptoms related to decreased cardiac output and hemodynamic instability is key, as is monitoring serum digoxin levels and electrolyte levels.

JUNCTIONAL TACHYCARDIA

In junctional tachycardia, three or more premature junctional contractions occur in a row. This supraventricular tachycardia generally occurs as a result of enhanced automaticity of the atrioventricular (AV) junction, which causes the AV junction to override the sinoatrial node. (See *Characteristics and interpretation of junctional tachycardia.*)

Digoxin toxicity is the most common cause of junctional tachycardia. Other causes include inferior or posterior myocardial infarction, heart failure, or electrolyte imbalances.

Intervention

Treatment aims to identify and manage the arrhythmia's primary cause. If the cause is digoxin toxici-

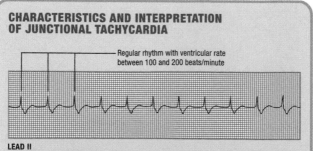

CHARACTERISTICS AND INTERPRETATION OF JUNCTIONAL TACHYCARDIA

Regular rhythm with ventricular rate between 100 and 200 beats/minute

LEAD II

Atrial rhythm: regular
Ventricular rhythm: regular
Atrial rate: if discernible, 100 to 200 beats/minute (On this strip, the rate isn't discernible.)
Ventricular rate: 100 to 200 beats/minute (115 beats/minute shown)
P wave: usually inverted; may precede, follow, or fall within the QRS complex; may be absent (On this strip, the P wave is inverted; follows QRS complex.)

PR interval: less than 0.12 second and constant if the P wave precedes the QRS complex; otherwise, not measurable (not measurable on this strip)
QRS complex: duration normal; configuration usually normal (0.08-second duration shown)
T wave: usually normal configuration
QT interval: usually normal (0.36-second duration shown)

ty, the drug should be discontinued. Drugs such as the calcium channel blocker verapamil may slow the heart rate for symptomatic patients.

PREMATURE JUNCTIONAL CONTRACTIONS

In premature junctional contractions (PJCs), a junctional beat occurs before the next normal sinus beat. Ectopic beats, PJCs commonly result from increased automaticity in the bundle of His or the surrounding junctional tissue, which interrupts the underlying rhythm. (See *Characteristics and interpretation of premature junctional contractions.*)

Digoxin toxicity is the most common cause of PJCs. Other causes include ischemia associated with an inferior wall myocardial infarction, excessive caffeine ingestion, and excessive levels of amphetamines.

Intervention

In most cases, treatment is directed at the underlying cause.

PREMATURE VENTRICULAR CONTRACTIONS

Among the most common arrhythmias, premature ventricular contractions (PVCs) occur in healthy and diseased hearts. These ectopic beats occur singly, in bigeminy,

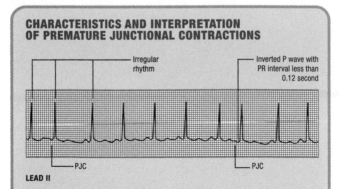

CHARACTERISTICS AND INTERPRETATION OF PREMATURE JUNCTIONAL CONTRACTIONS

LEAD II

Atrial rhythm: irregular with PJC, but underlying rhythm may be regular
Ventricular rhythm: irregular with PJC, but underlying rhythm may be regular
Atrial rate: follows the underlying rhythm (100 beats/minute shown)
Ventricular rate: follows the underlying rhythm (100 beats/minute shown)
P wave: usually inverted; may precede, follow, or fall within the QRS complex; may be absent (shown preceding the QRS complex)

PR interval: less than 0.12 second on the PJC if P wave precedes the QRS complex; otherwise, not measurable (On this strip, the PR interval is 0.14 second and constant on the underlying rhythm and 0.06 second on the PJC.)
QRS complex: normal duration and configuration (0.06-second duration shown)
T wave: usually normal configuration
QT interval: usually within normal limits (0.30-second interval shown)

trigeminy, quadrigeminy, or clusters. (See *Characteristics and interpretation of premature ventricular contractions*.)

PVCs may result from certain drugs, electrolyte imbalance, or stress.

When you detect PVCs, you must determine whether the pattern indicates danger. *Paired PVCs* can produce ventricular tachycardia because the second PVC usually meets refractory tissue. Three or more in a row is a run of ventricular tachycardia. *Multiform PVCs* look different from one another and may arise from different ventricular sites or be abnormally conducted. In *R-on-T phenomenon*, the PVC occurs so early that it falls on the downslope of the T wave of the preceding beat. Because the cells haven't fully depolarized, ventricular tachycardia or fibrillation can result.

The earlier the PVC, the shorter the diastolic filling time and the lower the stroke volume. Some patients complain of palpitations with frequent PVCs.

Intervention

If the PVCs are thought to result from a serious cardiac problem, an-

---

CHARACTERISTICS AND INTERPRETATION OF PREMATURE VENTRICULAR CONTRACTIONS

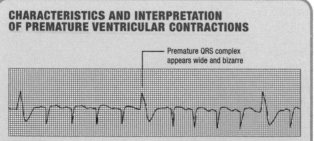

Premature QRS complex appears wide and bizarre

LEAD MCL₁

Atrial rhythm: irregular during premature ventricular contractions (PVC); underlying rhythm may be regular
Ventricular rhythm: irregular during PVC; underlying rhythm may be regular
Atrial rate: follows underlying rhythm (120 beats/minute shown)
Ventricular rate: follows underlying rhythm (120 beats/minute shown)
P wave: atrial activity independent of the PVC (If retrograde atrial depolarization exists, a retrograde P wave will distort the ST segment of the PVC. On this strip, no P wave appears before the PVC, but one occurs with each QRS complex.)

PR interval: determined by underlying rhythm; not associated with the PVC (0.12-second, constant interval shown)
QRS complex: occurs earlier than expected; duration exceeds 0.12 second and complex has a bizarre configuration; may be normal in the underlying rhythm (On this strip, it's 0.08 second in the normal beats; it's bizarre and 0.12 second in the PVC.)
T wave: occurs in the direction opposite that of the QRS complex; normal in the underlying complexes
QT interval: not usually measured in the PVC but may be within normal limits in the underlying rhythm (On this strip, the QT interval is 0.28 second in the underlying rhythm.)

tiarrhythmics such as lidocaine, procainamide, or amiodarone may be given to suppress ventricular irritability. When the PVCs are thought to result from a noncardiac problem, treatment aims at correcting the underlying cause — an acid-base or electrolyte imbalance, hypothermia, or high catecholamine levels.

VENTRICULAR TACHYCARDIA

The life-threatening arrhythmia ventricular tachycardia develops when three or more premature ventricular contractions occur in a row, and the rate exceeds 100 beats/minute. (See *Characteristics and interpretation of ventricular tachycardia.*) It may result from enhanced automaticity or reentry within the Purkinje system. The rapid ventricular rate reduces ventricular filling time, and because atrial kick is lost, cardiac output drops. This puts the patient at risk for ventricular fibrillation.

Ventricular tachycardia (VT) usually results from acute myocardial infarction, coronary artery disease, valvular heart disease, heart failure, or cardiomyopathy. The arrhythmia can also stem from an electrolyte imbalance or from toxic levels of a drug, such as digoxin, procainamide, or quinidine. You may detect two variations of this arrhythmia: ventricular flutter and torsades de pointes.

Intervention

Treatment depends on the patient's clinical status. This rhythm often degenerates into ventricular fibrillation and cardiovascular collapse, requiring immediate cardiopulmonary

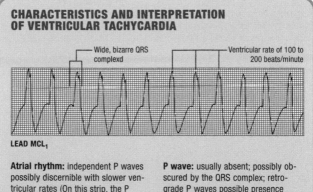

CHARACTERISTICS AND INTERPRETATION OF VENTRICULAR TACHYCARDIA

Wide, bizarre QRS complexd

Ventricular rate of 100 to 200 beats/minute

LEAD MCL₁

Atrial rhythm: independent P waves possibly discernible with slower ventricular rates (On this strip, the P waves aren't visible.)
Ventricular rhythm: usually regular but may be slightly irregular (On this strip, it's regular.)
Atrial rate: can't be determined
Ventricular rate: usually 100 to 200 beats/minute (120 beats/minute shown)

P wave: usually absent; possibly obscured by the QRS complex; retrograde P waves possible presence
PR interval: not measurable
QRS complex: duration greater than 0.12 second; bizarre appearance, usually with increased amplitude (0.16 second-duration shown)
T wave: opposite direction of the QRS complex
QT interval: not measurable

resuscitation and defibrillation. Patients with pulseless VT are treated the same as those with ventricular fibrillation and require immediate defibrillation. If the patient is unstable and has a pulse, prepare for immediate synchronized cardioversion followed by antiarrhythmic therapy. Drug therapy may include amiodarone, lidocaine, magnesium, or procainamide. Patients with chronic, recurrent episodes of VT unresponsive to drug therapy may need an implantable cardioverter-defibrillator.

VENTRICULAR FIBRILLATION

Defined as chaotic, asynchronous electrical activity within the ventricular tissue, ventricular fibrillation is a life-threatening arrhythmia that results in death if the rhythm isn't stopped immediately. (See *Characteristics and interpretation of ventricular fibrillation*.) Conditions leading to ventricular fibrillation include myocardial ischemia, hypokalemia, cocaine toxicity, hypoxia, hypothermia, severe acidosis, and severe alkalosis.

Patients with myocardial infarctions have the greatest risk of ventricular fibrillation during the initial 2 hours after the onset of chest pain.

In ventricular fibrillation, a lack of cardiac output results in a loss of consciousness, pulselessness, and respiratory arrest. Initially, you may see coarse fibrillatory waves on the electrocardiogram strip. As the acidosis develops, the waves become fine and progress to asystole unless defibrillation restores cardiac rhythm.

Intervention

Perform cardiopulmonary resuscitation until the patient can receive defibrillation. Administer epinephrine or vasopressin if the initial defibrillation series is unsuccessful. Other drugs that may be used include amiodarone, lidocaine, magnesium, and procainamide.

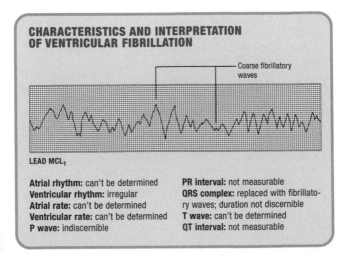

CHARACTERISTICS AND INTERPRETATION OF VENTRICULAR FIBRILLATION

Coarse fibrillatory waves

LEAD MCL₁

Atrial rhythm: can't be determined
Ventricular rhythm: irregular
Atrial rate: can't be determined
Ventricular rate: can't be determined
P wave: indiscernible

PR interval: not measurable
QRS complex: replaced with fibrillatory waves; duration not discernible
T wave: can't be determined
QT interval: not measurable

IDIOVENTRICULAR RHYTHM

Idioventricular rhythm, also referred to as *ventricular escape rhythm,* originates in an escape pacemaker site in the ventricles. The inherent firing rate of this ectopic pacemaker is less than 40 beats/minute. The rhythm acts as a safety mechanism when all potential pacemakers above the ventricles fail to discharge or when a block prevents supraventricular impulses from reaching the ventricles. (See *Characteristics and interpretation of idioventricular rhythm.*)

The slow ventricular rate and loss of atrial kick associated with this arrhythmia markedly reduce cardiac output. In turn, this causes hypotension, confusion, vertigo, and syncope. If not rapidly identified and appropriately managed, idioventricular rhythm may cause death.

Intervention

Treatment aims to identify and manage the primary problem that triggered the arrhythmia, and measures should be initiated to increase the patient's heart rate, improve cardiac output, and establish a normal rhythm. Atropine may be administered to increase the heart rate. If atropine isn't effective or if the patient develops hypotension or other signs of clinical instability, a pacemaker (transcutaneous or transvenous) may be needed to reestablish a heart rate that provides enough cardiac output to perfuse organs properly.

●●● **RED FLAG** *The goal of treating* ●●● *idioventricular rhythm doesn't include suppressing the rhythm because it acts as a safety mecha-*

CHARACTERISTICS AND INTERPRETATION OF IDIOVENTRICULAR RHYTHM

Irregular ventricular rhythm and ventricular rate less than 40 beats/minute

LEAD II

Atrial rhythm: can't be determined
Ventricular rhythm: usually regular, except with isolated escape beats (irregular rhythm shown)
Atrial rate: unable to be determined
Ventricular rate: less than 40 beats/minute (30 beats/minute shown)
P wave: absent
PR interval: usually not measurable

QRS complex: duration greater than 0.12 second; complex is wide and has a bizarre configuration (On this strip, the complex is 0.20 second and bizarre.)
T wave: abnormal; deflection usually opposite last part of QRS
QT interval: usually greater than 0.44 second (0.46-second interval shown)

nism to protect the heart from ventricular standstill. Idioventricular rhythm should never be treated with antiarrhythmics such as lidocaine that would suppress the escape beats.

ACCELERATED IDIOVENTRICULAR RHYTHM

When the pacemaker cells above the ventricles fail to generate an impulse or when a block prevents supraventricular impulses from reaching the ventricles, idioventricular rhythms result. When the rate of an idioventricular rhythm ranges from 40 to 100 beats/minute, it's considered accelerated idioventricular rhythm, denoting a rate greater than the inherent pacemaker. (See *Characteristics and interpretation of accelerated idioventricular rhythm.*)

In this life-threatening arrhythmia, the cells of the His-Purkinje system operate as pacemaker cells.

The characteristic waveform results from an area of enhanced automaticity within the ventricles, which may be associated with myocardial infarction, digoxin toxicity, or metabolic imbalances. In addition, the arrhythmia commonly occurs during myocardial reperfusion after thrombolytic therapy.

The patient may be symptomatic, depending on his heart rate and ability to compensate for the loss of the atrial kick. If symptomatic, he may experience signs and symptoms of decreased cardiac output, including hypotension, confusion, syncope, and loss of consciousness.

Intervention

An asymptomatic patient needs no treatment. For a symptomatic patient, treatment focuses on maintaining cardiac output and identifying the cause of the arrhythmia. The patient may require a pacemaker to enhance cardiac output. Remember, this rhythm protects the

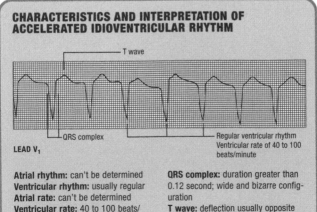

CHARACTERISTICS AND INTERPRETATION OF ACCELERATED IDIOVENTRICULAR RHYTHM

T wave

QRS complex

Regular ventricular rhythm
Ventricular rate of 40 to 100 beats/minute

LEAD V₁

Atrial rhythm: can't be determined
Ventricular rhythm: usually regular
Atrial rate: can't be determined
Ventricular rate: 40 to 100 beats/minute
P wave: absent
PR interval: not measurable

QRS complex: duration greater than 0.12 second; wide and bizarre configuration
T wave: deflection usually opposite that of QRS complex
QT interval: may be within normal limits or prolonged

heart from ventricular standstill and shouldn't be treated with antiarrhythmic agents.

FIRST-DEGREE AV BLOCK

First-degree atrioventricular (AV) block occurs when there's a delay in the conduction of electrical impulses from the atria to the ventricles. This delay usually occurs at the level of the AV node but may also be infranodal.

First-degree AV block is characterized by a constant PR interval greater than 0.20 second. (See *Characteristics and interpretation of first-degree atrioventricular block.*) It may result from myocardial ischemia, myocardial infarction, myocarditis, or degenerative changes in the heart associated with aging. Drugs, such as digoxin, beta-adrenergic blockers, and calcium channel blockers, may also cause this condition.

Most patients with first-degree AV block are asymptomatic.

Intervention

Management of first-degree AV block includes identifying and treating the underlying cause as well as monitoring the patient for signs of progressive AV block.

SECOND-DEGREE AV BLOCK, TYPE I

Type I (Wenckebach or Mobitz I) second-degree atrioventricular (AV) block occurs when each successive impulse from the sinoatrial node is delayed in the AV node slightly longer than the previous impulse. This pattern of progressive prolongation of the PR interval continues

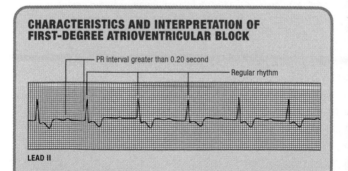

CHARACTERISTICS AND INTERPRETATION OF FIRST-DEGREE ATRIOVENTRICULAR BLOCK

PR interval greater than 0.20 second

Regular rhythm

LEAD II

Atrial rhythm: regular
Ventricular rhythm: regular
Atrial rate: usually within normal limits (60 beats/minute shown)
Ventricular rate: usually within normal limits (60 beats/minute shown)
P wave: normal size and configuration (One P wave precedes each QRS complex.)

PR interval: greater than 0.20 second and constant (0.32-second duration shown)
QRS complex: usually normal duration and configuration (0.08-second duration and normal configuration shown)
T wave: normal size and configuration
QT interval: usually within normal limits (0.32-second interval shown)

until an impulse fails to be conducted to the ventricles.

Type I block most commonly occurs at the level of the AV node and is caused by an inferior wall myocardial infarction, vagal stimulation, or digoxin toxicity. The arrhythmia usually doesn't cause symptoms; however, a patient may have signs and symptoms of decreased cardiac output, such as hypotension, confusion, and syncope. These effects occur especially if the patient's ventricular rate is slow.

Intervention

If the patient is asymptomatic, no intervention is required other than monitoring the electrocardiogram frequently to see if a more serious form of AV block develops.

If the patient is symptomatic, atropine may be ordered to increase the rate. Treatment may also in-clude a temporary pacemaker (transcutaneous or transvenous) to maintain an effective cardiac output. (See *Characteristics and interpretation of second-degree atrioventricular block, type I*.)

SECOND-DEGREE AV BLOCK, TYPE II

Produced by a conduction disturbance in the His-Purkinje system, a type II (Mobitz II) second-degree atrioventricular (AV) block causes an intermittent absence of conduction. In type II block, two or more atrial impulses are conducted to the ventricles with constant PR intervals, when suddenly, without warning, the atrial impulse is blocked. This type of block occurs in an anterior wall myocardial infarction (MI), severe coronary artery dis-

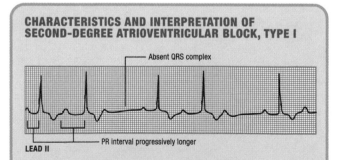

CHARACTERISTICS AND INTERPRETATION OF SECOND-DEGREE ATRIOVENTRICULAR BLOCK, TYPE I

— Absent QRS complex

LEAD II
— PR interval progressively longer

Atrial rhythm: regular
Ventricular rhythm: irregular
Atrial rate: determined by the underlying rhythm (80 beats/minute shown)
Ventricular rate: slower than the atrial rate (50 beats/minute shown)
P wave: normal size and configuration
PR interval: progressively prolonged with each beat until a P wave appears without a QRS complex

QRS complex: normal duration and configuration; periodically absent (0.08-second duration shown)
T wave: normal size and configuration
QT interval: usually within normal limits (0.46-second, constant interval shown)
Other: usually distinguished by a pattern of group beating, referred to as the footprints of Wenckebach

ease, and chronic degeneration of the conduction system.

Type II second-degree AV block is more serious than type I and can be a life-threatening arrhythmia; it requires prompt intervention.

Intervention

If the patient is hypotensive, treatment aims at increasing his heart rate to improve cardiac output. Because the conduction block occurs in the His-Purkinje system, drugs that act directly on the myocardium usually prove more effective than those that increase the atrial rate. As a result, dopamine or epinephrine instead of atropine may be ordered to increase the ventricular rate.

If the patient has an anterior wall MI, the physician will immediately insert a temporary pacemaker to prevent ventricular asystole. A transcutaneous pacemaker should be used until a transvenous pacemaker is placed. For long-term management, the patient may need a permanent pacemaker. (See *Characteristics and interpretation of second-degree atrioventricular block, type II*.)

THIRD-DEGREE AV BLOCK

Also called *complete heart block*, third-degree atrioventricular (AV) block indicates the complete absence of impulse conduction be-

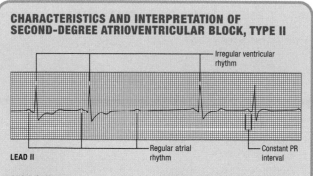

CHARACTERISTICS AND INTERPRETATION OF SECOND-DEGREE ATRIOVENTRICULAR BLOCK, TYPE II

Irregular ventricular rhythm

LEAD II

Regular atrial rhythm — Constant PR interval

Atrial rhythm: regular
Ventricular rhythm: regular or irregular
Atrial rate: usually within normal limits (60 beats/minute shown)
Ventricular rate: may be within normal limits but less than the atrial rate (40 beats/minute shown)
P wave: normal size and configuration (Not all P waves are followed by a QRS complex.)

PR interval: constant and frequently within normal limits for all conducted beats
QRS complex: duration within normal limits if the block occurs at the bundle of His and is greater than 0.16 second if the block occurs at the bundle branches (0.12-second complex shown)
T wave: usually normal size and configuration
QT interval: usually within normal limits (0.44-second interval shown)

tween the atria and ventricles. The atrial rate is generally equal to or faster than the ventricular rate. Third-degree AV block may occur at the level of the AV node, the bundle of His, or the bundle branches. The patient's treatment and prognosis vary depending on the anatomic level of the block.

If this type of block originates at the AV node, a junctional escape rhythm occurs; if it originates below the AV node, an idioventricular escape rhythm occurs. (See *Characteristics and interpretation of third-degree atrioventricular block.*)

Third-degree AV block involving the AV node may result from an inferior wall myocardial infarction (MI) or drug toxicity (cardiac glycosides, beta-adrenergic blockers, calcium channel blockers). Third-

degree AV block below the AV node may result from an anterior wall MI or chronic degeneration of the conduction system.

Some patients with complete heart block will be relatively free from symptoms, complaining only that they can't tolerate exercise or increased activity. However, most patients will experience significant signs and symptoms, including severe fatigue, dyspnea, chest pain, light-headedness, and changes in mental status. The severity of symptoms depends on the ventricular rate and the patient's ability to compensate for decreased cardiac output.

Intervention

Third-degree AV block can be a life-threatening arrhythmia; it requires

CHARACTERISTICS AND INTERPRETATION OF THIRD-DEGREE ATRIOVENTRICULAR BLOCK

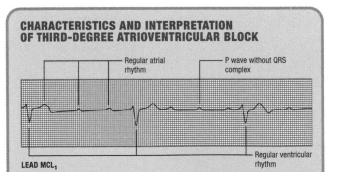

LEAD MCL₁

Atrial rhythm: usually regular
Ventricular rhythm: usually regular
Atrial rate: usually within normal limits (90 beats/minute shown)
Ventricular rate: slow (30 beats/minute shown)
P wave: normal size and configuration
PR interval: not measurable because the atria and ventricles beat independently of each other
QRS complex: determined by the site of the escape rhythm (With a junction-

al escape rhythm, the duration and configuration are normal; with an idioventricular escape rhythm, the duration is greater than 0.12 second and the complex is distorted. In the complex shown, the duration is 0.16 second, the configuration is abnormal, and the complex is distorted.)
T wave: normal size and configuration
QT interval: may or may not be within normal limits (0.56-second interval shown)

prompt intervention. If the patient is experiencing serious signs and symptoms, and cardiac output isn't adequate, interventions may include transcutaneous or transvenous pacing or I.V. atropine, dopamine, or epinephrine. Patients with third-degree AV block occurring at the infranodal level and associated with an extensive anterior MI usually require a permanent pacemaker.

●●● RED FLAG *Atropine isn't indicated for third-degree AV block with new wide QRS complexes. In such cases, a pacemaker is indicated because atropine rarely increase sinus rate and AV node conduction when AV block is at the His-Purkinje level.*

12-lead ECGs

BASIC COMPONENTS AND PRINCIPLES

Whereas rhythm strips are used to detect arrhythmias, the 12-lead or standard electrocardiogram (ECG) has a different purpose. The most common procedure for evaluating cardiac status, this diagnostic test helps identify various pathological conditions — most commonly, acute myocardial infarction.

The 12-lead ECG provides 12 views of the heart's electrical activity. (See *12 views of the heart,* page 114.) The 12 leads include:

▸ three bipolar limb leads (I, II, and III)
▸ three unipolar augmented limb leads (aV_R, aV_L, and aV_F)
▸ six unipolar precordial, or chest, leads (V_1, V_2, V_3, V_4, V_5, and V_6).

Leads

The six limb leads record electrical potential from the frontal plane, and the six precordial leads record electrical potential from the horizontal plane. Each waveform reflects the orientation of a lead to the wave of depolarization passing through the myocardium. Normally, this wave moves through the heart from right to left and from top to bottom.

Bipolar leads

Bipolar leads record the electrical potential difference between two points on the patient's body where you place electrodes.

▸ Lead I goes from the right arm (–) to the left arm (+).
▸ Lead II goes from the right arm (–) to the left leg (+).
▸ Lead III goes from the left arm (–) to the left leg (+).

Because of the orientation of these leads to the wave of depolarization, the QRS complexes typically appear upright. In lead II, these complexes are usually the tallest because this lead parallels the wave of depolarization.

Unipolar leads

Unipolar leads (the augmented limb leads and the precordial leads) have only one electrode, which represents the positive pole. The negative pole is computed by the ECG. Lead aV_R typically records negative QRS complex deflections because the wave of depolarization moves away from it. In the aV_F lead, QRS complexes are positive; in the aV_L lead, they're biphasic.

Unipolar precordial leads V_1 and V_2 usually have a small R wave because the direction of ventricular activation is left to right initially. That's because conduction time is normally faster down the left bundle branch than down the right. The wave of depolarization, however, moves toward the left ventricle and away from these leads, causing a low S wave.

In leads V_3 and V_4, the R and S waves may have the same ampli-

12 VIEWS OF THE HEART

Each of the leads on a 12-lead electrocardiogram (ECG) views the heart from a different angle. These illustrations show the direction of electrical activity (depolarization) monitored by each lead and the 12 views of the heart.

Views reflected on a 12-lead ECG

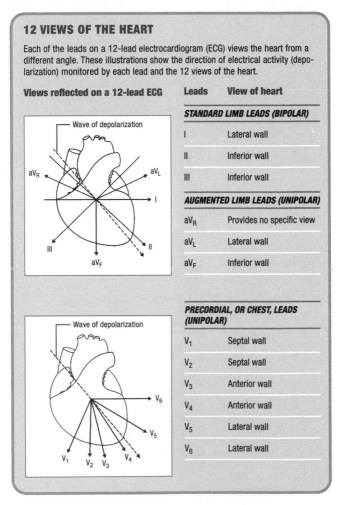

Leads	View of heart
STANDARD LIMB LEADS (BIPOLAR)	
I	Lateral wall
II	Inferior wall
III	Inferior wall
AUGMENTED LIMB LEADS (UNIPOLAR)	
aV$_R$	Provides no specific view
aV$_L$	Lateral wall
aV$_F$	Inferior wall
PRECORDIAL, OR CHEST, LEADS (UNIPOLAR)	
V$_1$	Septal wall
V$_2$	Septal wall
V$_3$	Anterior wall
V$_4$	Anterior wall
V$_5$	Lateral wall
V$_6$	Lateral wall

tude, and you won't see a Q wave. In leads V$_5$ and V$_6$, the initial ventricular activation appears as a small Q wave; the following tall R wave represents the strong wave of depolarization moving toward the left ventricle. These leads record a small or absent S wave.

DETERMINING ELECTRICAL AXIS

As electrical impulses travel through the heart, they generate small electrical forces called *instant-to-instant vectors*. The mean of these vectors represents the direction and force of the wave of depolarization, also known as the heart's electrical axis.

In a healthy heart, the wave of depolarization originates in the sinoatrial node and travels through the atria and the atrioventricular node and on to the ventricles. The normal movement is downward and to the left.

In an unhealthy heart, the wave of depolarization varies. That's because the direction of electrical activity swings away from areas of damage or necrosis.

A simple method to determine the direction of your patient's electrical axis is the quadrant method. Before you use this method, you need to understand the hexaxial reference system — a schematic view of the heart that uses the six limb leads. These leads include the three standard limb leads (I, II, and III), which are bipolar, and the three augmented limb leads (aV$_R$, aV$_L$, and aV$_F$), which are unipolar. Combined, these leads give a view of the wave of depolarization in the frontal plane, including the right, left, inferior, and superior portions of the heart.

Hexaxial reference system

The axes of the six limb leads also make up the hexaxial reference system, which divides the heart into six equal areas. To use the hexaxial reference system, picture in your mind the position of each lead: lead I connects the right arm (negative pole) with the left arm (positive pole); lead II connects the right arm (negative pole) with the left leg (positive pole); and lead III connects the left arm (negative pole) with the left leg (positive pole). The augmented limb leads have only one electrode, which represents the positive pole. As a result, lead aV$_R$

goes from the heart toward the right arm (positive pole); aV$_L$ goes from the heart toward the left arm (positive pole); and aV$_F$ goes from the heart to the left leg (positive pole).

Now, draw an imaginary line to illustrate the axis of each lead. For example, for lead I, you'd draw a horizontal line between the right and left arms; for lead II, between the right arm and left leg; and so on. All the lines should intersect near the center, somewhere over the heart. If you draw a circle to represent the heart, you'd end up with a rough pie shape, with each wedge representing a portion of the heart monitored by each lead. (See *Understanding the hexaxial reference system*, page 116.)

This schematic representation of the heart allows you to plot your patient's electrical axis. If his axis falls in the right lower quadrant, between 0 degrees and +90 degrees, it's considered normal. (Several sources consider the normal axis to be between –30 and +90 degrees.) An axis between +90 degrees and +180 degrees indicates right axis deviation; one between 0 degrees and –90 degrees, left axis deviation; and one between –180 degrees and –90 degrees, extreme axis deviation, which is sometimes called the *no-man's-land axis* or *indeterminate axis*. (Several sources consider left axis deviation to be between –30 degrees and –90 degrees.)

Quadrant method

A simple, rapid method for determining the heart's axis is the quadrant method, in which you observe the main deflection of the QRS complex in leads I and aV$_F$. The QRS complex serves as the traditional marker for determining the electrical axis because the ventricles produce the greatest amount of electrical force when they contract.

UNDERSTANDING THE HEXAXIAL REFERENCE SYSTEM

The hexaxial reference system consists of six bisecting lines, each representing one of the six limb leads, and a circle, representing the heart. The intersection of these lines divides the circle into equal 30-degree segments.

Note that 0 degrees appears at the 3 o'clock position. Moving counterclockwise, the degrees become increasingly negative, until reaching ±180 degrees at the 9 o'clock position. The bottom half of the circle contains the corresponding positive degrees. A positive-degree designation doesn't necessarily mean that the pole is positive.

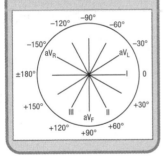

Lead I indicates whether impulses are moving to the right or left; lead aV_F indicates whether they're moving up or down. (See *Using the quadrant method.*)

On the waveform for lead I, a positive main deflection of the QRS complex indicates that the electrical impulses are moving to the right, toward the positive pole of the lead, which is at the 0-degree position on the hexaxial reference system. Conversely, a negative deflection indicates that the impulses are moving to the left, toward the negative pole

of the lead, which is at the ±180-degree position on the hexaxial reference system. On the waveform for lead aV_F, a positive deflection of the QRS complex indicates that the electrical impulses are traveling downward, toward the positive pole of the lead, which is at the +90-degree position of the hexaxial reference system. A negative deflection indicates that impulses are traveling upward, toward the negative pole of the lead, which is at the −90-degree position of the hexaxial reference system.

Plotting this information on the hexaxial reference system (with the horizontal axis representing lead I and the vertical axis representing lead aV_F) will reveal the patient's electrical axis. For example, if lead I shows a positive deflection of the QRS complex, darken the horizontal axis between the center of the hexaxial reference system and the 0-degree position. If lead aV_F also shows a positive deflection of the QRS complex, darken the vertical axis between the center of the reference system and the +90-degree position. The quadrant between the two axes you've darkened indicates the patient's electrical axis. In this case, it's the left lower quadrant, which indicates a normal electrical axis.

Causes of axis deviation

Determining the electrical axis can help confirm a diagnosis or narrow possibilities. Many factors influence the electrical axis, including the position of the heart within the chest, the size of the heart, the conduction pathways, and the force of electrical generation.

As you know, cardiac electrical activity swings away from areas of damage or necrosis. More specifically, electrical forces in the healthy portion of the heart take over for

USING THE QUADRANT METHOD

This chart will help you quickly determine the direction of a patient's electrical axis. Observe the deflections of the QRS complexes in leads I and aV_F. Then check the chart to determine whether the patient's axis is normal or has a left, right, or extreme axis deviation.

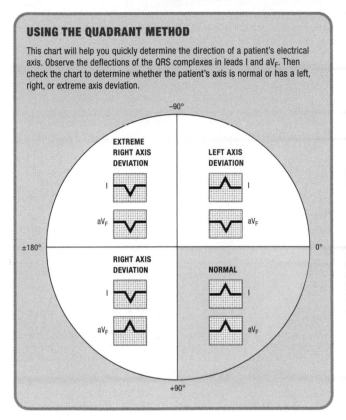

weak, or even absent, electrical forces in the damaged portion. For instance, after an inferior wall myocardial infarction, portions of the inferior wall can no longer conduct electricity. As a result, the major electrical vectors shift to the left, resulting in a left axis deviation.

Typically, the damaged portion of the heart is the last area to be depolarized. For example, in a left anterior hemiblock, the left anterior fascicle of the left bundle branch can no longer conduct electricity. Therefore, the portion normally

served by the left bundle branch is the last portion of the heart to be depolarized. This shifts electrical forces to the left; consequently, the electrocardiogram shows left axis deviation.

An opposite shift occurs with right bundle-branch block. In this condition, the wave of impulse travels quickly down the normal left side but much more slowly down the damaged right side. This shifts the electrical forces to the right, causing a right axis deviation.

An axis shift also takes place when the right or left ventricle is being paced artificially. It likewise takes place when the ventricles are depolarizing abnormally such as occurs in ventricular tachycardia. Both of these conditions can cause a left axis deviation or, occasionally, an extreme axis deviation.

Axis deviation may also result from ventricular hypertrophy. For example, an enlarged right ventricle generates greater electrical forces than normal and would consequently shift the electrical axis to the right. Wolff-Parkinson-White syndrome may produce a right, left, or extreme axis deviation, depending on which part of the ventricle is activated early.

LIFE SPAN *Sometimes axis deviation may be a normal variation, as in infants and children who normally experience right axis deviation. It may also stem from noncardiac causes. For example, if the heart is shifted in the chest cavity because of a high diaphragm from pregnancy, expect to find a left axis deviation.*

If a patient's heart is situated on the right side of his chest instead of the left (a condition called *dextrocardia*), expect to find right axis deviation.

HOW TO INTERPRET A 12-LEAD ECG

To interpret a 12-lead electrocardiogram (ECG), use a systematic approach. Compare the patient's previous ECG, if available, with the current one. This will help you identify changes. You can use various methods to interpret a 12-lead ECG. Here's a logical, easy-to-follow method that will help ensure that you're interpreting it accurately.

1. Check the ECG tracing to see if it's technically correct. Make sure

the baseline is free from electrical interference and drift.

2. Scan the limb leads I, II, and III. The R-wave voltage in lead II should equal the sum of the R-wave voltage in leads I and III. Lead aV_R is typically negative. If these rules aren't met, the tracing may be recorded incorrectly.

3. Locate the lead markers on the waveform. Lead markers are the points where one lead changes to another.

4. Check the standardization markings to make sure all leads were recorded with the ECG machine's amplitude at the same setting. Standardization markings are usually located at the beginning of the strip.

5. Assess the heart's rate and rhythm.

6. Determine the heart's electrical axis using the quadrant method.

7. Examine limb leads I, II, and III. The R wave in lead II should be taller than in lead I. The R wave in lead III should be a smaller version of the R wave in lead I. The P wave or QRS complex may be inverted. Each lead should have flat ST segments and upright T waves. Pathologic Q waves should be absent.

8. Examine limb leads aV_L, aV_F, and aV_R. The tracings from lead aV_L and aV_F should be similar, but lead aV_F should have taller P and R waves. Lead aV_R has little diagnostic value. Its P wave, QRS complex, and T wave should be deflected downward.

9. Examine the R wave in the precordial leads. Normally, the R wave — the first positive deflection of the QRS complex — gets progressively taller from lead V_1 to V_5. It gets slightly smaller in lead V_6. (See *12-lead ECG: Normal findings*.)

10. Examine the S wave (the negative deflection after an R wave) in the precordial leads. It should

12-LEAD ECG: NORMAL FINDINGS

LEAD I

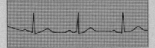

P wave: upright
Q wave: small or none
R wave: large wave
S wave: none present, or smaller than R wave
T wave: upright
U wave: none present
ST segment: may vary from +1 to −0.5 mm

LEAD II

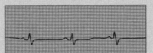

P wave: upright
Q wave: small or none
R wave: largest wave
S wave: none present, or smaller than R wave
T wave: upright
U wave: none present
ST segment: may vary from +1 to −0.5 mm

LEAD III

P wave: upright, diphasic, or inverted
Q wave: usually small or none
R wave: none present to large wave
S wave: none present to large wave, indicating horizontal heart
T wave: upright, diphasic, or inverted
U wave: none present
ST segment: may vary from +1 to −0.5 mm

LEAD AV_R

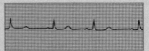

P wave: inverted
Q wave: none, small wave, or large wave present
R wave: none or small wave present
S wave: large wave (may be QS)
T wave: inverted
U wave: none present
ST segment: may vary from +1 to −0.5 mm

LEAD AV_L

P wave: upright, diphasic, or inverted
Q wave: none, small wave, or large wave present (Q wave must also be present in lead I or precordial leads to be considered diagnostic.)
R wave: none, small wave, or large wave present (A large wave indicates horizontal heart.)
S wave: none present to large wave (A large wave indicates vertical heart.)
T wave: upright, diphasic, or inverted
U wave: none present
ST segment: may vary from +1 to −0.5 mm

(continued)

12-LEAD ECG: NORMAL FINDINGS *(continued)*

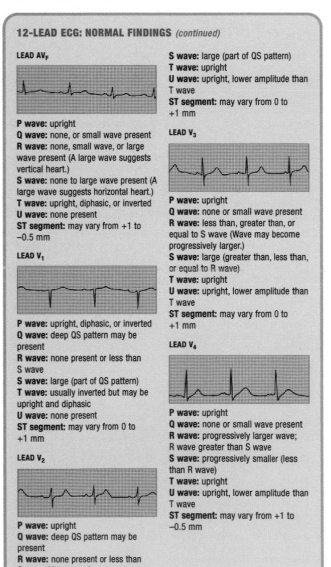

LEAD AV$_F$

P wave: upright
Q wave: none, or small wave present
R wave: none, small wave, or large wave present (A large wave suggests vertical heart.)
S wave: none to large wave present (A large wave suggests horizontal heart.)
T wave: upright, diphasic, or inverted
U wave: none present
ST segment: may vary from +1 to –0.5 mm

LEAD V$_1$

P wave: upright, diphasic, or inverted
Q wave: deep QS pattern may be present
R wave: none present or less than S wave
S wave: large (part of QS pattern)
T wave: usually inverted but may be upright and diphasic
U wave: none present
ST segment: may vary from 0 to +1 mm

LEAD V$_2$

P wave: upright
Q wave: deep QS pattern may be present
R wave: none present or less than S wave (Wave may become progressively larger.)

S wave: large (part of QS pattern)
T wave: upright
U wave: upright, lower amplitude than T wave
ST segment: may vary from 0 to +1 mm

LEAD V$_3$

P wave: upright
Q wave: none or small wave present
R wave: less than, greater than, or equal to S wave (Wave may become progressively larger.)
S wave: large (greater than, less than, or equal to R wave)
T wave: upright
U wave: upright, lower amplitude than T wave
ST segment: may vary from 0 to +1 mm

LEAD V$_4$

P wave: upright
Q wave: none or small wave present
R wave: progressively larger wave; R wave greater than S wave
S wave: progressively smaller (less than R wave)
T wave: upright
U wave: upright, lower amplitude than T wave
ST segment: may vary from +1 to –0.5 mm

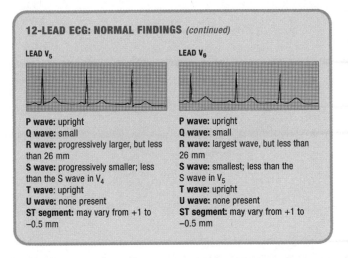

12-LEAD ECG: NORMAL FINDINGS *(continued)*

LEAD V₅

P wave: upright
Q wave: small
R wave: progressively larger, but less than 26 mm
S wave: progressively smaller; less than the S wave in V₄
T wave: upright
U wave: none present
ST segment: may vary from +1 to −0.5 mm

LEAD V₆

P wave: upright
Q wave: small
R wave: largest wave, but less than 26 mm
S wave: smallest; less than the S wave in V₅
T wave: upright
U wave: none present
ST segment: may vary from +1 to −0.5 mm

appear extremely deep in lead V₁ and become progressively more shallow, usually disappearing by lead V₅.

11. If you suspect myocardial infarction (MI), start with lead I and continue through to lead V₆, observing the waveforms for changes in ECG characteristics that can indicate acute MI, such as T-wave inversion, ST-segment elevation, and pathological Q waves. Note the leads in which you see such changes and describe the changes. When first learning to interpret the 12-lead ECG, ignore lead aV_R because it won't provide clues to left ventricular infarction or injury.

12. Determine the site and extent of myocardial damage. To do so, use the chart *Locating myocardial damage,* on page 122, and follow these steps:

▶ Identify the leads recording pathological Q waves. Look at the second column of the chart for those leads. Then look at the first column to find the corresponding myocardial wall, where infarction has occurred. Keep in mind that this chart serves as a guideline only. Actual areas of infarction may overlap or be larger or smaller than listed.

▶ Identify the leads recording ST-segment elevation (or depression for reciprocal leads), and use the chart to locate the corresponding areas of myocardial injury.

▶ Identify the leads recording T-wave inversion, and locate the corresponding areas of ischemia.

ACUTE MYOCARDIAL INFARCTION

An acute myocardial infarction (MI) can arise from any condition in which myocardial oxygen supply can't meet oxygen demand. Starved of oxygen, the myocardium suffers progressive ischemia, leading to injury and, eventually, to infarction.

In most cases, an acute MI involves the left ventricle, although it

LOCATING MYOCARDIAL DAMAGE

After you've noted characteristic lead changes in an acute myocardial infarction, use this chart to identify the areas of damage. Match the lead changes (ST elevation, abnormal Q waves) in the second column with the affected wall in the first column and the artery involved in the third column. The fourth column shows reciprocal lead changes.

Wall affected	Leads	Artery involved	Reciprocal changes
Anterior	V_2, V_3, V_4	Left coronary artery, left anterior descending (LAD)	II, III, aV_F
Anterolateral	I, aV_L, V_3, V_4, V_5, V_6	LAD and diagonal branches, circumflex and marginal branches	II, III, aV_F
Anteroseptal	V_1, V_2, V_3, V_4	LAD	None
Inferior	II, III, aV_F	Right coronary artery (RCA)	I, aV_L
Lateral	I, aV_L, V_5, V_6	Circumflex branch of left coronary artery	II, III, aV_F
Posterior	None	RCA or circumflex	V_1, V_2, V_3, V_4 (R greater than S in V_1 and V_2, ST-segment depression, elevated T wave)
Right ventricular	V_{4R}, V_{5R}, V_{6R}	RCA	None

can also involve the right ventricle or the atria. Typically, acute MIs are classified as either Q wave or non–Q wave.

In an acute MI, the characteristic electrocardiogram (ECG) changes result from the three I's (ischemia, injury, and infarction).

▶ Ischemia results from a temporary interruption of the myocardial blood supply. Its characteristic ECG change is T-wave inversion, a result of altered tissue repolarization. ST-segment depression may also occur.

Ischemia

Ischemia produces T-wave inversion

▶ Injury to myocardial cells results from a prolonged interruption of blood flow. Its characteristic ECG change, ST-segment elevation, reflects altered depolarization. Usually, you'll consider an elevation greater than 0.1 mV significant.

Injury

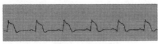

Injury produces ST-segment elevation

▶ Infarction results from an absence of blood flow to myocardial tissue, leading to necrosis. The ECG shows pathological Q waves, reflecting abnormal depolarization in damaged tissue or absent depolarization in scar tissue. The characteristic of a pathological Q wave is a duration of 0.04 second or an amplitude measuring at least one-third the height of the entire QRS complex.

Infarction

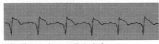

Infarction produces pathologic Q waves

Besides these three characteristic ECG changes, you may see reciprocal (or mirror image) changes. Reciprocal changes — most commonly ST-segment depression or tall R waves — occur in the leads opposite those reflecting the area of ischemia, injury, or infarction.

Acute MI phases

To detect an acute MI, you'll look for ST-segment elevation first, followed by T-wave inversion and pathological Q waves.

Serial ECG recordings yield the best evidence of an MI. Normally, an acute MI progresses through the following phases.

Hyperacute phase
The hyperacute phase begins a few hours after the onset of acute MI. You'll see ST-segment elevation and upright (usually peaked) T waves.

Fully evolved phase
The fully evolved phase starts several hours after MI onset. You'll see deep T-wave inversion and pathological Q waves.

Resolution phase
The resolution phase appears within a few weeks of acute MI. You'll see normal T waves.

Stabilized chronic phase
After the resolution phase, you'll see permanent pathological Q waves revealing an old infarction.

With an acute non–Q wave MI, you may see persistent ST-segment depression, T-wave inversion, or both; however, pathological Q waves may not appear. To differentiate an acute non–Q wave MI from myocardial ischemia, cardiac enzyme tests must be performed.

It's important to remember that for a true clinical diagnosis of an acute MI, a patient must have symptoms, ECG changes, and elevated cardiac enzyme levels. If the patient shows such signs and symptoms as chest pain, left arm pain, diaphoresis, and nausea, proceed as if he has had an acute MI until this possibility has been ruled out.

RIGHT-SIDED ECG, LEADS V_{4R} TO V_{6R}

A right-sided electrocardiogram (ECG) provides information about the extent of damage to the right ventricle, especially during the first 12 hours of MI. Right-sided ECG

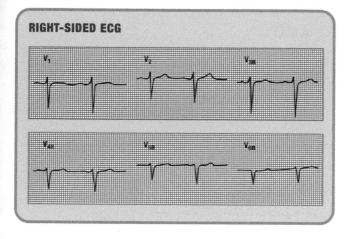

RIGHT-SIDED ECG

leads, placed over the right chest in similar but reversed positions from the left precordial leads, are called unipolar right-sided chest leads. (See *Right-sided ECG*.)

Placing electrodes

Right-sided ECG leads are precordial leads designated by the letter V, a number representing the electrode position, and the letter R, indicating right chest lead placement. Lead positions are:

▶ V_1: fourth intercostal space, right sternal border
▶ V_2: fourth intercostal space, left sternal border
▶ V_{3R}: midway between V_1 and V_{4R}, on a line joining these two locations
▶ V_{4R}: fifth intercostal space, right midclavicular line
▶ V_{5R}: fifth intercostal space, right anterior axillary line
▶ V_{6R}: fifth intercostal space, right midaxillary line.

Viewing the heart

Chest leads, whether on the left or the right chest, view the horizontal plane of the heart. The placement of left precordial leads gives a good picture of the electrical activity within the left ventricle. Because the right ventricle lies behind the left ventricle, the ability to evaluate right ventricular electrical activity when using only left precordial leads is limited. Right-sided ECG leads better visualize the right ventricular wall. This may be especially useful when evaluating a patient for a right ventricular MI.

POSTERIOR-LEAD ECG, LEADS V_7, V_8, V_9

Because of lung and muscle barriers, the usual chest leads can't "see" the heart's posterior to record myocardial damage there. To compensate for this, some practitioners add three posterior leads to the 12-lead electrocardiogram (ECG): leads

POSTERIOR ECG

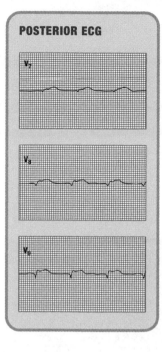

V_7, V_8, and V_9. The addition of the posterior leads to the 12-lead ECG increases the sensitivity of identifying posterior wall infarction so that appropriate treatment can begin. (See *Posterior ECG*.)

Placing electrodes

To ensure an accurate ECG reading, make sure the posterior electrodes V_7, V_8, and V_9 are placed at the same level horizontally as the V_6 lead at the fifth intercostal space. Lead positions are:
▶ V_7: posterior axillary line
▶ V_8: halfway between V_7 and V_9
▶ V_9: at the paraspinal line.

LEFT BUNDLE-BRANCH BLOCK

In left bundle-branch block, a conduction delay or block occurs in both the left posterior and the left anterior fascicles of the left bundle. This delay or block disrupts the normal left-to-right direction of depolarization. As a result, normal septal Q waves are absent. Because of the block, the wave of depolarization must move down the right bundle first and then spread from right to left. (See *Characteristics and interpretation of left bundle-branch block*, page 126.)

This arrhythmia may indicate underlying heart disease such as coronary artery disease. It carries a more serious prognosis than right bundle-branch block because of its close correlation with organic heart disease, and it requires a large lesion to block the thick, broad left bundle branch.

Intervention

When left bundle-branch block occurs along with an anterior wall myocardial infarction, it usually signals complete heart block, which requires insertion of a pacemaker.

RIGHT BUNDLE-BRANCH BLOCK

In the conduction delay or block associated with right bundle-branch block, the initial left-to-right direction of depolarization isn't affected. The left ventricle depolarizes on time, so the intrinsic deflection in leads V_5 and V_6 (the left precordial leads) takes place on time as well; however, the right ventricle depolarizes late, causing a late intrinsic deflection in leads V_1 and V_2 (the right precordial leads). This late de-

CHARACTERISTICS AND INTERPRETATION OF LEFT BUNDLE-BRANCH BLOCK

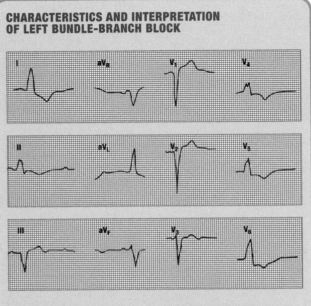

Rhythm: regular atrial and ventricular rhythms
Rate: atrial and ventricular rates within normal limits
P wave: normal size and configuration
PR interval: within normal limits
QRS complex: duration that varies from 0.10 to 0.12 second in incomplete left bundle-branch block (It's at least 0.12 second in complete block. Lead V_1 shows a wide, entirely negative rS or QS complex. Leads I, aV_L, and V_6 show a wide, tall R wave without a Q or S wave.)
T wave: deflection opposite that of the QRS complex in most leads
QT interval: may be prolonged or within normal limits
Other: magnitude of changes paralleling the magnitude of the QRS complex aberration, with normal axis or left-axis deviation; delayed intrinsic deflection over the left ventricle (lead V_6)

polarization also causes the axis to deviate to the right. (See *Characteristics and interpretation of right bundle-branch block.*)

Intervention

One potential complication of a myocardial infarction is a bundle-branch block. Some blocks require treatment with a temporary pacemaker. Others are monitored only to detect progression to a more complete block.

CHARACTERISTICS AND INTERPRETATION OF RIGHT BUNDLE-BRANCH BLOCK

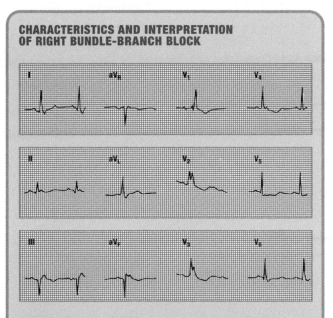

Rhythm: regular atrial and ventricular rhythms

Rate: atrial and ventricular rates within normal limits; P wave of normal size and configuration

PR interval: within normal limits

QRS complex: duration of at least 0.12 second in complete block and 0.10 to 0.12 second in incomplete block (In lead V_1, the QRS complex is wide and can appear in one of several patterns: an rSR' complex with a wide S and rSR' wave; an rS complex with a wide R wave; and a wide R wave with an M-shaped pattern. The complex is mainly positive, with the R wave occurring late. In leads I, aV_L, V_5, and V_6, a broad S wave can be seen.)

T wave: in most leads, deflection opposite that of the QRS deflection

QT interval: may be prolonged or within normal limits

Other: in the precordial leads, occurrence of triphasic complexes because the right ventricle continues to depolarize after the left ventricle depolarizes, thereby producing a third phase of ventricular stimulation

PERICARDITIS

An inflammation of the pericardium, the fibroserous sac that envelops the heart, pericarditis can be acute or chronic. The acute form may be fibrinous or effusive, with a purulent serous or hemorrhagic exudate. Chronic constrictive pericarditis causes dense fibrous pericardial thickening. Regardless of the form, pericarditis can cause cardiac tamponade if fluid accumulates too

CHARACTERISTICS AND INTERPRETATION OF PERICARDITIS

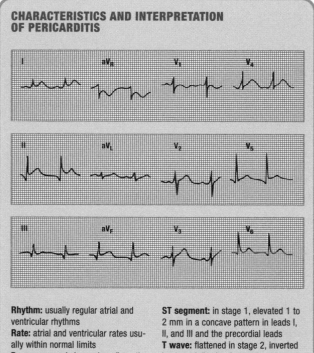

Rhythm: usually regular atrial and ventricular rhythms
Rate: atrial and ventricular rates usually within normal limits
P wave: normal size and configuration
PR interval: usually depressed in all leads except V_1 and aV_R, in which it may be elevated
QRS complex: within normal limits, but with a possible decrease in amplitude

ST segment: in stage 1, elevated 1 to 2 mm in a concave pattern in leads I, II, and III and the precordial leads
T wave: flattened in stage 2, inverted in stage 3 (lasting for weeks or months), and returning to normal in stage 4 (although sometimes becoming deeply inverted)
QT interval: within normal limits
Other: possible atrial fibrillation or tachycardia from sinoatrial node irritation

quickly. It can also cause heart failure if constriction occurs.

In pericarditis, ECG changes occur in four stages. Stage 1 coincides with the onset of chest pain. Stage 2 begins within several days. Stage 3 starts several days after stage 2. Stage 4 occurs weeks later. (See *Characteristics and interpretation of pericarditis.*)

Intervention

Pericarditis is usually treated with aspirin or nonsteroidal anti-inflammatory drugs. A last resort is prednisone, quickly tapered over 3 days.

5
Dermatologic disorders
Managing common skin problems

Selected skin problems

INTRODUCTION

More than 50% of all patients with skin problems receive treatment in a primary care setting, and this number is expected to increase. Because it's impossible to be familiar with the thousands of skin disorders and lesions, it's important to know when to refer or consult. In addition, it takes specialized training to differentiate which treatment plan will be most effective for a specific malignant lesion. This chapter explores some commonly seen lesions, how to manage them, and when to refer or consult.

ACNE VULGARIS

ICD-9-CM 706.1
An androgenically stimulated, inflammatory disease of the sebaceous follicles, acne vulgaris primarily affects adolescents, although lesions can appear as early as age 8. Although acne strikes boys more commonly and more severely, it usually occurs in girls at an earlier age and tends to last longer, sometimes into adulthood. Manifested as comedones, papules, pustules, and cysts, it can cause scarring. The prognosis is good with treatment.

Contagion

Acne vulgaris isn't contagious.

Causes

The cause of acne is multifactorial but isn't caused by any dietary factor. An overproduction of androgen or an increased response by the sebaceous glands can lead to acne. Also, hypersensitivity to *Propionibacterium acnes* and its metabolic byproducts can cause acne. It results from a complex interaction between androgen and bacteria in the hair follicles.

CULTURAL KEY *Acne vulgaris can occur in all adolescents, but incidence and severity are lower in people of African and Asian descent. Acne rosacea is more common in people of European and especially Celtic descent.*

Predisposing factors include heredity; adolescence; male sex; hormonal contraceptive use (many females experience an acne flare-up during their first few menses after starting or discontinuing hormonal contraceptives); androgen stimulation; certain drugs, including corticosteroids, corticotropin, androgens, iodides, phenytoin, isoniazid, and lithium; cobalt irradiation; and hyperalimentation.

Other precipitating factors include exposure to heavy oils, greases, or tars; trauma or rubbing from tight clothing; oily cosmetics; emotional stress; and a hot, humid climate. Also, check the patient's drug history because certain medications may cause an acne flare-up.

More is known about the pathogenesis of acne. Androgens stimulate sebaceous gland growth and production of sebum, which is secreted into dilated hair follicles that contain bacteria. The bacteria, usually *P. acnes* and *Staphylococcus epidermidis* — which are normal skin flora — secrete lipase. This enzyme interacts with sebum to produce free fatty acids, which provoke inflammation. Also, the hair follicles produce more keratin, which joins with the sebum to form a plug in the dilated follicle.

Clinical presentation

The appearance of characteristic acne lesions, especially in an adolescent patient, confirms the presence of acne vulgaris. The acne plug may appear as a closed comedone, or whitehead (if it doesn't protrude from the follicle and is covered by the epidermis), or as an open comedone, or blackhead (if it does protrude and isn't covered by the epidermis). The black coloration is caused by oxidation of tyrosine to melanin in the hair follicle.

Rupture or leakage of an enlarged plug into the dermis produces inflammation and characteristic acne pustules, papules or, in severe forms, acne cysts or abscesses. Chronic, recurring lesions produce acne scars.

Differential diagnosis

Conditions to consider before diagnosing acne vulgaris include folliculitis, rosacea, perioral dermatitis, steroid-induced acne, pseudofolliculitis barbae, staphylococcal infection (which may cause folliculitis or abscess), molluscum contagiosum, and ruptured inclusion cyst.

Diagnostic tests

▶ This condition is commonly diagnosed solely by clinical presentation.

▶ Consider ordering metabolite tests and testosterone levels when acne starts in a previously unaffected adult.

Management

▶ Be aware that acne can cause psychological problems, including depression and withdrawal from social situations. Pay special attention to the patient's perception of his physical appearance, and offer emotional support.

Drugs

▶ Frequently, acne is treated topically with benzoyl peroxide, a powerful antibacterial, alone or in combination with a keratin stabilizer (tretinoin) or another antiacne drug (such as azelaic acid).

▶ Systemic therapy consists primarily of antibiotics from the tetracycline or erythromycin families. It's used to decrease skin's bacteria and inflammation. Usual doses are given but frequency is decreased to twice daily rather than four times per day. When the condition improves, a lower daily dosage is used for long-term maintenance. Metronidazole gel is used topically to treat acne rosacea.

✳ **LIFE SPAN** *Tetracycline is contraindicated during pregnancy because it discolors the teeth of the fetus. Erythromycin may be substituted for these patients.*

▶ Exacerbation of pustules or abscesses during topical or systemic therapy requires a culture to identify a possible secondary bacterial infection.

▶ Oral isotretinoin combats acne by inhibiting sebaceous gland function and keratinization. Because of its severe adverse effects, the 16- to 20-week course of isotretinoin is limited to those with severe papulopustular or cystic acne that doesn't respond to conventional therapy. To prescribe oral isotretinoin, the provider must complete the booklet "System to Manage Accutane-Related Teratogenicity (S.M.A.R.T.) Guide to Best Practices" and obtain the qualification stickers, which must be placed on the prescription.

Before prescribing isotretinoin, refer to the complete product information. The drug is contraindicated during pregnancy and in women who are breast-feeding (pregnancy category X). It also has several drug warnings, including the risk of developing acute pancreatitis and psychiatric disorders, such as depression and suicidal ideations.

▶ Hormonal contraceptives are effective in improving acne in adult female patients. Hormonal contraceptives with estrogen and progestins of low androgenic activity are the most useful and may be used alone or in combination with other topical or oral medications. In many cases, acne flares after discontinuation of hormonal contraceptives.

Collaborative practice

Consult with a dermatologist for cases that are severe or nonresponsive after 12 weeks of treatment or if considering isotretinoin (Accutane).

Follow-up

Two or three visits in a 12-week period are needed to evaluate treatment and adjust it according to the patient's response. Try to quantify skin eruptions to allow a more accurate evaluation of therapy. Advise monthly visits until an adequate response is obtained.

These visits can serve a second purpose in a population that doesn't frequently visit the primary care provider — to address high-risk behaviors, such as drugs, unprotected sex, and reckless or impaired driving.

Complications

▸ Facial scarring
▸ Psychological effects
▸ Severe, confluent, inflammatory acne (acne conglobata)

Patient teaching

▸ Try to identify predisposing factors that can be eliminated or modified.
▸ Emphasize that acne isn't caused or exacerbated by too much or too little sex, masturbation, dirty skin, or various foods.
▸ Explain the causes of acne to the patient and his family. Make sure they understand that the prescribed treatment is more likely to improve acne than a strict diet and continual scrubbing with soap and water. Provide written instructions regarding treatment.

▸ Advise the patient to avoid exposure to sunlight or to use a sunscreen. If the prescribed regimen includes tretinoin and benzoyl peroxide, tell the patient to avoid skin irritation by using one preparation in the morning and the other at night.
▸ Instruct the patient to take tetracycline on an empty stomach and to avoid taking it with antacids or milk, which inhibit drug absorption.
▸ Tell the patient who is taking isotretinoin to avoid vitamin A supplements, which can worsen adverse effects. Also, discuss how to deal with the dry skin and mucous membranes that usually occur during treatment.

🌸 **LIFE SPAN** *Warn the female patient of child-bearing age about the severe risk of teratogenicity with isotretinoin. In addition to signing a special permission form, she'll need monthly measurement of lipid levels and liver function as well as monthly pregnancy tests.*

▸ Inform the patient that acne takes a long time — sometimes years — for complete resolution. Encourage continued local skin care even after acne clears. Explain the adverse effects of all drugs.

Resources

▸ American Academy of Dermatology: (847) 330-0230; *www.aad.org*

BASAL CELL CARCINOMA

ICD-9-CM facial 173.3; scalp or neck 173.4; trunk 173.5; upper limb 173.6; lower limb 173.7

A slow-growing, destructive skin tumor, basal cell carcinoma usually occurs in people older than age 40.

🔱 **CULTURAL KEY** *Basal cell carcinoma is more prevalent in blond, fair-skinned men and is the* most common malignant tumor affecting whites.

Contagion

Basal cell carcinoma isn't contagious.

Causes

Prolonged sun exposure is the most common cause of basal cell carcinoma. Other possible causes include arsenic ingestion, radiation exposure, burns, immunosuppression and, rarely, vaccinations.

Although the pathogenesis of basal cell carcinoma is uncertain, some experts now hypothesize that it originates when, under certain conditions, undifferentiated basal cells become neoplastic instead of differentiating into sweat glands, sebum, and hair.

Clinical presentation

Four types of basal cell carcinoma occur:
▶ *Nodular carcinomas* present as shiny translucent lesions.
▶ *Ulcerative carcinomas* are often covered with a dry crust and appear as an ulcerated nodule.
▶ *Rodent ulcerative carcinomas* have an elevated skin border or rolled appearance. These lesions occur most often on the face, particularly the forehead, eyelid margins, and nasolabial folds. Telangiectatic vessels cross the surface, and the lesions are occasionally pigmented. As the lesions enlarge, their centers become depressed and their borders become firm and elevated. Ulceration and local invasion eventually occur. Rodent ulcers rarely metastasize; however, if untreated, they can spread to vital areas and become infected. If they invade large blood vessels, they can cause massive hemorrhage.
▶ *Sclerosing basal cell carcinomas (morphea-like)* are waxy, sclerotic, yellow to white plaques with indistinct borders. Occurring on the trunk, sclerosing basal cell carcinomas often look like small patches of scleroderma. They commonly appear as multiple erythematous lesions with occasional pearly papules at the periphery and typically have variegated pigmentation.

Basal cell carcinomas are usually detected on examination with good lighting, a hand lens, and careful palpation.

Differential diagnosis

▶ Actinic keratosis
▶ Benign mole
▶ Hyperpigmentation
▶ Intradermal nevi
▶ Molluscum contagiosum
▶ Sebaceous hyperplasia

Diagnostic tests

Biopsy and histologic study confirm the diagnosis by showing basal cells extending into the dermis.

Management

▶ In all physical examinations, look for unusual nevi or other skin lesions.

⚫⚫⚫ RED FLAG *If melanoma is suspected, the lesion should never be curetted, shaved, or electrodesiccated. Refer all suspicious lesions to a dermatologist, not just for identification but also for determination of the most effective treatment plan. When a biopsy is taken, it's best to take detailed notes, including what the lesion looks like and why melanoma is suspected, in order to help the pathology laboratory correlate the clinical presentation with the biopsy outcome.*

▶ Depending on the size, location, and depth of the lesion, expected treatment may include curettage and electrodesiccation, chemotherapy, surgical excision, irradiation, or chemosurgery.

WARNING SIGNS OF LESIONS

Use this mnemonic device to help evaluate basal cell carcinoma or epithelioma.
Asymmetrical
Bleeding
Color variegated within lesion
Diameter greater than 6 mm (pencil eraser)
Edges irregular
Feeling (sensitive to touch, burning, itching)
Growing in height or diameter

▶ Curettage and electrodesiccation offer good cosmetic results for small lesions.
▶ Topical fluorouracil is commonly used for superficial lesions. This medication produces marked local irritation or inflammation in the involved tissue but no systemic effects.
▶ Moh's surgery is a microscopically controlled surgical excision that carefully removes recurrent lesions until a tumor-free plane is achieved. After removal of large lesions, skin grafting may be required.

✳ **LIFE SPAN** *Irradiation is used if the tumor location requires it and for elderly or debilitated patients who might not withstand surgery. It may cause disfigurement.*
▶ Cryotherapy with liquid nitrogen freezes and kills the cells.
▶ Chemosurgery is usually necessary for persistent or recurrent lesions. It consists of periodic applications of a fixative paste (such as zinc chloride) and subsequent removal of fixed pathologic tissue. Treatment continues until tumor removal is complete.

Collaborative practice
Consult a dermatologist for suspicious lesions and for biopsy.

Follow-up
Visits are needed monthly for 3 months, then every 3 months for 9 months, and then every 6 months for 5 years. After that, an annual visit is required.

Complications
▶ Metastasis (rare)
▶ Recurrences and new lesions (usually occur within 5 years)
▶ Scarring

Patient teaching
▶ Most skin cancers are curable, particularly if caught in early stages. Discuss diagnosis and treatment options. Warn the patient that it's common to have recurrences or new lesions within 5 years.
▶ Instruct the patient to eat frequent, small meals that are high in protein. Suggest eggnog, pureed foods, and liquid protein supplements if the lesion has invaded the oral cavity and caused eating problems.
▶ Stress the importance of routinely examining the skin, becoming familiar with the body, and focusing on moles and new lesions to detect changes early.
▶ Tell the patient that to prevent disease recurrence, he must avoid excessive sun exposure, use a strong sunscreen, and wear a wide-brimmed hat and long-sleeved shirts to protect his skin from damage by ultraviolet rays.
▶ Advise the patient to relieve local inflammation from topical fluorouracil with cool compresses or corticosteroid ointment.
▶ Instruct the patient with noduloulcerative basal cell carcinoma to wash his face gently when ulcera-

tions and crusting occur; scrubbing too vigorously may cause bleeding.

▶ To help prevent malignant melanoma, stress the detrimental effects of overexposure to solar radiation, especially to fair-skinned, blonde, blue-eyed patients. Recommend that all patients use a sunscreen.

●●● **RED FLAG** *Tell the patient to call* ●●● *his primary care provider if he experiences persistent, changing, worsening, anxiety-producing, or specific signs and symptoms, including lesions that fit the mnemonic ABCDEFG. (See* Warning signs of lesions.*)*

Resources

▶ Skin Cancer Foundation: 1-800-SKIN-490; *www.skincancer.org*
▶ American Cancer Society: 1-800-ACS-2345; *www.cancer.org*
▶ Cancer Information Service: 1-800-4-CANCER; *http://cis.nci.nih.gov*
▶ Cancer Care: 1-800-813-HOPE; *www.cancercare.org*
▶ Association of Cancer Online Resources: (212) 226-5525; *www.acor.org*

CONTACT DERMATITIS

ICD-9-CM 692.9

Contact dermatitis is a general term describing inflammatory skin reactions after contact with specific antigens. It's the most common skin disease attributed to the workplace and is the cause of a considerable portion of disability in industry. Contact dermatitis can be divided into two categories: nonallergic and allergic. Nonallergic dermatitis (such as reaction to poison ivy) is caused by chemical irritation and tends to develop more rapidly. The reaction depends on the concentration of the irritant. Conversely, al-

lergic dermatitis (such as reaction to a specific brand of soap) is caused by an antigen (also called an *allergen*) that evokes a cell-mediated hypersensitivity reaction only in people who are sensitized to it. The reaction occurs even with small amounts of exposure, takes longer to appear, and occurs after each exposure. (See *Types of dermatitis*, pages 136 to 139.)

Contagion

Contact dermatitis isn't contagious.

Causes

Contact dermatitis is a delayed hypersensitivity reaction and appears several hours to a week (and rarely even longer) after exposure to the antigen. The time delay is caused by the *cell-mediated immune cascade*. When immunoglobulin (Ig) G or IgM reacts with antigens as part of the body's immune response, complement factors are activated that move through the epidermis to the lymph nodes to stimulate T-cell proliferation. From the lymph nodes, T cells move by way of the bloodstream to tissues and then to the dermal layers to produce the dermatitis. Consequently, chronic skin irritation usually continues even after exposure to the allergen has ended or after the irritation has been systemically controlled. In addition, because of the cell-mediated pathway, all skin becomes hypersensitive to the antigen.

Clinical presentation

The acute stage can occur over a few days and is characterized by well-demarcated, erythematous, edematous lesions that may be superimposed on other lesions, with skin erosions. Crusting, oozing, and pruritus may be present.

(Text continues on page 138.)

TYPES OF DERMATITIS

Type	Causes	Signs and symptoms
Exfoliative dermatitis Severe, chronic noninfectious inflammation characterized by redness and widespread erythema and scaling	▸ Preexisting lesions progressing to exfoliative stage, such as in contact dermatitis, drug reaction, lymphoma, leukemia, or atopic dermatitis ▸ May be idiopathic	▸ Generalized dermatitis, with acute loss of stratum corneum, and erythema and scaling ▸ Sensation of tight skin ▸ Hair loss ▸ Possible fever, sensitivity to cold, shivering, gynecomastia, and lymphadenopathy
Hand or foot dermatitis Noninfectious disease characterized by inflammatory eruptions on the hands or feet	▸ Usually unknown but may result from progressive contact dermatitis ▸ Excessive skin dryness commonly a contributing factor ▸ 50% of patients atopic	▸ Redness and scaling of the palms or soles ▸ May produce painful fissures ▸ Some cases present with blisters (dyshidrotic eczema)
Localized neurodermatitis (lichen simplex chronicus, essential pruritus) Superficial inflammation characterized by itching and papular eruptions that appear on thickened, hyperpigmented skin	▸ Chronic scratching or rubbing of a primary lesion or insect bite or other skin irritation ▸ May be psychogenic	▸ Intense, sometimes continual scratching ▸ Thick, sharp-bordered, possibly dry, scaly lesions with raised papules and accentuated skin lines (lichenification) ▸ Usually affects easily reached areas, such as ankles, lower legs, anogenital area, back of neck, and ears ▸ One or a few lesions present; asymmetrical distribution
Nummular dermatitis A chronic form of dermatitis characterized by inflammation of coin-shaped, scaling, or vesicular patches; usually quite pruritic	▸ Possibly precipitated by stress, skin dryness, irritants, or scratching	▸ Round, nummular (coin-shaped), red lesions, usually on arms and legs, with distinct borders of crusts and scales ▸ Possible oozing and severe itching ▸ Summertime remissions common, with wintertime recurrence

Diagnosis	Treatment and interventions
▶ Diagnosis requires identification of the underlying cause.	▶ Hospitalization, with protective isolation and hygienic measures to prevent secondary bacterial infection ▶ Open wet dressings with colloidal baths ▶ Bland lotions over topical corticosteroids ▶ Maintenance of constant environmental temperature to prevent chilling or overheating ▶ Careful monitoring of renal and cardiac status ▶ Systemic antibiotics and steroids
▶ Patient history and physical findings (distribution of eruption on palms and soles) confirm diagnosis.	▶ Antibiotics for secondary infection ▶ Avoidance of excessive hand washing and drying and of accumulation of soaps and detergents under rings ▶ Use of emollients with topical corticosteroids
▶ Physical findings confirm diagnosis.	▶ Cessation of scratching (Lesions disappear in about 2 weeks.) ▶ Fixed dressings or Unna's boot to cover affected areas ▶ Topical corticosteroids under occlusive dressing or by intralesional injection ▶ Antihistamines and open wet dressings ▶ Emollients ▶ Patient informed about underlying cause
▶ Physical findings and patient history confirm nummular dermatitis. ▶ Diagnosis must rule out fungal infections, atopic or contact dermatitis, and psoriasis.	▶ Elimination of known irritants ▶ Measures to relieve dry skin: increased humidification, limited frequency of baths, use of bland soap and bath oils, and application of emollients ▶ Application of wet dressings in acute phase ▶ Topical corticosteroids (occlusive dressing or intralesional injection) for persistent lesions ▶ Tar preparations and antihistamines to control itching ▶ Antibiotics for secondary infection

(continued)

TYPES OF DERMATITIS *(continued)*

Type	Causes	Signs and symptoms
Seborrheic dermatitis A subacute skin disease that affects the scalp, face and, occasionally, other areas; characterized by lesions covered with yellow or brownish gray scales	▶ Unknown; stress, immunodeficiency, and neurologic conditions may be predisposing factors; related to the yeast *Pityrosporum ovale*	▶ Eruptions in areas with many sebaceous glands (usually scalp, face, chest, axillae, and groin) and in skin folds ▶ Itching, redness, and inflammation of affected areas; lesions may appear greasy; fissures may occur ▶ Indistinct, occasionally yellowish, scaly patches from excess stratum corneum (dandruff may be a mild seborrheic dermatitis)
Stasis dermatitis A condition usually caused by impaired circulation and characterized by eczema of the legs with edema, hyperpigmentation, and persistent inflammation	▶ Secondary to peripheral vascular diseases affecting legs, such as recurrent thrombophlebitis and resultant chronic venous insufficiency	▶ Varicosities and edema common, but obvious vasular insufficiency not always present ▶ Usually affects the lower leg, just above internal malleolus, or sites of trauma or irritation ▶ Early signs: dusky red deposits of hemosiderin in skin, with itching and dimpling of subcutaneous tissue ▶ Later signs: edema, redness, and scaling of large areas of legs ▶ Possibly fissures, crusts, and ulcers

Subacute cases present with mildly erythematous lesions with small, dry scaling or exfoliation and, occasionally, small, firm papules.

Chronic dermatitis can last for months or years. It also has a mildly erythematous base, but thickening, scaling, excoriations, and fissuring predominate. Skin that's thinner or has more contact with the irritant is more strongly affected. Constitutional symptoms (such as fever) may occur in severe cases of acute dermatitis.

Common secondary conditions associated with contact dermatitis include viral, fungal, or bacterial infections and ocular disorders, probably due to scratching.

Differential diagnosis

▶ Bullous pemphigoid
▶ Herpes simplex
▶ Photoallergy
▶ Scabies
▶ Tinea

Diagnosis	Treatment and interventions
▸ Patient history and physical findings, especially distribution of lesions in sebaceous gland areas, confirm seborrheic dermatitis. ▸ Diagnosis must rule out psoriasis.	▸ Removal of scales with frequent washing and shampooing with selenium sulfide suspension, zinc pyrithione, ketoconazole 2%, or tar and salicylic acid shampoo ▸ Application of topical corticosteroids and antifungals to involved areas
▸ Diagnosis requires positive history of venous insufficiency and physical findings such as varicosities.	▸ Measures to prevent venous stasis: avoidance of prolonged sitting or standing, use of support stockings, weight reduction in obesity, and leg elevation ▸ Corrective surgery for underlying cause ▸ After ulcer develops: rest periods with legs elevated; open wet dressings; Unna's boot; and antibiotics for secondary infection after wound culture

CLINICAL PEARL *Typical distribution of skin lesions rules out other inflammatory skin lesions, such as diaper rash (lesions confined to the diapered area), seborrheic dermatitis (no pigmentation changes or lichenification in chronic lesions), or atopic dermatitis (antecubital, groin, facial areas).*

Diagnostic tests

▸ The diagnosis is based on physical examination and patient history.
▸ A *skin patch test* confirms identity of the allergen.

Management

▸ Effective treatment of contact dermatitis consists of eliminating allergens and avoiding irritants. Local and systemic measures aim to relieve itching and inflammation.
▸ Large vesicles may be drained; however, to reduce the chance of infection, their tops shouldn't be removed.

LIFE SPAN *Remember that coping with disfigurement is extremely difficult, especially for children and adolescents. Be careful not* *to show anxiety or revulsion when touching the lesions during examination. Help the patient accept his altered body image, and encourage him to verbalize his feelings.*

▶ Although the patient can help clear lichenified skin by applying occlusive dressings such as plastic film, this should be done only after consulting with a dermatologist because the dressing increases the potency of the corticosteroid cream.

Drugs

▶ A combination of zinc oxide, talc, menthol, and phenol reduces dryness and is protective.

▶ A high-potency corticosteroid ointment (fluocinonide, triamcinolone) may be applied thinly twice daily, especially after bathing, until lesions are controlled to alleviate inflammation. Avoid using corticosteroids (particularly high-potency types) on thin-skinned areas (face, skin folds) because they thin the skin over time.

▶ Calamine can alleviate pruritus.

▶ Systemic corticosteroids should be used only during extreme exacerbations and after consultation or referral with a dermatologist.

✿ **LIFE SPAN** *In infants and children, use hydrocortisone ointment 2.5% (1% for face and intertriginous areas).*

▶ Antibiotics (erythromycin) are used for secondary infections.

Collaborative practice

For severe, refractory, or complex cases and before using systemic corticosteroids, refer the patient to a primary care physician or dermatologist.

Refer the patient to a psychologist or psychiatrist as needed for counseling due to altered body image, particularly in adolescents and children.

Follow-up

Although the clinical picture may vary, generally follow up in 1 week

to assess response. If nonresponsive to treatment, seek consultation. Two weeks after resolution of symptoms, consider patch testing to determine the causative agent.

Complications

▶ Generalized dermatitis

▶ Secondary bacterial infections

Patient teaching

▶ Instruct the patient to avoid contact with known allergens; if the patient develops a chronic problem of unknown cause, advise keeping a symptom diary to try to identify allergens.

▶ Advise the patient to set up an individual schedule and plan for daily skin care.

▶ Advise the patient to bathe in plain water. (He may have to limit bathing, according to the severity of the lesions.) Tell him to bathe with a nonfatty soap and tepid water (96° F [35.6° C]) but to avoid using soap when lesions are acutely inflamed.

▶ For acute pruritus, tell the patient to apply moisturizer immediately after bathing if skin is dry.

▶ Advise the patient that soaking in cool water with Burow's solution, Aveeno, or baking soda is helpful. A cool compress or ice cube can provide local relief.

▶ Caution the patient that extended periods in a hot environment will exacerbate symptoms.

▶ Advise the patient to shampoo frequently (no more than once daily) and apply corticosteroid solution to the scalp afterward.

▶ As indicated, recommend hypoallergenic cosmetics, decreased use of milder deodorants, and use of mild detergents without fragrance. Advise the patient to check for the words "hypoallergenic" and "dye and perfume free."

❯ Daytime drowsiness is possible with the use of antihistamines to relieve itching. This may interfere with sleep. Advise the patient to use alternate methods for inducing natural sleep, such as drinking a glass of warm milk, to help prevent overuse of sedatives.

❯ Advise the patient that applying a moisturizing cream between steroid doses can help retain lubricant in the skin, particularly if applied during and after a tub bath.

❯ Instruct the patient to keep fingernails short to limit excoriation and secondary infections caused by scratching.

❯ Advise the patient that irritants, such as detergents and wool, exacerbate dermatitis.

⚫⚫⚫ RED FLAG *Tell the patient to call* **⚫⚫⚫** *the primary care provider and report persistent, changing, worsening, anxiety-producing, or specific signs and symptoms, including:*

❯ *signs of infection (redness, edema, or drainage, especially if cloudy, thick, or colored), fever (greater than 102.5° F [39.2° C]), and large, painful open areas*

❯ *itching or rash nonresponsive to management plan after 3 days*

❯ *signs of serious allergic reaction (lesions around or in eyes and mouth).*

❯ Tell the patient to call emergency medical services if he experiences difficulty breathing, shortness of breath, wheezing, swelling of tongue or throat, abdominal or chest pain, confusion, or loss of consciousness.

Resources

❯ American Academy of Allergy, Asthma & Immunology: 1-800-822-2762; *www.aaaai.org*

❯ Asthma and Allergy Foundation of America: 1-800-7-ASTHMA; *www.aafa.org*

❯ American Academy of Dermatology: 1-888-462-DERM; *www.aad.org*

⚫ ECZEMA

ICD-9-CM Atopic dermatitis (acute, allergic, chronic, erythematous, fissum, occupational, rubrum, squamous) 692.9, atopic 691.8, external ear 380.22, flexural 691.8, gouty 274.89, infantile (acute or chronic) 690.12

Eczema (also known as *atopic dermatitis*) is a chronic skin disorder that's characterized by superficial skin inflammation and intense itching. Scratching causes weeping and skin infection that crusts over, progressing to thick, roughened skin. This condition can flare up intermittently throughout a person's lifetime.

☀ LIFE SPAN *Ninety percent of people with eczema have the characteristic rash by age 5.*

Contagion

Eczema isn't contagious.

Causes

The skin is unable to retain adequate water, and the dryness causes itching. Constant scratching leads to a vicious cycle: itch-scratch-rash-itch. Eczema is chronic and has a strong genetic component. More than two-thirds of patients have a personal or family history of asthma, eczema, hay fever, or other allergies. Increasing prevalence is thought to be due to increased exposure to allergens, a decline in breast-feeding, and heightened parental and clinician awareness.

Clinical presentation

Pruritus is the hallmark symptom of eczema. Scratching can cause weeping, infected skin, and crusting. When acute, lesions are poorly defined erythematous and edematous papules and plaques with tiny vesicles, exudation, crusting, and excoriation. Chronic lesions are lichenified, hyperpigmented, and thickened, with fissured skin folds. Presentation generally differs by age. In infants, it affects the face. In children, it affects the antecubital and popliteal fossae. In adults, it's more generalized and often more severe.

Differential diagnosis

▶ Contact dermatitis
▶ Dermatophytosis
▶ Early-stage mycosis fungoides
▶ Nummular eczema
▶ Photosensitivity
▶ Psoriasis
▶ Scabies
▶ Seborrheic dermatitis

Diagnostic tests

▶ Diagnosis is made on clinical grounds. Typically, the patient has a history of atopy.
▶ *Bacterial culture* is indicated because almost 90% of patients are secondarily colonized.
▶ *Viral culture* rules out herpes simplex virus in crusted lesions.
▶ *Radioallergosorbent testing* is rarely helpful.

Management

Drugs

▶ *Topical corticosteroids* decrease erythema, inflammation, and pruritus and are the most commonly used agents. Adverse effects include adrenal suppression with chronic use, permanent thinning of the skin, and striae formation.
▶ *Menthol* and *camphor lotions* help control itching.
▶ *Topical anesthetics* alone or with hydrocortisone (Aveeno Anti-Itch, PrameGel, Epifoam) may be used for itching. Avoid benzocaine because of allergic reactions.
▶ *Nonsedating antihistamines,* such as loratadine (Claritin), are good for daytime itch.
▶ *Sedating antihistamines* (hydroxyzine or doxepin) can be used daily at bedtime.

▶ *Topical antibacterials* are used for excoriations and crusted areas. Avoid neomycin-containing topicals because of sensitization.
▶ *Topical and oral antibiotics* are used for secondary infections.
▶ *Systemic corticosteroids* help acute flares, but recurrence after discontinuation is common.
▶ *Ultraviolet B* and *psoralen plus ultraviolet A* may be useful in refractory disease after age 10.
▶ *Acyclovir* (I.V. or by mouth) is used for secondary infection by herpes simplex. Eczema herpeticum requires immediate treatment; it has a punched-out appearance and occurs in grouped and disseminated crusted erosions. Daily acyclovir for suppressive therapy may be needed.

Collaborative practice

Consult a dermatologist for refractory lesions, disease complicated by herpes simplex infection, or when allergic contact dermatitis is suspected. Refer or consult before using occlusive dressings with corticosteroids, systemic corticosteroids, or cyclosporine. Refer the patient to an allergist or immunologist in cases with congenital immunodeficiency or significant respiratory atopy or when an environmental allergen is suspected.

Follow-up

Generally, follow up in 1 week to assess response and then in 1 month or as otherwise ordered.

Complications

▶ Skin atrophy
▶ Skin infections
▶ Striae
▶ Systemic effects

Patient teaching

Preventive measures

▶ Advise the patient to wear loose-fitting soft fabrics and to minimize skin irritants (clothes made of coarse fabric, harsh soaps, pro-longed hot baths or showers).

▶ Instruct the patient to minimize drying of the skin and loss of epithelium, which lowers defenses and increases risk of infection. Tell him he should avoid bathing more than once per day; take lukewarm baths or showers using moisturizing soaps (Dove, Aveeno Oilated Bath) or colloidal oatmeal (Aveeno); use soap to wash body folds, but on other parts of the body use only as needed; and pat dry and apply moisturizer (hydrated petroleum moisture creams) while skin is damp. Advise him to avoid ointments because they clog pores and increase itching.

▶ Teach the patient to reduce stress, which may cause exacerbations.

▶ Advise the patient to try not to scratch or rub. If he must do so, advise using pads of fingers, not nails.

✿ LIFE SPAN *Tell parents that children's nails should be trimmed to minimize damage from scratching.*

▶ Tell the patient that wet-work activities such as dishwashing should be done while wearing white cotton gloves under rubber gloves. Contact with chlorine (in swimming pools as well as when cleaning) should be avoided.

▶ Tell the patient to call his primary care provider if he experiences persistent, changing, worsening, anxiety-producing, or specific signs and symptoms, including:
– signs of infection (increased redness of lesions, swelling, cloudy or odorous drainage, and temperature above 102° F [38.9° C])
– itching unrelieved by management plan
– rash not much improved after 1 week of management.

Resources

▶ American Academy of Dermatology: 1-888-462-DERM; *www.aad.org*

FUNGAL INFECTIONS

ICD-9-CM Tinea corporis 110.5, pedis 110.4, capitis/barbae 110.0, unguium 110.1, cruris 110.3

Also called *tinea, ringworm,* or *dermatophytosis,* fungal infections can affect the scalp (tinea capitis), body (tinea corporis), nails (tinea unguium), feet (tinea pedis), groin (tinea cruris), and bearded skin (tinea barbae).

Tinea infections are quite prevalent in the United States and are usually more common in males than in females. With effective treatment, the cure rate is high, although about 20% of people with infected feet or nails develop chronic conditions.

Contagion

Fungal infections are contagious. Transmission can occur directly (through contact with infected lesions) or indirectly (through contact with contaminated articles, such as shoes, towels, and shower stalls). Some infections come from contact with animals or soil.
Incubation period: 10 to 14 days.
Isolation: No direct contact.
Communicable period: In humans, as long as lesions are present; on fomites (objects contaminated with causative organisms), extended time.

Causes

Tinea infections (except for tinea versicolor, which is caused by overgrowth of normal skin flora and isn't transmittable) result from infection with dermatophytes (fungi) of the genera *Trichophyton, Microsporum,* and *Epidermophyton.*

Clinical presentation

Lesions vary in appearance and duration with the type of infection.

▶ *Tinea capitis,* which mainly affects children, is characterized by round erythematous patches on the scalp, causing hair loss with scaling. In some children, a hypersensitivity reaction develops, leading to boggy, inflamed, commonly pus-filled lesions (kerions).

▶ *Tinea corporis* produces flat lesions on the skin except the scalp, bearded skin, groin, palms, or soles. The lesions may be dry and scaly or moist and crusty; as they enlarge, their centers heal, causing the classic ring-shaped appearance.

▶ *Tinea unguium* (onychomycosis) infection typically starts at the tip of one or more toenails (fingernail infection is less common) and produces gradual thickening, discoloration, and crumbling of the nail, with accumulation of subungual debris. Eventually, the nail may be destroyed completely.

▶ *Tinea pedis* causes scaling and blisters between the toes. Severe infection may result in inflammation, with severe itching and pain on walking. A dry, squamous inflammation may affect the entire sole.

▶ *Tinea cruris* (jock itch) produces red, raised, sharply defined, itchy lesions in the groin that may extend to the buttocks, inner thighs, and external genitalia. Warm weather and tight clothing encourage fungus growth.

▶ *Tinea barbae* is an uncommon infection that affects the bearded facial area of men.

▶ *Tinea versicolor,* also called *pityriasis versicolor,* is a chronic, asymptomatic, hypopigmented, scaling, macular rash with sharp margins. It's caused by opportunistic overgrowth of a lipophilic yeast that's normally present on the skin. High-risk factors include high humidity, excessive sebum production, and application of grease or corticosteroids for extended periods.

Differential diagnosis

▶ Alopecia areata
▶ Dermatitis (atopic, contact, seborrheic)
▶ Pityriasis alba
▶ Psoriasis
▶ Vitiligo

Diagnostic tests

▶ *Microscopic examination of lesion scrapings prepared in potassium hydroxide solution* usually confirms tinea infection, detecting arthrospores within hair shafts.

▶ Other diagnostic procedures include Wood's light examination (which is useful in only 10% of cases of tinea capitis and further identifies the dermatophyte but doesn't affect treatment) and culture of the infecting organism.

Management
Drugs

▶ Tinea infections usually respond to *topical antifungals* such as clotrimazole (Lotrimin) used twice daily for 3 to 6 weeks. Topical therapy is ineffective for tinea capitis; griseofulvin is the treatment of choice.

▶ *Oral griseofulvin* (250 to 500 mg twice daily for 1 to 3 months) is especially effective in tinea infections of the skin and hair but requires baseline complete blood count (CBC) and liver function tests (LFTs).

▶ *Pulse therapy with oral terbinafine* (250 mg) daily for 3 months or itraconazole (200 mg) by mouth twice per day for 1 week, repeated monthly for 3 to 6 months for fingernails and 8 to 12 months for toenails, depending on extent of infection is helpful in nail infections. Remember, the effect will continue after treatment because the drug is absorbed into the nail, and as the nail slowly grows out, the drug will continue to kill fungus.

▶ Other antifungals *include naftifine, ciclopirox olamine, tolnaftate, ketoconazole* (baseline CBC and LFTs required), and numerous others. Topical treatments should continue for 2 weeks after lesions resolve.

▶ Tinea versicolor responds to *selenium sulfide (2.5%) shampoo*. The shampoo is applied to affected sites daily for 1 week, allowed to remain for 15 minutes, and then rinsed out.

▶ Supportive measures include open wet dressings, removal of scabs and scales, and application of keratolytics such as salicylic acid to soften and remove hyperkeratotic lesions of the heels or soles.

▶ For tinea corporis, use abdominal pads between skin folds for the patient with excessive abdominal girth; change pads frequently. Check daily for excoriated, newly denuded areas of skin. If the involved area is moist, apply open wet dressings two or three times daily to decrease inflammation and help remove scales.

Collaborative practice
Refer to or consult with a primary care physician or dermatologist if the patient is nonresponsive in 2 weeks.

Follow-up
Evaluate the patient's response to the drug every 2 weeks and then monthly for the duration of treatment (for nail involvement). If prescribing griseofulvin or ketoconazole, monitor with CBC and LFTs every 3 months.

Complications
▶ Hair loss
▶ Permanent scarring

Patient teaching

✿ **LIFE SPAN** *For tinea corporis or tinea capitis, remind parents to check with the school or day-care facility for its policy on tinea. Many children may attend with some restrictions, such as no swimming, gym, or activities likely to lead to close physical contact. Restrictions for younger children may be stricter because of their inability to avoid intimate contact.*

▶ For all tinea infections except those of the hair and nails, first line therapy is topical. Advise the patient to watch for sensitivity reactions and secondary bacterial infections. Tell him to continue topical treatments for 2 weeks after lesions are completely gone.

▶ Advise the patient to use good hand-washing technique. To prevent spreading the infection to others, advise washing towels, bedclothes, and combs frequently in hot water and avoiding sharing them. Suggest that family members be checked (particularly for tinea capitis).

▶ For tinea unguium, advise the patient to keep nails short and straight and to gently remove debris from under the nails with an emery board.

▶ For tinea pedis, encourage the patient to expose his feet to air whenever possible and to wear sandals or leather shoes and clean cotton socks. Instruct the patient to wash the feet twice daily and, after drying them thoroughly, to apply the antifungal cream followed by antifungal powder to absorb perspiration and prevent excoriation.

▶ For tinea cruris, instruct the patient to dry the affected area thoroughly after bathing and to apply antifungal powder evenly after applying the topical antifungal agent. Advise the patient to wear loose-fitting clothing, which should be changed frequently and washed in hot water.

▶ For tinea barbae, suggest that the patient let his beard grow. (Whiskers should be trimmed with scissors, not a razor.) If the patient insists that he must shave, advise him to use an electric razor instead of a blade.

▶ Tell the patient to call the primary care provider and report persistent, changing, worsening, anxiety-producing, or specific signs and symptoms, including:

– no improvement after 1 week of management plan (1 month for nails)

– lesions spreading to the scalp or nails

– lesions appearing infected (fever, increased redness, swelling, cloudy or colored drainage).

Resources

▶ National Library of Medicine: *www.nlm.nih.gov* (search "fungal infections")

HERPES SIMPLEX

ICD-9-CM Herpes simplex 054.73, conjunctiva simplex 054.43, genital 054.10, whitlow 054.6

Herpes simplex is a recurring viral infection. Herpes simplex type 1 (HSV-1) may affect the mucous membranes, oropharynx, conjunctiva, and skin and most commonly produces cold sores and fever blisters. It may also infect the genital area.

Herpes simplex type 2 (HSV-2) primarily affects the genital area but may involve the anus, buttocks, and legs.

The usual course of primary infection is 2 weeks; recurrences are less severe with less viral shedding. The infection may disseminate, however, causing encephalitis or pneumonia.

Primary herpesvirus hominis (HVH) is the leading cause of gingivostomatitis in children ages 1 to 3 and causes the most common nonepidemic encephalitis. It's the second most common viral infection in pregnant women, and vertical transmission may cause spontaneous abortion.

Contagion

Herpes simplex is contagious. It's spread by skin-skin or mucosa-skin contact.

HSV-1 is spread in oral and respiratory secretions and can also be sexually transmitted.

HSV-2 is usually spread by sexual contact but is also vertically transmitted.

Incubation period: 2 to 12 days.

Communicable period: During viral shedding. This is generally 1 week after mouth lesions resolve, up to 12 days after genital lesions resolve in primary infection, and up to 7 days after genital lesions resolve in recurrences; however, reactivations may be asymptomatic and consist of viral shedding only.

Isolation: Avoid contact with infants under 4 months, people who are immunosuppressed, and children with eczema.

Causes

Most HVH infections are subclinical. The remainder produce localized lesions and systemic reactions. After the first infection, a patient is a carrier susceptible to reactivation, which may be provoked by physical or emotional stress; however, in recurrences, the patient usually has no constitutional symptoms.

Saliva, feces, urine, skin lesions, and purulent eye exudate are potential sources of infection.

Clinical presentation

Infection causes perioral (most common site), clustered, uniform vesicles on erythematous base, which crust over before resolving.

Primary infection

▶ Prodrome of local pain, tender lymphadenopathy, headache, generalized ache, fevers

▶ Located on mucous membranes

▶ Clustered, often umbilicated vesicles on an erythematous base

▶ Lesions eroding, forming moist erosions or yellowish crusts that last 2 to 4 weeks

▶ Virus traveling to dorsal root ganglia and entering latent stage

Recurrent infection

▶ Reduced severity and duration but still infectious

▶ Prodrome of constitutional symptoms less common

▶ Dome-shaped lesions opening and crusting in 2 to 4 days

▶ Yellowish crust shedding in 8 days

In neonates, HVH symptoms usually appear 1 or 2 weeks after birth. They range from localized skin lesions to a disseminated infection of such organs as the liver, lungs, and brain. The death rate of infants with disseminated disease is 90%. Herpetic stomatitis may lead to severe dehydration in children.

Vesicles may form on the oral mucosa, especially the tongue, gingiva, and cheeks, and is usually HSV-1. In generalized infection, vesicles occur with submaxillary lymphadenopathy. Other symptoms include increased salivation, halitosis, anorexia, and temperature of up to 105° F (40.6° C).

Genital herpes usually affects adolescents and young adults and most commonly is HSV-2. Typically painful, the initial attack produces fluid-filled vesicles that ulcerate and heal in 1 to 3 weeks. Fever, regional lymphadenopathy, and dysuria may also occur.

Herpetic keratoconjunctivitis is usually unilateral, causing local symptoms: conjunctivitis, regional adenopathy, blepharitis, and vesicles on the lid. Other ocular symptoms may include excessive lacrimation, edema, chemosis, photophobia, and purulent exudate. Uveitis may cause permanent vision loss.

Differential diagnosis

Infection is diagnosed by clinical appearance.

▶ *Impetigo crusts and exudate* are straw-colored.

▶ *Aphthous stomatitis* exhibits gray, shallow erosions with a ring of hyperemia on the anterior mouth and lips.

▶ *Hand-foot-and-mouth disease* presents with lesions on distal extremities.

▶ *Herpes zoster* appears on unilateral dermatome.

▶ *Syphilitic chancre* is a painless ulcer.

▶ *Herpangina* appears on the posterior buccal mucosa (soft palate, oropharynx) but not the anterior gums and on lips; Stevens-Johnson syndrome is suspected if the person recently started on a new medication.

▶ *Herpetic whitlow,* a primary finger infection, commonly affects health care workers. First, the finger tingles or itches, and then it becomes inflamed with neuralgia. Herpetic whitlow may also present with satellite vesicles, fever, chills, malaise, and a red streak up the arm.

Diagnostic tests

▶ *Tzanck smear* shows multinucleated giant cells. (Herpes zoster has identical findings.)

▶ *HSV culture* takes from 2 to 6 days to get results.

▶ *Herpes antibody titers* don't differentiate HSV-1 from HSV-2.

▶ Screen for other sexually transmitted diseases with primary genital herpes.

Management

▶ There's no cure for herpes; however, symptomatic therapy and supportive therapy are essential to the patient's treatment.

Drugs

▸ *Topical antiviral agents* (Penciclovir cream) to reduce pain and shorten healing time for lesions on the lip and face
▸ *Systemic antivirals* (acyclovir, valacyclovir, famciclovir)
▸ *Analgesic-antipyretics* (acetaminophen, ibuprofen) for fever and pain
▸ *Local anesthetics* (viscous lidocaine) for the pain of gingivostomatitis, enabling the patient to eat and preventing dehydration
▸ *Drying agents* (calamine lotion) to make labial lesions less painful
▸ *Optional daily suppressive therapy* for patients with more than six recurrences each year (After 1 year, discontinue drug and reevaluate.)

Collaborative practice
Consult with a physician for extensive lesions.

RED FLAG *Consult an ophthalmologist for eye involvement.*

Follow-up
Follow up in 1 week after treatment is initiated and then every 2 weeks until lesions heal. For pregnant women with HSV infection, follow up as ordered by the obstetrician.

Complications
▸ Aseptic meningitis
▸ Encephalitis
▸ Ocular involvement
▸ Pneumonia
▸ Viremia

LIFE SPAN *In infants, systemic complications are severe, with a 90% mortality.*

Patient teaching
▸ Explain to the patient that this disease isn't curable and recurrence rates vary widely.
▸ Advise the patient to seek treatment at the first sign of recurrence.
▸ Tell the patient to apply analgesic spray (Americaine) to the genital area and to keep the area dry.
▸ Tell the patient that painful urination can be eased by pouring 1 cup of warm water over the genitals while urinating.
▸ Tell the parents to monitor children older than age 3 months for dehydration: less than three voids in 24 hours, cotton mouth, tenting skin, no tears when crying.
▸ For oral pain, advise the patient to use a soft toothbrush, eat a soft-diet, drink plenty of clear liquids, and avoid irritating foods.
▸ Tell the patient to rinse with warm water after meals.
▸ For mouthwash, advise saline (¼ tsp salt in 8 oz of warm water).
▸ Advise the patient to avoid immunocompromised people and practice safer sex. (Herpes can be transmitted even when no lesions are present.) Explain condom usage and teach avoidance of sexual contact during active periods.
▸ Advise the patient to wash his hands frequently.

RED FLAG *Tell the patient to call his primary care provider if he experiences persistent, changing, worsening, anxiety-producing, or specific signs and symptoms, including:*
▸ *worsening of sores*
▸ *high fever nonresponsive to antipyretics*
▸ *signs of dehydration (less than three voids in 24 hours; dark, foul-smelling urine; skin tenting; crying without tearing)*
▸ *severe mouth pain*
▸ *difficulty awakening or stiff neck.*

Resources
▸ National Herpes Hotline: (919) 361-8488
▸ National STD Hotline: 1-800-227-8922
▸ Planned Parenthood Federation of America: (212) 541-7800; *www.plannedparenthood.org*

HERPES ZOSTER

ICD-9-CM Herpes zoster 053.9, eye zoster 053.29

Also called *shingles*, herpes zoster is an acute, unilateral and segmental inflammation of the dorsal root ganglia. The virus continues to multiply in the ganglia, destroys the host neuron, and spreads down the sensory nerves to the skin.

Although herpes zoster is less contagious than varicella zoster (V-Z), contact with the vesicle fluid can cause chickenpox in V-Z-negative people. Shingles usually occurs in those ages 50 and older and seldom recurs. It may be activated by emotional or physical stress, immunocompromise, or immunosuppressive therapy. It produces localized vesicular skin lesions confined to a dermatome and severe neuralgia. Occasionally, postherpetic neuralgia (PHN) may persist for months or years.

Contagion

Herpes zoster is contagious. It doesn't cause shingles but may cause chickenpox (V-Z) if the patient isn't immune. Herpes zoster is much less infectious than V-Z. Transmission is by contact with fluid from the vesicles, which can also become airborne. Vertical transmission is possible.

Incubation period: 2 to 3 weeks.
Communicable period: Infectious from up to 5 days before rash appears until 7 days after lesions first appeared and up to 21 days after rash appears in an immunocompromised person.
Isolation: Make sure lesions are covered (as with a shirt) when in public. Avoid immunocompromised and pregnant people for 7 or 21 days after lesions appeared (depending on the patient's immunocompetence).

Causes

This condition is caused by infection with the herpesvirus V-Z, a local reactivation of latent varicella infection.

Clinical presentation

Prodrome: itching, burning, stabbing pain; usually involving one dermatome more common on the trunk

Eruptions

▶ Red clustered lesions of varied size become edematous vesicles on an erythematous base, filled with cloudy fluid; they continue to appear for 7 days.
▶ About 10 days after they appear, the vesicles dry and form scabs. Compared to V-Z, they're unilateral, more deeply seated, more closely aggregated, and restricted to the area supplied by the dorsal root ganglia that contains the reactivated V-Z.

Postherpetic neuralgia

▶ Risk increases with age, may last, and can be severe.

Differential diagnosis

Diagnosis is made by patient history and physical examination.

Diagnostic tests

Diagnostic testing is rarely indicated, but may include the following:
▶ *Viral culture* is an expensive test but shows varicella isolate.
▶ *Tzanck smear* shows multinucleated giant cells but doesn't differentiate from herpes simplex.
▶ *Staining antibodies* from vesicular fluid and identification under fluorescent light differentiate herpes zoster from localized herpes simplex.

Management

Drugs

Consider the following drugs for the management of herpes zoster:

150 ● *Dermatologic disorders*

● *analgesics and antipyretics:* acetaminophen and nonsteroidal anti-
inflammatory drugs (NSAIDs)
● *systemic antivirals,* such as valacyclovir, famciclovir, or acyclovir (to
prevent disseminated, life-threatening disease in immunocompromised
patients and those with encephalitis
or pneumonitis)
● systemic antivirals, such as acyclovir, for 1 week (to reduce illness
severity)
● *systemic antibiotics* (for bacterial
infection).
   For PHN, consider:
● *NSAIDs* as a first-line therapy
● *opioid analgesia* (codeine) as
needed for short-term pain management
● *topical analgesic* (capsaicin
cream) to delete pain impulse trans-
mitter substance P and prevent its
resynthesis
● *5% lidocaine patch* (Lidoderm)
extended-release topical analgesic
● *tricyclic antidepressant* (amitriptyline) for neurogenic pain.
   Researchers are trying to prove
the efficacy of primary prevention
with *varicella vaccine* (VZV) in patients older than age 65 (primarily
for immunocompromised people).
VZV has an established 80% prevention rate for varicella zoster.
When varicella zoster rash develops, patients average 50 lesions instead of 400.
   Collaborative practice
Consult with a physician if the patient is immunocompromised.
● ● ● RED FLAG *Refer the patient to*
● ● ● *an ophthalmologist for lesions
affecting the eyes.*
   Follow-up
Follow up in 2 weeks to verify resolution and check for PHN.

Complications
● Corneal ulceration
● Cranial nerve syndromes
● Cutaneous dissemination

● Guillain-Barré syndrome
● Hepatitis
● Meningoencephalitis
● Ocular involvement
● Peripheral motor weakness
● PHN
● Pneumonitis
● Segmental myelitis
● Superinfection of lesions

Patient teaching
● Advise the patient to get adequate
rest during the acute phase.
● Teach the patient to apply a drying agent (calamine lotion) liberally
to lesions.
● For itch relief, suggest that the
patient soak in a tepid water bath
with ½ cup baking soda.
● Instruct the patient to avoid
scratching the lesions and to trim
fingernails to decrease superinfection from scratching.
● Tell the patient to wash his hands
frequently and to wash lesions gently with antibacterial soap and
warm water without rubbing or
scrubbing.
● Tell the patient to apply a cold
compress if vesicles rupture.
● Tell the patient that the rash usually resolves in 2 to 3 weeks.
● If the patient believes he has been
in proximity to an immunocompromised person, he should notify the
person.
● To minimize PHN, teach the patient not to delay analgesics because the pain is severe. Teach that
antidepressant drugs are used for
their effect on nerve endings, not as
antidepressants.
● Repeatedly reassure the patient
that herpetic pain will eventually
subside but may take months to
years.
● ● ● RED FLAG *Tell the patient to call*
● ● ● *the primary care provider and
report persistent, changing, worsening, anxiety-producing, or specific
signs and symptoms, including:*

▸ *visual changes and pain*
▸ *signs of infection or scabs changing from soft brown to soft golden yellow*
▸ *development of cough*
▸ *temperature above 101° F (38.3° C).*

Resources

▸ American Chronic Pain Association: 1-800-533-3231; *www.theacpa.org*

LYME DISEASE

ICD-9-CM 088.81
A multisystemic disorder, Lyme disease is caused by the spirochete *Borrelia burgdorferi*, which is carried by the minute tick *Ixodes dammini* or another tick in the Ixodidae family. It often begins in the summer with the classic skin lesion called *erythema migrans* (EM). (Although EM is the classic early sign of Lyme disease, about 25% of patients don't develop this skin manifestation.) Weeks or months later, cardiac or neurologic abnormalities sometimes develop, possibly followed by arthritis.

Initially, Lyme disease was identified in a group of children in Lyme, Connecticut. Now Lyme disease is known to occur primarily in three parts of the United States:
▸ Northeast — Massachusetts to Maryland
▸ Midwest — Wisconsin and Minnesota
▸ West — California and Oregon.

Although Lyme disease is endemic to these areas, cases have been reported in 43 states and 20 other countries, including Germany, Switzerland, France, and Australia.

Contagion

Lyme disease isn't contagious. It's transmitted by ticks only. (Animal studies show a tick must be attached for 24 hours to transmit; this may also be true for humans.)
Incubation period: 3 to 32 days.
Communicable period: None.
Isolation: None.

Causes

Lyme disease occurs when a tick injects spirochete-laden saliva into the bloodstream or deposits fecal matter on the skin. After incubating for 3 to 32 days, the spirochetes migrate out to the skin, causing EM. They then disseminate to other skin sites or organs by way of the bloodstream or lymph system. The spirochetes' life cycle isn't completely clear; they may survive for years in the joints or they may trigger an inflammatory response in the host and then die.

Clinical presentation

Typically, Lyme disease has three stages.
Stage 1
EM heralds stage 1 with a red macule or papule, often at the site of a tick bite. This lesion often feels hot and itchy and may grow to more than 20″ (50 cm) in diameter. Within a few days, more lesions may erupt along with a malar rash, conjunctivitis, or diffuse urticaria. In 3 to 4 weeks, lesions are replaced by small, red blotches, which persist for several more weeks.

Malaise and fatigue are constant, but other findings (headache, fever, chills, myalgias, and regional lymphadenopathy) are intermittent. Less common effects are meningeal irritation, mild encephalopathy, migrating musculoskeletal pain, and hepatitis. A persistent sore throat and dry cough may appear several days before EM.
Stage 2
Weeks to months later, the second stage begins with neurologic abnormalities — fluctuating meningoen-

cephalitis with peripheral and cranial neuropathy — that usually resolve after days or months. Facial palsy is especially noticeable. Cardiac abnormalities, such as a brief, fluctuating atrioventricular heart block, may also develop.

Stage 3

Characterized by arthritis, stage 3 begins weeks or years later. Migrating musculoskeletal pain leads to frank arthritis with marked swelling, especially in the large joints. Recurrent attacks may precede chronic arthritis with severe cartilage and bone erosion.

Differential diagnosis

Because isolation of *B. burgdorferi* is unusual in humans and because indirect immunofluorescent antibody tests are marginally sensitive, diagnosis often rests on the characteristic EM lesion and related clinical findings, especially in endemic areas. This is important because early treatment is most beneficial in preventing long-term sequelae.

Conditions to consider when making the diagnosis for constitutional symptoms include viral syndromes, rheumatoid arthritis, tularemia, lupus, Bell's palsy, Reiter's syndrome, encephalitis, Rocky Mountain spotted fever, and rheumatic fever. When classifying the lesion, consider tinea corporis, herald patch of pityriasis rosea, insect bite, cellulitis, urticaria, erythema multiforme, drug eruption, syphilis, and cutaneous lymphomas.

Diagnostic tests

▶ *Enzyme-linked immunosorbent assay* may be positive for immunoglobulin G and M. *B. burgdorferi* antibodies; however, false-negatives can arise in first-stage infection or in late stages where patients received early antibiotic treatment. False-positives have been seen with Rocky Mountain spotted fever,

syphilis, lupus, and rheumatoid arthritis.

▶ *Cerebrospinal fluid and synovial fluid analyses* can be cultured for *B. burgdorferi.*

▶ *Blood culture* or *skin biopsy* has less than a 40% detection rate for *B. burgdorferi* spirochetes and must be placed on Kelly's medium.

▶ *Complete blood count* and *erythrocyte sedimentation rate (ESR)* may detect mild anemia, an elevated ESR and leukocyte count, and elevated aspartate aminotransferase levels, all supporting the diagnosis.

The PreVue *B. burgdorferi* antibody detection assay can be performed and read in 1 hour. Positive results must be confirmed by the Western blot test.

Management

Urgent

Stage 2 and stage 3 Lyme disease may require inpatient care, determined by the clinical picture. Treatment involves either high-dose penicillin (penicillin G) or third-generation cephalosporins (ceftriaxone, cefotaxime) for 2 to 4 weeks I.V.

General

▶ Take a detailed patient history, asking about travel to endemic areas and exposure to ticks.

▶ Check for drug allergies, and check for adverse effects when starting an antibiotic the patient hasn't been exposed to before.

✹ **LIFE SPAN** *Education regarding avoidance and detection is paramount to preventing infection, particularly for children.*

✹ **LIFE SPAN** B. burgdorferi *can cross the placenta; therefore pregnant patients with active infection require parenteral antibiotics.*

Drugs

▶ A 14- to 21-day course of *oral tetracycline* (doxycycline) is the treatment of choice for adults. *Beta-*

lactamase-inhibiting penicillins (amoxicillin) and *second-generation cephalosporins* (cefuroxime) are alternates. Oral amoxicillin is usually prescribed for children. When given in the early stages, these drugs can minimize later complications.

▸ A short course of *corticosteroids* (prednisone) may be helpful.

Collaborative practice

Consult with a physician, especially for disease stages 2 and 3 or severe manifestations. Refer the patient to a physical therapist for arthritis to increase range of motion (ROM) and strength.

✦ **LIFE SPAN** *Consult with an obstetrician if the patient is pregnant. Expect no treatment if the patient is asymptomatic. For early disease, drugs are administered by mouth; for later stages, the parenteral route is used.*

Follow-up

Follow-up is determined by clinical presentation. Reevaluate mild cases at the end of oral treatment. Stages 2 and 3 require careful monitoring over months to years. At each visit, focus on the patient's neurologic system; check for signs of increased intracranial pressure and cranial nerve involvement, such as ptosis, strabismus, and diplopia; also check for cardiac abnormalities, such as arrhythmias and heart block.

Complications

▸ Bursitis
▸ Chronic lyme disease (arthritis, meningitis, and carditis)
▸ Chronic neurologic systems
▸ Peripheral neuropathies
▸ Recurrent synovitis
▸ Tendinitis

Patient teaching

▸ Emphasize the importance of ROM and strengthening exercises, and avoiding overexertion.

Preventive measures

▸ Stress that prevention of Lyme disease is possible by early detection and prompt removal of ticks. (Removal within 24 hours may preclude transmission of spirochete.)

▸ Explain that *B. burgdorferi* is carried by deer ticks, but despite the name, the ticks occur on mice and vegetation as well as on deer. They are about the size of the period at the end of this sentence. Teach the patient to try to walk in the center of paths to avoid brushing against vegetation, to cover all skin with brightly colored clothes so that ticks are seen easily, and to tuck his pants inside boots or socks.

▸ Advise the patient to use insect repellents containing N,N-diethyl-m-toluamide (DEET) on clothing and exposed skin surfaces sparingly but as often as every 2 hours. (Follow product instructions.) Advise him to examine his skin carefully after outdoor activities, especially around vegetation, and to wash repellent off when inside.

▰▰▰ **RED FLAG** *Tell the patient to call the primary care provider and report persistent, changing, worsening, anxiety-producing, or specific signs and symptoms, including:*

▸ *inability to remove whole tick (including the head)*
▸ *whole tick removed, but duration of presence unknown or more than 18 hours*
▸ *development of an expanding circular lesion (bull's-eye appearance of red border with clear center); flu-like symptoms, rash, or headaches 3 to 32 days after known or possible tick bite; high fever; paralysis of part of the body; palpitations; pain and swelling of more than one joint.*

Resources

▸ Lyme Disease Foundation: (860) 525-2000; *www.lyme.org*
▸ Arthritis Foundation: 1-800-283-7800; *www.arthritis.org*

PEDICULOSIS

ICD-9-CM Pediculosis infestation 132.9, corporis 132.1, capitis 132.0, eyelid 373.6, more than one site 132.3, pubic 132.2

Pediculosis is the clinical term for lice infestation. The presence of lice means a cutaneous parasitic infestation with lice and eggs. Head lice (*Pediculus humanus capitis*), body lice (*P. humanus corporis*), and pubic or crab lice (*Phthirus pubis*) are tiny (less than 2 mm) parasitic insects that suck blood from the skin. Female lice live for approximately 1 month and deposit up to 10 eggs per day on the host. Eggs (nits) hatch in 7 to 10 days and are mature at 2 weeks. Capitis and corporis are more likely in children; pubis are more common in young adults.

Contagion

Pediculosis is highly contagious. Lice are spread by personal contact. Fomites are commonly implicated in the transmission of body lice; culprits include infested clothing, combs, brushes, bedding, and upholstered chairs. Overcrowding increases transmission. Fever of the host encourages lice to migrate to new host.

Incubation period: Eggs hatch in 7 to 10 days.

Communicable period: Until insecticide is applied to skin. On fomites: lice can survive 10 days away from a host before starving to death; eggs survive less than 2 weeks.

Isolation: Contact isolation for 24 hours after insecticide is applied; fomites, 3 weeks.

School or day-care staff should be notified if evidence of lice is found on children.

Causes

Causative organisms of pediculosis are *P. humanus captitis* (head lice), *P. humanus corporis* (body lice), and *P. pubis* (crab lice). Risk factors for infestation include close, crowded living conditions; close person-to-person contact; and situations in which washing and changing clothing isn't possible.

Clinical presentation

All lice cause intense itching. The nits, or clusters of louse eggs, are seen as tiny, grayish white or honey-colored ovals glued to hair shafts. Body lice are difficult to find because they burrow under the skin. A secondary excoriation or infection may be caused by scratching.

Differential diagnosis

Rule out scabies and other mites that cause cutaneous reactions in humans. Dandruff, hair lacquer, and hair gel droplets may be mistaken for head lice. The diagnosis is made on clinical grounds. No testing is indicated.

Management

▶ Pubic lice have a 90% sexual transmission rate. About one-third of these patients have another sexually transmitted disease.

▶ Eyelash lice on a child may indicate sexual abuse and must be evaluated.

Drugs

▶ *Permethrin* (Nix) is used as a one-time treatment.

▶ *Pyrethrins* and *lindane* aren't totally ovicidal; thus it's often necessary to re-treat in 7 to 14 days because of the 7- to 10-day incubation period.

▶ *Antibiotics* (usually erythromycin or dicloxacillin) can be used in treatment of secondary infection.

▸ *Over-the-counter preparations,* such as calamine lotion, hydrocortisone cream, and topical antihistamines, can be used to control itching.

Collaborative practice

Consult with a primary care physician or dermatologist if the patient is unresponsive to treatment.

Follow-up

Follow up as needed for persistent or recurring symptoms.

Complications

▸ Secondary skin infections

Patient teaching

▸ Teach the patient that poor hygiene isn't a risk factor in acquiring pediculosis.

▸ Advise the patient that the dead nits remain in the scalp or pubic hair after treatment with shampoo or lotion. Nits are best removed with a very fine comb. (A nit comb is included in the RID package.) Tell the patient that soaking the hair in a solution of equal parts water and white vinegar and wrapping wet hair and scalp in a towel for 15 minutes eases removal.

▸ Instruct the patient that all family members and close contacts should be treated concomitantly to prevent recurrence or reinfection.

LIFE SPAN *Tell parents to keep children's fingernails short to minimize damage from scratching.*

▸ Teach the patient that linens, clothing, and close contact items such as bed decorations must be washed in hot water (140° F [60° C]) or dry-cleaned; carpets and rugs should be well vacuumed and the bags disposed of immediately; brushes and combs should be soaked in rubbing alcohol for 1 hour; and anything that can't be cleaned in this manner (hats, upholstery, stuffed animals) should be put in a sealed plastic bag and set aside for 3 weeks (2 week incubation period, 1 week starvation period).

▸ Tell the patient to remove eyelash lice by applying petroleum jelly (Vaseline) to lashes (eyelid margins) twice daily for 8 days, followed by removal of nits.

▸ Warn the patient that persistent itching may be caused by too-frequent use of pediculicide.

RED FLAG *Tell the patient to call his primary care provider if he experiences persistent, changing, worsening, anxiety-producing, or specific signs and symptoms, including:*

▸ *signs of infection (redness of lesions, edema, drainage from sites, temperature above 101° F [38.3° C])*

▸ *itching that isn't relieved within 3 days.*

Resources

▸ National Pediculosis Foundation: (781) 449-NITS; *www.headlice.org*

PSORIASIS

ICD-9-CM 696.1

Psoriasis is a chronic, recurrent disease marked by epidermal proliferation. Its lesions, which appear as sharply demarcated papules and plaques covered with silver scales or as erythematous pustules, vary widely in severity and distribution.

CULTURAL KEY *Psoriasis affects about 2% of the population in the United States, and incidence is higher among whites than other races. Incidence is low in West Africans, Japanese, Inuits, and Native Americans.*

Although this disorder commonly presents in young adults, it may strike at any age, including infancy.

Recurring partial remissions and exacerbations characterize psoriasis. Flare-ups are usually related to specific systemic and environmental factors but may be unpredictable;

they can usually be controlled with therapy. The disease is more common in colder areas.

Contagion

Psoriasis isn't contagious.

Causes

The tendency to develop psoriasis is genetically determined. Researchers have discovered a significantly higher-than-normal incidence of certain human leukocyte antigens in families with psoriasis, suggesting a possible immune disorder. This theory is supported by the presence of many T cells in psoriatic lesions and successful treatment with cyclosporine. Another theory is that psoriasis results from a genetic error of mitotic control. Onset of the disease is also influenced by environmental factors.

Trauma can trigger the isomorphic effect (Koebner's phenomenon) in which lesions develop at sites of injury. Rubbing and scratching stimulate the proliferative process. Infections, especially those resulting from beta-hemolytic streptococci, may cause a flare-up of guttate (drop-shaped) lesions. Other contributing factors include pregnancy, endocrine changes, climate (cold weather tends to exacerbate), and emotional stress.

Generally, a skin cell takes 14 days to move from the basal layer to the stratum corneum where, after 14 days of normal wear and tear, it's sloughed off. The life cycle of a normal skin cell is 28 days, compared with only 4 days for a psoriatic skin cell. This markedly shortened cycle doesn't allow time for the cell to mature. Consequently, the stratum corneum becomes thick and flaky, producing the cardinal manifestations of psoriasis.

Clinical presentation

The most common complaint of the patient with psoriasis is itching and occasional pain from dry, cracked, encrusted lesions.

Plaques

Psoriatic lesions are erythematous and usually form well-defined plaques, sometimes covering large areas of the body. Such lesions most commonly appear on the scalp, chest, elbows, knees, back, and buttocks. The plaques consist of characteristic silver scales that either flake off easily or thicken, covering the lesion. Removal of psoriatic scales frequently produces fine bleeding points (Auspitz sign). Occasionally, small guttate lesions appear, either alone or with plaques; these lesions are typically thin and erythematous with few scales.

Widespread shedding of scales is common in exfoliative or erythrodermic psoriasis and may also develop in chronic psoriasis.

In about 25% of patients, psoriasis spreads to the fingernails, producing small indentations and yellow or brown discolorations. In severe cases, the accumulation of thick, crumbly debris under the nail causes it to separate from the nail bed.

Pustular psoriasis

Rarely, psoriasis becomes pustular, taking one of two forms. In localized pustular (Barber) psoriasis, pustules appear on the palms and soles and remain sterile until opened. In generalized pustular (von Zumbusch) psoriasis, which often occurs with fever, leukocytosis, and malaise, groups of pustules coalesce to form lakes of pus on red skin. These pustules also remain sterile until opened and commonly involve the tongue and oral mucosa.

Arthritic symptoms

Some patients with psoriasis develop arthritic symptoms, usually in one or more joints of the fingers or toes or sometimes in the sacroiliac joints, which may progress to spondylitis. Such patients may complain of morning stiffness. Joint symptoms show no consistent linkage to the course of the cutaneous manifestations of psoriasis; they demonstrate remissions and exacerbations similar to those of rheumatoid arthritis.

Differential diagnosis

Conditions to consider when making the diagnosis include tinea, pityriasis, syphilis, Reiter's disease, pustular eruptions, drug eruptions (such as beta blockers, gold, methyldopa), lichen planus, and cancer. The distribution and shape of lesions commonly confirm the diagnosis, with some consideration of patient history. Some conditions to consider include:

▶ cancer
▶ candidiasis
▶ dermatitis (seborrheic, nummular, atopic, or hand)
▶ drug eruptions
▶ eczema
▶ lichen planus
▶ pityriasis
▶ pustular eruptions
▶ Reiter's disease
▶ syphilis
▶ tinea.

Diagnostic tests

▶ *Skin biopsy* on microscopic examination may detect thickened stratum corneum, epidermal hyperplasia, and minimal inflammation.
▶ *Serum uric acid levels, leukocytes,* and *sedimentation rates* may be elevated because of accelerated nucleic acid degradation, but indications of gout are absent.

▶ *Human leukocyte antigen (HLA)-Cw6, B-13, and B-w57* may be present in early-onset psoriasis.
▶ *Rheumatoid factor* isn't present.
▶ *Complete blood count with differential* may indicate anemia and vitamin B_{12}, folate, and iron deficiencies.

Management

⬤ **CLINICAL PEARL** *Severe and unstable forms, such as acute pustular psoriasis (von Zumbusch's) and acute erythroderma, may require emergency inpatient treatment. Symptoms include frightened appearance, tachycardia, tachypnea, fever that may be high, and burning erythema preceding clusters of tiny pustules that become confluent, forming "lakes" of pus. Treatment includes bed rest, isolation, fluid replacement, and repeated blood cultures for early diagnosis and treatment of secondary infection. Medication options include I.V. antibiotics, retinoids, methotrexate, and psoralen plus ultraviolet–A (PUVA) when tolerated.*

▶ Appropriate treatment depends on the type of psoriasis, the extent of the disease, the patient's response to it, and what effect the disease has on the patient's lifestyle. No permanent cure exists, and all methods of treatment are palliative.
▶ Be aware that psoriasis can cause psychological problems, including depression and withdrawal from social situations. Pay special attention to the patient's perception of his physical appearance, and offer emotional support.
▶ To remove psoriatic scales, the patient must apply an occlusive ointment, such as petroleum jelly, salicylic acid preparations, or preparations containing urea. These medications soften the scales, which can then be removed by

scrubbing them carefully with a soft brush while bathing.

UVB exposure or solar radiation

Methods to retard rapid cell production include exposure to ultraviolet B (UVB) or natural sunlight to the point of minimal erythema.

A thin layer of petroleum jelly may be applied before UVB exposure (the most common treatment for generalized psoriasis). Exposure time can increase gradually. Outpatient or day treatment with UVB avoids long hospitalizations and prolongs remission.

Drugs

▶ A *potent fluorinated steroid ointment* (betamethasone valerate or fluocinolone acetonide) works well except on the face and intertriginous areas. These ointments are applied twice daily, preferably after bathing to facilitate absorption, and with overnight use of occlusive dressings, such as plastic wrap, plastic gloves and booties, a vinyl exercise suit, or corticosteroid-impregnated tape (Cordran tape), under direct medical or nursing supervision. Switching products prevents tachyphylaxis.

▶ Limit *high-potency topical steroids* to 2 weeks, avoid occlusive dressings, and taper applications to prevent rebound.

▶ Small (less than 4.1 cm), stubborn plaques may require *intralesional steroid injections* (2 to 5 mg/ml triamcinolone acetonide). Injection is intradermal, not subcutaneous (requires pressure to inject, otherwise needle is in subcutaneous tissue).

Hypopigmentation at the site can result from steroid injection and is more apparent in darker-pigmented patients.

▶ *Anthralin*, combined with a paste mixture, may be used for well-defined plaques but must not be ap-plied to unaffected areas because it causes injury and stains normal skin. Apply petroleum jelly around the affected skin before applying anthralin. Anthralin is commonly used concurrently with steroids; anthralin is applied at night and steroids are used during the day

▶ *Topical vitamin D analogue* (calcipotriene) is slower acting (2 months) than steroids but does last. Apply to less than 40% of body surface (not to facial area) and less than 100 g/week.

▶ *TAZORAC* is a water-based topical retinoid (a synthetic vitamin A derivative) that improves psoriasis by slowing the growth of skin cells, normalizing their shape, and reducing inflammation.

Goeckerman, Ingram, and PUVA

In a patient with severe chronic psoriasis, the Goeckerman regimen, which combines tar baths and UVB treatments, may help achieve remission and clear the skin in 3 to 5 weeks. The Ingram technique is a variation of this treatment, using anthralin instead of tar. PUVA therapy combines administration of psoralens with exposure to high-intensity UVA.

Other treatments

▶ *Low-dose antihistamines, oatmeal baths, emollients,* and *open wet dressings* may help relieve pruritus. *Aspirin* and *local heat* help alleviate the pain of psoriatic arthritis; severe cases may require *nonsteroidal anti-inflammatory agents.*

▶ Therapy for psoriasis of the scalp consists of a *tar shampoo* followed by application of a *steroid lotion.* No effective treatment exists for psoriasis of the nails.

▶ An *immunosuppressant* (cyclosporine or tacrolimus) is indicated as short-term treatment for recalcitrant psoriases.

▶ As a last resort, a *cytotoxin* (usually methotrexate) may help severe, refractory psoriasis.

▶ The FDA recently approved *Alefacept*, the first biologic therapy for psoriasis. It works by simultaneously blocking and reducing the cellular component (activated T cells) of the immune system that play a role in the psoriasis disease process.

❋ **LIFE SPAN** *Isotretinoin (Accutane), a retinoid acid derivative, is effective in treating extensive cases of psoriasis. Warn the female patient of child-bearing age about the severe risk of teratogenicity. In addition to signing a special permission form, she'll need monthly measurements of lipid levels and liver function as well as monthly pregnancy tests.*

▶ Many common drugs can exacerbate psoriasis. Monitor hepatic and renal function when using cytotoxic drugs.

Collaborative practice

Refer patients with extensive disease to a dermatologist who specializes in UV therapy. Also refer patients to a dermatologist before using systemic steroids, before using occlusive dressings with high-potency topical steroids, and for scalp or perineal involvement.

Consult with a physician for nonresponsiveness to treatment within 2 months, extensive disease, psoriatic arthritis, or inflammatory disease.

Consult with a psychologist or psychiatrist for counseling and coping mechanisms.

Follow-up

Follow up with a monthly focus on examination of skin, effectiveness of treatment, evaluation of psychological health, and adverse drug effects. Monitor for adverse reactions, especially allergic reactions to anthralin, atrophy and acne from steroids, and burning, itching, nausea, and squamous cell carcinomas from PUVA.

Evaluate the patient on methotrexate pretreatment weekly and then monthly for red blood cell, white blood cell, and platelet counts; aspartate aminotransferase; and albumin because cytotoxins may cause hepatic or bone marrow toxicity.

Liver biopsies may be done to assess the effects of methotrexate (pretreatment, after 3 months, and then with every cumulative methotrexate dose of 1.5 g; usually about every 2 years).

Complications

▶ Continuous chronic flare-ups
▶ Exfoliative erythrodermatitis
▶ Hypopigmentation
▶ Immunocompromise
▶ Psychological distress
▶ Pustular psoriasis
▶ Rebound after stopping corticosteroids (especially oral corticosteroids)
▶ Secondary infection
▶ Striae
▶ Tachyphylaxis from topical corticosteroids
▶ Thinning of skin

Patient teaching

▶ Teach correct application of prescribed ointments, creams, and lotions. A steroid cream, for example, should be applied in a thin film and rubbed gently into the skin until the cream disappears.

▶ Instruct the patient to apply all topical medications, especially those containing anthralin and tar, with a downward motion to avoid rubbing them into the follicles. He must wear gloves because anthralin stains and injures the skin. After application, the patient may dust himself with powder to prevent anthralin from rubbing off on his clothes.

● Warn the patient never to put an occlusive dressing over anthralin. Suggest the use of mineral oil and then soap and water to remove anthralin.

● Caution the patient to avoid scrubbing his skin vigorously, to prevent Koebner's phenomenon (appearance of isomorphic lesions). If a medication has been applied to the scales to soften them, suggest that the patient use a soft brush to remove them.

● Caution the patient receiving PUVA therapy to stay out of the sun on the day of treatment and to protect his eyes with sunglasses that screen UVA rays for 24 hours after treatment. Tell him to wear goggles during exposure to this light.

● Assure the patient that psoriasis isn't contagious and, although exacerbations and remissions occur, they're controllable with treatment; however, there's no cure.

● Because stressful situations tend to exacerbate psoriasis, help the patient learn to cope with stress.

● Explain the relationship between psoriasis and arthritis, but point out that psoriasis causes no other systemic disturbances.

●●● **RED FLAG** *Tell the patient to call his primary care provider if he experiences persistent, changing, worsening, anxiety-producing, or specific signs and symptoms, including:*

● *symptoms of acute erythroderma (frightened appearance, racing heartbeat, rapid breathing or shortness of breath, fever that may be high, burning erythema preceding clusters of tiny pustules that run together, forming "lakes" of pus)*

● *depression*

● *flare-up*

● *signs of infection (increasing redness, cloudy or colored drainage, large open areas, swelling).*

● Make sure the patient understands his prescribed therapy; provide written instructions to avoid confusion.

Resources
● National Psoriasis Foundation: 1-800-723-9166; *www.psoriasis.org*

SCABIES

ICD-9-CM 133.0

Scabies is a parasitic skin infection by a mite (*Sarcoptes scabiei*) that causes intense itching. A secondary eczematous dermatitis usually occurs. (Classic itch causes scratching, which exacerbates itching, which increases scratching.)

Contagion

Scabies skin infestation usually spreads by skin-to-skin contact but also by contact with clothing or bedding. It's usually spread by sexual contact, contact with mite-infested sheets in institutionalized individuals, and close contact (frequently among children younger than age 6). It's transmitted rarely by fomites because the mite survives only 4 days apart from the host.

Incubation: No symptoms in primary infection for 2 to 6 weeks. Because of prior sensitization, recurrent infestations cause symptoms in 1 to 4 days.

Communicable period: Until after effective application of insecticide. On fomites: 10 days (time for eggs to hatch and mites to starve).

Isolation: Exclude from school or work for 24 hours after effective treatment (5% of infestations require a second treatment after 1 week to eliminate scabies).

School or day-care staff should be notified.

Causes

Scabies is caused by the itch mite, *S. scabiei*. Risk factors include close person-to-person contact and contact with fomites carrying *S. scabiei*.

Clinical presentation

Generalized itching, mostly at night when mites feed, is almost always present. Lesions, burrows, vesicles, and nodules may occur in the web spaces of fingers and toes, on the wrists and axillae, and in the groin or buttock areas.

LIFE SPAN *In elderly people, scabies may be found on the back, and skin may appear to be simply excoriated. Patients with human immunodeficiency virus infection may present with crusted scabies that look like psoriasis.*

Differential diagnosis

▶ Atopic dermatitis
▶ Dermatitis herpetiformis
▶ Insect bites
▶ Pediculosis
▶ Pityriasis rosea
▶ Seborrheic dermatitis
▶ Secondary syphilis

Diagnostic tests

▶ *Magnifying lens examination* may detect a dark point at the end of the burrow (the mite). Place a drop of mineral oil over a lesion and scrape and examine under a microscope for mites, eggs, egg casings, and feces. Scraping from under fingernails may be positive.
▶ If burrows aren't visible, apply ink to an area of rash and then wipe off with alcohol. Burrows become more distinct as the ink gets under the skin.

Management

▶ It's usually necessary to treat close family members and those with whom the patient has had close contact within the past month.

▶ If treatment is unsuccessful after 2 applications 1 week apart, consider poor application technique or another diagnosis.

Drugs

▶ *Scabicides* (permethrin or crotamiton creams or lotions) are left on 8 to 12 hours (follow product instructions), washed off, and repeated after 1 week if indicated.
▶ Another scabicide (lindane) may be used; however, some lindane resistant scabies have been reported. This drug shouldn't be used after a bath or by those with extensive dermatitis because of extensive absorption and increased risk of seizures. Lindane can also cause aplastic anemia.
▶ *Antihistamines* are used for symptomatic relief of itching only.
▶ *Mupirocin ointment* or *systemic antimicrobials* are used for secondary bacterial infections.

Follow-up

Follow up weekly as needed for persistent or recurring symptoms.

Complications

▶ Eczema
▶ Secondary infections

Patient teaching

▶ Tell the patient to wash all clothes, bedding, hats, belts, and scarves in hot water and to dry them in a hot dryer. If an article can't be washed, put it in a plastic bag, tie off the bag, and set it aside for 10 days.
▶ Advise the patient to check all household members for symptoms (itching, burrows in the skin).
▶ Explain to the patient that itching is an allergic response to excrement, so itching may persist for several weeks after effective treatment.
▶ Advise the patient not to self-treat more than twice with scabicides unless advised by a clinician. These

medications are harmful when used excessively.

●●● **RED FLAG** *Tell the patient to call*
●●● *the primary care provider and report persistent, changing, worsening, anxiety-producing, or specific signs and symptoms, including no improvement within 3 days.*

Resources

▶ National Library of Medicine: *www.nlm.nih.gov* (search "scabies")

URTICARIA AND ANGIOEDEMA

ICD-9-CM Urticaria 708.9, hereditary 277.6, allergic 708.0, due to cold/heat 708.2, idiopathic/nonallergic 708.1, larynx 995.1, recurrent periodic 708.8 (480)

Commonly known as *hives*, urticaria is a raised skin lesion secondary to edema of the superficial dermis. Angioedema describes deeper swellings with poorly defined borders that are slightly painful or pruritic. Angioedema often involves eyelids, lips, tongue, genitalia, hands, and feet.

Contagion

These conditions aren't contagious.

Causes

Usually immunoglobulin (Ig) E-mediated, hives are caused by numerous factors, both immunologic and nonimmunologic, that result in edema. The most common causes are food and medications. Other causes are hard to identify absolutely but include physical agents (such as heat, cold, and light), infection, insect bites, and idiopathic processes.

Clinical presentation

Transient wheals (irregular borders, bright to light pink, some with central clearing) with larger edematous areas appear and are frequently pruritic. Each lesion resolves in less than 24 hours. Angioedema involves subcutaneous tissue as well as the dermis.

Diagnosis is made by checking the history for possible causes and by physical examination. For acute episodes, screening laboratory tests and a radioallergosorbent test (RAST) are of little value. For lack of expected response to antihistamines, reevaluate the diagnosis.

Differential diagnosis

It's important to quickly differentiate a severe allergic reaction that may be life-threatening from one that isn't. Most commonly, insect bites and adverse drug reactions can cause this reaction. Other conditions to consider include:

▶ contact dermatitis
▶ lupus
▶ lymphoma
▶ mononucleosis
▶ vasculitis.

Diagnostic tests

▶ For chronic urticaria, consider a *hepatitis test panel.* (See chapter 2.)
▶ *RAST* identifies IgE antibodies (for allergies).
▶ *Erythrocyte sedimentation rate* may indicate necrotizing vasculitis if elevation is persistent.
▶ *Complete blood count* reveals high eosinophils in a patient with a fever and suggests angioedema-urticaria-eosinophilia syndrome. It may detect transient eosinophilia from reaction to foods, parasites, and drugs.

Management

Treatment aims to prevent or limit contact with the triggering factors or desensitize the patient to help relieve symptoms.

Drugs

▶ *Antihistamine therapy* is the therapy of choice. Hydroxyzine is used to help ease itching and decrease swelling; diphenhydramine may also be used.

▶ *Epinephrine* (subcutaneous form) is indicated in emergency situations for severe acute episodes. Clinical effects last a few hours, so this is an adjunct to an antihistamine. In some cases, especially with food allergies, the patient may be given an EpiPen to carry with him at all times. Follow up at each visit to reinforce avoidance behavior of known triggers and check the expiration date on the EpiPen.

▶ *Corticosteroids* (prednisone) are reserved for refractory or unresponsive cases.

▶ Many patients won't have a detectable cause for chronic urticaria or angioedema. In this case, it's important to offer support and medication, combined with realistic expectations.

Collaborative practice

Consult with a dermatologist for a patient with acute angioedema if symptoms aren't relieved with antihistamines and for patients with chronic urticaria lasting more than 6 weeks.

Follow-up

Follow up with the patient daily, weekly, or monthly according to his response to treatment.

Complications

▶ Respiratory collapse
▶ Respiratory distress
▶ Severe systemic allergic reaction

Patient teaching

▶ Give the patient a thorough explanation of the disorder so he can control the frequency and severity of symptomatic episodes by adjusting his lifestyle.

▶ Patients with severe allergies should carry an emergency anaphylaxis kit. Advise the patient to wear medical identification jewelry if he has a history of anaphylaxis.

▶ Teach the patient to eliminate triggers if known.

▶ Suggest baking soda (½ cup per tub) or Aveeno baths with cool water to relieve itching. For temporary relief, suggest cool showers and compresses.

▶ In cold-induced urticaria, warn the patient that vascular collapse is possible if he jumps into a cool pool.

▶ If food allergies are strongly suspected, teach the patient about an elimination diet. The patient eats basically rice and chicken for several days; after hives have resolved, foods are reintroduced one at a time.

▶ Tell patients with ultraviolet B-induced solar urticaria that sun avoidance and the use of sunscreens may be adequate; however, sunscreens may be insufficient for those sensitive to ultraviolet A and visible light. Some patients with solar urticaria improve by gradually increasing their exposure to natural or artificial light.

●●● **RED FLAG** *Tell the patient to call*
●●● *his primary care provider if he experiences persistent, changing, worsening, anxiety-producing, or specific signs and symptoms, including:*

▶ *symptoms that aren't mostly gone within 24 hours of following management plan*

▶ *signs of infection (increased redness of lesions, swelling, cloudy or odorous drainage, temperature above 102° F [38.9° C])*

▶ *hives that develop shortly after beginning a new medication.*

▶ Warn the patient to call emergency medical services for a severe reaction (shortness of breath, difficulty swallowing, wheezing, swelling of tongue or throat, severe abdominal or chest pain, cold sweats, pallor, or strong feelings of impending doom).

Resources
▶ National Library of Medicine: *www.nlm.nih.gov* (search "urticaria and angioedema")

VIRAL RASHES

Many viral infections are accompanied by generalized rashes (exanthems) and mucous membrane eruptions (enanthems). They're all contagious and may be difficult to differentiate. Treatment and complications are, however, similar for most viral rashes.

●●● **RED FLAG** *For all viral rashes*
●●● *with fever, tell the patient to call the primary care provider for a rash that turns purple or looks like spots of blood under the skin, rash that lasts longer than 3 days, ear pain or tugging on ears, change in mental status (such as increasing sleepiness), and fever that isn't controlled with medication.*

Enteroviral rashes
ICD-9-CM coxsackievirus 079.2, echovirus 079.1
▶ Cause virtually all types of rash, most commonly hand-foot-mouth disease (especially in children) caused by coxsackievirus A16
▶ Responsible for most viral rashes in late summer and early fall

Transmission and precautions
Transmission: Mostly by the fecal-oral route; also in droplet spray and by direct contact with respiratory secretions
Incubation: 3 to 7 days
Communicable period: Present in feces for several weeks

Isolation: Enteric precautions, prompt hand washing after diaper change and other contact; hot water and soap for soiled items

Signs and symptoms
▶ Infection may begin with abrupt onset of fever, often along with pharyngitis, cervical lymphadenopathy, myalgia, abdominal pain, and GI symptoms.
▶ Rash usually begins on the face and, within hours, spreads to the trunk and limbs. Lesions persist for up to 7 days and may be erythematous, macular, papular, and urticarial. Some echoviruses produce small blanchable papules with a white halo.
▶ Hand-foot-and-mouth disease begins with up to 2 days of low-grade fever and malaise before the appearance of small red 1- to 3-cm macules that vesiculate and ulcerate in the mouth, usually sparing the lips; pain may interfere with eating. Dorsal and volar aspects of the hands and feet may be involved. Rash usually resolves in 7 to 10 days.

Treatment and complications
▶ No antiviral therapy exists.
▶ For symptomatic relief, give antipyretics and analgesics or nonsteroidal anti-inflammatory drugs but *never* aspirin.
▶ Encourage fluid intake to prevent dehydration, including cool liquids or dairy products that are soothing and nutritious.
▶ Avoid hot, spicy, salty, or acidic foods to decrease local irritation.
▶ Advise good oral hygiene, including careful brushing twice daily to decrease the risk of secondary infection. Suggest a mouth rinse of ¼ tsp of salt in a glass of warm water.

● Comfort measures for children include holding, rocking, and distraction.

● Complications aren't common or life-threatening.

Erythema infectiosum

ICD-9-CM 057.0

● Called "slapped cheek" because of its appearance

● Common, benign, self-limited, highly contagious; affects mainly children younger than age 12

● Caused by human parvovirus B19

Transmission and precautions

Transmission: Primarily by direct contact with respiratory secretions

Incubation: 2 weeks

Communicable period: Highest rate of transmission precedes rash onset; immunocompromised people may remain contagious for months or longer.

Isolation: Most transmission occurs before symptoms occur, and exclusion isn't indicated. However, exclude children from school or day care until fever dissipates.

Signs and symptoms

● A fine, lacy rash appears abruptly on the cheeks, causing a "slapped cheek" or "sunburn" appearance. It intensifies with heat, friction, exercise, or emotional outbursts and disappears in less than 4 days.

● Over a few days, the rash spreads to the rest of the body. Around day six, fading begins with central clearing, leading to a marbled appearance. This may last from 1 to several weeks or may subside and recur intermittently over a 2-month period.

● Other symptoms may include pruritus and arthralgias (more common in adults).

Treatment and complications

● No treatment is necessary except antipyretics for fever and nonsteroidal anti-inflammatories (*never* aspirin) for arthralgias.

● Complications are uncommon except in patients with hemolytic anemias or hydrops fetalis. These patients are at risk for aplastic crisis (symptoms include dyspnea, fatigue, ecchymoses, pallor, and palpitations) and may require transfusion.

Roseola infantum

ICD-9-CM Rose, infantile 057.8, epidemic 056.9

● Common, benign, self-limited; most common viral rash in children younger than age 3

● Caused by human herpes virus 6

Transmission and precautions

Transmission: Uncertain; believed to be in salivary secretions, primarily by adults

Incubation: 5 to 15 days

Communicable period: Until rash resolves

Isolation: Not recommended

Signs and symptoms

● The prodrome may consist of 3 to 5 days of high fever, mild constitutional symptoms, and pharyngitis, or the patient may be asymptomatic.

● A rash appears abruptly up to 2 days after fever breaks, generally as the patient is feeling better. Lesions are nonpruritic, discrete pink macules and papules, 2 to 5 mm in diameter, mainly on the trunk and neck.

● The rash resolves within hours or up to 2 days; lesions aren't itchy or uncomfortable.

● History and physical examination rule out other sources of fever including otitis media, urinary tract infection, meningitis, and occult bacteremia.

Treatment and complications

▶ No treatment is necessary except antipyretics (*never* aspirin) for fever.
▶ Recommend tepid sponge baths for fever that isn't controlled with medication.

Rubella

ICD-9-CM 056

▶ Also called *German measles* or *3-day measles*
▶ Typically occurs in childhood or early adulthood
▶ Dangerous for pregnant women; causes birth defects
▶ Mild, self-limited, highly contagious
▶ Caused by rubella virus

Transmission and precautions

Transmission: In droplet spray, by direct contact with respiratory secretions, in urine of infants, and on items soiled with these secretions
Incubation: 14 to 23 days
Communicable period: 1 week before to at least 4 days after rash appears
Isolation: Avoid contact with soiled articles, prevent exposure of nonimmune pregnant women, and exclude children from school and adults from work for 7 days after onset of rash.

Signs and symptoms

▶ 80% of cases are asymptomatic.
▶ Mild upper respiratory and constitutional symptoms may occur, most commonly pain on lateral and upward eye movement.
▶ Lesions appear as discrete pink-red macules and papules that start on the face, begin clearing within a day, and resolve by day three. They're differentiated from rubeola by pink-red color (rather than

purplish-red) and rapid appearance changes, commonly within hours.
▶ Other symptoms include petechiae on the soft palate and tender lymphadenopathy.

Treatment and complications

▶ No antiviral treatment exists, but prevention is possible with vaccination.
▶ Complications include congenital birth defects if a pregnant patient contracts the virus, particularly during the first trimester.
▶ Report all cases to local health authorities.

Rubeola

ICD-9-CM 055

▶ Also called *measles*
▶ Self-limited, systemic, highly contagious
▶ Caused by a paramyxovirus

Transmission and precautions

Transmission: In droplet spray, by direct contact with respiratory secretions, and on items freshly soiled with these secretions
Incubation: 7 to 18 days
Communicable period: 2 to 3 days before to 4 days after rash appears
Isolation: Respiratory isolation for 4 days after rash appears (Keep children home for at least 4 days after rash appears.)

Signs and symptoms

▶ Stage 1: The patient is asymptomatic or shows mild prodromal symptoms.
▶ Stage 2 (prodrome): Transient Koplik's spots appear, usually preceding rash by 2 days, along with brassy cough, coryza, conjunctivitis, fever, photophobia, and constitutional symptoms.
▶ Stage 3: Erythematous, macular, but nonpruritic lesions appear at the hairline and spread downward, generally reaching the feet by day

two or three and becoming increasingly papular and confluent.

▶ Fever and constitutional symptoms peak as rash starts spreading down the body.

▶ Lesions fade in order of appearance over 3 to 6 days and may leave desquamated areas.

Treatment and complications

▶ No antiviral therapy exists, but prevention is possible with vaccination.

▶ Symptomatic relief includes antipyretics and analgesics (but *never* aspirin).

▶ Encourage fluids to prevent dehydration.

▶ Complications include otitis media, pneumonia, and encephalitis. Compared to all viral rashes, neurologic complications are most common in rubeola (approximately 2:1,000 cases).

▶ Report all cases to local health authorities.

6

Disease management

Initiating a treatment plan

Selected disorders   169

Selected disorders

ACUTE CORONARY SYNDROMES

ICD–9-CM anterolateral MI 410.0, anterior wall MI 410.1, inferior wall MI 410.4, posterior wall MI 410.6, unstable angina 411.1, Prinzmetal's 413.1

A patient with an acute coronary syndrome (ACS) has some degree of coronary artery occlusion. The degree of occlusion defines whether the ACS is:
◗ unstable angina
◗ Q-wave myocardial infarction (MI)
◗ non–Q-wave MI.

Causes

The development of any ACS begins with a disturbance (rupture or erosion) of plaque — an unstable, lipid-rich substance. The disturbance results in platelet adhesions, fibrin clot formation, activation of thrombin, and subsequent occlusion of a coronary artery. The severity and outcome of the episode depends on several factors:
◗ the site and size of the plaque disturbance
◗ the resulting disturbance in blood flow
◗ the duration of thrombotic occlusion
◗ whether or not there's adequate collateral coronary circulation.

Risk factors for development of ACS include hypertension; smoking; obesity or excessive intake of saturated fats, carbohydrates, or salt; sedentary lifestyle; menopause; stress or type A personality; diabetes mellitus; elevated serum triglycerides, total cholesterol, and low-density lipoprotein levels; and a family history of heart disease.

Clinical presentation

Angina

A patient with angina typically experiences burning, squeezing, and crushing tightness in the substernal or precordial chest that may radiate to the left arm, neck, jaw, or shoulder blade.

● **CLINICAL PEARL** *Women with ACS commonly experience atypical chest pain, vague pain, or no pain at all. Women are more likely than men to experience a toothache or pain in the arm, shoulder, jaw, neck, throat, back, breast, or stomach.*

Angina, which is less severe and of shorter duration than the pain of acute MI, most frequently follows physical exertion but may also follow emotional excitement, exposure to cold, or a large meal. It's commonly relieved by nitroglycerin.

Angina has four major forms:
◗ *microvascular* — angina-like chest pain due to impairment of vasodilator reserve in a patient with normal coronary arteries
◗ *Prinzmetal's (or variant)* — pain from unpredictable coronary artery spasm
◗ *stable* — predictable pain, in frequency and duration, that can be relieved with nitrates and rest
◗ *unstable* — increased pain that's easily induced.

MI

A patient with MI experiences severe, persistent chest pain that isn't relieved by rest or nitroglycerin. He may describe pain as crushing or squeezing. The pain is usually substernal, but may radiate to the left arm, jaw, neck, or shoulder blades.

Other signs and symptoms of MI include:
◗ a feeling of impending doom
◗ fatigue
◗ nausea and vomiting
◗ shortness of breath
◗ cool extremities

▶ perspiration
▶ anxiety
▶ hypotension or hypertension
▶ palpable precordial pulse
▶ muffled heart sounds.

Differential diagnosis

▶ Acute aortic dissection
▶ Acute cholecystitis
▶ Acute pericarditis
▶ Esophageal spasm or reflex disease
▶ Myocarditis
▶ Pneumothorax
▶ Pulmonary embolism

Diagnostic tests

▶ *Electrocardiogram (ECG)* during an anginal episode shows ischemia. Serial 12-lead ECGs may be normal or inconclusive during the first few hours after an MI. Abnormalities include serial ST-segment depression in non–Q-wave MI and ST-segment elevation and Q waves, representing scarring and necrosis, in a Q-wave MI. (See *Zones of myocardial infarction.*)
▶ *Coronary angiography* reveals coronary artery stenosis or obstruction and collateral circulation and shows the condition of the arteries beyond the narrowing.
▶ *Myocardial perfusion imaging* with thallium-201 during treadmill exercise discloses ischemic areas of the myocardium, visualized as "cold spots."
▶ With MI, *serial serum cardiac marker measurements* show elevated creatine kinase, especially the CK-MB isoenzyme (the cardiac muscle fraction of CK), troponin T and I, and myoglobin.
▶ With a *Q-wave MI,* echocardiography shows ventricular wall dyskinesia.

Management

Acute

Hospitalize patients with unstable angina and acute MI. The goal of treatment includes:
▶ reducing the amount of myocardial necrosis in those with ongoing infarction
▶ preventing major adverse cardiac events
▶ providing for rapid defibrillation when ventricular fibrillation is present.

During anginal episodes, monitor blood pressure and heart rate. Obtain a 12-lead ECG and assess heart rate and blood pressure when the patient experiences acute chest pain. If possible, perform the ECG before administering nitroglycerin or other nitrates. Record duration of pain, amount of medication required to relieve it, and accompanying symptoms.

Monitor the patient's hemodynamic status closely. Be alert for indicators suggesting decreased cardiac output, such as decreased blood pressure, increased heart rate, and increased pulmonary artery pressure readings.

Obstructive lesions may necessitate coronary artery bypass surgery or percutaneous transluminal coronary angioplasty. Other alternatives include laser angioplasty, minimally invasive surgery, rotational atherectomy, or stent placement.

General

For patients with angina, the goal of treatment is to reduce myocardial oxygen demand or increase oxygen supply. The goals of treatment for patients with MI are to relieve pain, stabilize heart rhythm, revascularize the coronary artery, preserve myocardial tissue, and reduce cardiac workload.

ZONES OF MYOCARDIAL INFARCTION

Myocardial infarction has a central area of necrosis surrounded by a zone of injury that may recover if revascularization occurs. This zone of injury is surrounded by an outer ring of reversible ischemia. Characteristic electrocardiographic changes are associated with each zone.

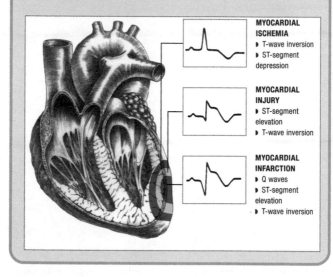

MYOCARDIAL ISCHEMIA
▶ T-wave inversion
▶ ST-segment depression

MYOCARDIAL INJURY
▶ ST-segment elevation
▶ T-wave inversion

MYOCARDIAL INFARCTION
▶ Q waves
▶ ST-segment elevation
▶ T-wave inversion

Medication
Angina
▶ *Nitrates* reduce myocardial oxygen consumption.

▶ *Beta-adrenergic blockers* may be administered to reduce the workload and oxygen demands of the heart.

▶ If angina is caused by coronary artery spasm, *calcium channel blockers* may be given.

▶ *Antiplatelet drugs* minimize platelet aggregation and the danger of coronary occlusion.

▶ *Antilipemic drugs* can reduce elevated serum cholesterol or triglyceride levels.

MI
▶ *Thrombolytic therapy* should be started within 3 hours of the onset of symptoms (unless contraindications exist). Thrombolytic therapy involves administration of streptokinase, alteplase, or reteplase.

▶ *Nitroglycerin* is administered sublingually to relieve chest pain, unless systolic blood pressure is less than 90 mm Hg or heart rate is less than 50 or greater than 100 beats/minute.

▶ *Morphine* is administered as analgesia because pain stimulates the sympathetic nervous system, leading to increased heart rate and vasoconstriction.

▶ *Aspirin* is administered to inhibit platelet aggregation.

▶ *I.V. heparin* is given to patients who have received tissue plasminogen activator to increase the chances of patency in the affected coronary artery.

● *Lidocaine, transcutaneous pacing patches* (or a *transvenous pacemaker*), *defibrillation,* or *epinephrine* may be used if arrhythmias are present.

● *I.V. nitroglycerin* is administered for 24 to 48 hours in patients without hypotension, bradycardia, or excessive tachycardia to reduce afterload and preload and relieve chest pain.

● *Glycoprotein IIb/IIIa inhibitors* are administered to patients with continued unstable angina or acute chest pain, or following invasive cardiac procedures, to reduce platelet aggregation.

● *I.V. beta-adrenergic blocker* is administered early to patients with evolving acute MI; it's followed by oral therapy to reduce heart rate and contractibility and myocardial oxygen requirements.

● *Angiotensin-converting enzyme inhibitors* are administered to those with evolving MI with ST-segment elevation or left bundle-branch block, to reduce afterload and preload and prevent remodeling.

● *Lipid-lowering drugs* are administered to patients with elevated low-density lipoprotein and cholesterol levels.

Collaborative practice

●●● **RED FLAG** *Refer the patient*
●●● *immediately to the physician for suspected MI and unstable angina. Activate the emergency medical system if necessary, and make arrangements for immediate transfer to the hospital. A patient is typically treated by the cardiologist during hospitalization. After discharge from the hospital, the patient should be referred to a cardiac rehabilitation exercise program after clearance by the cardiologist.*

Follow-up

Follow-up is every 3 to 6 months for stable angina, but more frequently for changes in the clinical picture. A patient who experienced MI should be reevaluated 3 to 6 weeks after discharge from the hospital.

Complications

● Arrhythmias
● Cardiogenic shock
● Death
● Extension of original infarction
● Heart failure
● Myocardial rupture
● Pericarditis
● Rupture of the atrial or ventricular septum, ventricular wall or valves
● Ventricular aneurysms

Patient teaching

● Stress to the patient the need to follow the prescribed drug regimen and to eat a low-fat, low-cholesterol diet.
● Encourage regular, moderate exercise.
● Refer the patient to a smoking-cessation program if appropriate.
● Advise the patient to minimize stress, and instruct him in relaxation techniques.
● Instruct the patient to have nitroglycerin available for immediate use and to keep it in an airtight, dark, lightproof container. Tell him to discard and replace this medication every 3 to 6 months or as otherwise instructed by the pharmacist.
● Tell the patient to call the primary care provider to report chest, arm, and neck pain; dyspnea; diaphoresis; sudden change in mental status; and sudden weakness.

Resources

● American Heart Association: 1-800-AHA-USA-1; *www.americanheart.org*

▶ National Heart, Lung, and Blood Institute: (301) 592-8573; *www.nhlbi.nih.gov*

ALZHEIMER'S DISEASE

ICD-9-CM 331.0

Alzheimer's disease, also called primary degenerative dementia, accounts for more than 50% of all dementias. This disease isn't found exclusively in the elder population. Its onset begins in middle age in 1% to 10% of cases. Because this is a primary progressive dementia, the prognosis for a patient with this disease is poor.

Causes

The cause of Alzheimer's disease is unknown; however, researchers have implicated several factors. These include neurochemical factors, such as deficiencies in the neurotransmitter acetylcholine, somatostatin, substance P, and norepinephrine; environmental factors, such as repeated head trauma or exposure to aluminum or manganese; and genetic immunologic factors. Genetic studies show that an autosomal dominant form of Alzheimer's disease is associated with early onset and early death.

A family history of Alzheimer's disease and the presence of Down syndrome are two established risk factors.

The brain tissue of patients with Alzheimer's disease has three hallmark features: neurofibrillary tangles, neuritic plaques, and granulovascular degeneration. Examination of the brain after death also finds that it's atrophic, commonly weighing less than 1,000 g, compared with a normal brain weight of about 1,380 g.

Clinical presentation

The onset of Alzheimer's disease is insidious. Initially, the patient undergoes almost imperceptible changes, including forgetfulness, recent memory loss, difficulty learning and remembering new information, deterioration in personal hygiene and appearance, and an inability to concentrate.

Gradually, tasks that require abstract thinking and activities that require judgment become more difficult. Progressive communication difficulties and severe deterioration in memory, language, and motor function result in a loss of coordination and an inability to write or speak. Personality changes (restlessness, irritability) and nocturnal awakenings are common.

Patients with Alzheimer's disease also exhibit a loss of eye contact, fearful look, wringing of hands, and other signs of anxiety; when overwhelmed with anxiety, they become dysfunctional, acutely confused, agitated, compulsive, and fearful.

Eventually, the patient becomes disoriented. Emotional lability and physical and intellectual disability also progress. The patient becomes susceptible to infection and accidents. Usually, death results from infection.

Differential diagnosis

▶ Demyelinating disease
▶ Depression
▶ Epilepsy
▶ Head trauma
▶ Toxin exposure
▶ Tumor

Diagnostic tests

Early diagnosis of Alzheimer's disease is difficult because the patient's signs and symptoms are subtle. Diagnosis relies on an accurate history from a reliable family member, mental status and neurologic examinations, and psychometric testing. A positron emission tomography scan measures the metabolic activity of the cerebral cortex and may help in early diagnosis. An EEG and a computed tomography scan may help in later diagnosis.

Currently, the disease is diagnosed by exclusion; that is, tests are performed to rule out other disorders. The presence of Alzheimer's disease can't be confirmed until death, when pathologic findings are revealed during an autopsy. Cognitive function can be determined by performing the Folstein Mini–Mental Status Examination. Symptoms and history are compared with the criteria in the *Diagnostic and Statistical Manual of Mental Disorders,* Fourth edition.

Management
General
Overall care focuses on supporting the patient's remaining abilities and compensating for ones he has lost.

Medication
▶ *Antidepressants,* such as fluoxetine, may be given if depression seems to exacerbate the patient's dementia.
▶ *Anticholinesterase agents,* such as donepezil, galantamine, rivastigmine, and tacrine, are given to help stabilize cognitive function.
▶ *Antioxidant therapy,* such as with vitamin E therapy, is currently under study for its delaying effect on the disease and its symptoms.
▶ *Memantine (namenda),* an N-methyl D-aspartate receptor antagonist, was approved in October 2003 for the treatment of moderate to severe Alzheimer's disease.
▶ Another approved treatment includes avoiding the use of antacids containing aluminum to help decrease aluminum intake.

● **CLINICAL PEARL** *Patients with Alzheimer's disease may also wish to refrain from using aluminum cooking utensils and aluminum-containing deodorants.*

Collaborative practice
▶ Refer the patient and his family to a support group, such as the National Alzheimer's Association. Support groups may be able to help caregivers deal with the emotional burden and multiple care-related issues placed upon them as the disease progresses.
▶ Refer the patient's family to social service and community resources for legal and financial advice and support.
▶ If additional care that the family can't provide is required, refer the patient to a home health agency or discuss the option of nursing home placement.

Follow-up
The patient should be seen as frequently as necessary to monitor medication usage and assess mental status. Serial mental status testing should be done. Coexisting medical conditions need to be monitored.

Complications
▶ Depression
▶ Hostile, uncontrollable behavior
▶ Infection
▶ Injury (related to disease progression affecting psychomotor skills)
▶ Pneumonia

Patient teaching
▶ Teach the patient's family to provide him a safe environment.
▶ Encourage exercise to help maintain mobility.
▶ Advise the family to establish durable power of attorney and advance directives as early as possible.

Resources
▶ The Alzheimer's Association: 1-800-272-3900; *www.alz.org*
▶ The Alzheimer's Association's Benjamin B. Green-Field Library and Resource Center: 1-800-272-

3900; *www.alz.org/ResourceCenter/ Programs/LibraryServices.htm*
▸ Alzheimer's Disease Education & Referral Center: 1-800-438-4380; *www.alzheimers.org*

ASTHMA

ICD-9-CM extrinsic 493.0, intrinsic 493.1

Asthma is a chronic inflammatory disorder of the airways characterized by airflow obstruction and airway hyperresponsiveness to multiple stimuli. This widespread but variable airflow obstruction is caused by bronchospasm, edema of the airway mucosa, increased mucus production with plugging, and airway remodeling. Symptoms usually show a high degree of reversibility — either spontaneously or with treatment — and vary from mild wheezing to life-threatening respiratory failure. Typically, the untreated patient may experience periods of symptom-free days with intermittent exacerbations of dyspnea, cough, chest tightness, and wheezing.

Causes

Although asthma can strike at any age, half of all cases first occur in children younger than age 10; in this age-group, asthma affects twice as many boys as girls. Asthma is increasing in prevalence and severity in Black and Hispanic patients.

Extrinsic and intrinsic asthma

Asthma that results from a sensitivity to specific external allergens is known as *extrinsic* or atopic asthma. In cases in which the allergen isn't obvious, asthma is referred to as *intrinsic* or nonatopic. Allergens that cause extrinsic asthma include pollen, animal dander, house dust or mold, kapok or feather pillows, and food additives containing sulfites.

Extrinsic asthma usually begins in childhood and is accompanied by other manifestations of atopy (type 1, immunoglobulin [Ig] E–mediated allergy), such as eczema and allergic rhinitis.

In intrinsic asthma, no extrinsic allergen can be identified. Most cases are preceded by a severe respiratory infection. Irritants, emotional stress, fatigue, exposure to noxious fumes, and endocrine, temperature, and humidity changes may aggravate intrinsic asthma attacks. In many asthmatic patients, intrinsic and extrinsic asthma coexist.

Other asthma triggers

Several drugs and chemicals may provoke an asthma attack without involving the IgE pathway. Apparently, they trigger release of mast-cell mediators through prostaglandin inhibition. Examples of these substances include aspirin, various nonsteroidal anti-inflammatory drugs (such as indomethacin and mefenamic acid), and tartrazine, a yellow food dye.

Exercise may also provoke an asthma attack. In exercise-induced asthma, bronchospasm may follow heat and moisture loss in the upper airways.

Two-phase allergic response

When the patient inhales an allergenic substance, sensitized IgE antibodies trigger mast-cell degranulation in the lung interstitium, thereby releasing histamine, cytokines, prostaglandins, thromboxanes, leukotrienes, and eosinophil chemotactic factors. Histamine then attaches to receptor sites in the larger bronchi, causing irritation, inflammation, and edema. In the late phase, an influx of inflammatory cells and eosinophils provides additional inflammatory mediators and contributes to local injury.

Clinical presentation

An asthma attack may begin dramatically, with simultaneous onset of many severe symptoms, or insidiously, with gradually increasing respiratory distress. It typically includes progressively worsening shortness of breath, cough, wheezing, and chest tightness or some combination of these symptoms.

During an acute attack, the cough sounds tight and dry. As the attack subsides, tenacious mucoid sputum is produced (except in young children, who don't expectorate). Characteristic wheezing may be accompanied by coarse rhonchi, but fine crackles aren't heard unless they're associated with a related complication. Between acute attacks, breath sounds may be normal.

The intensity of breath sounds in symptomatic asthma is typically reduced. A prolonged phase of forced expiration is typical of airflow obstruction. Evidence of lung hyperinflation (use of accessory muscles, for example) is particularly common in children. Acute attacks may be accompanied by tachycardia, tachypnea, and diaphoresis. In severe attacks, the patient may be unable to speak more than a few words without pausing for breath. Cyanosis, confusion, and lethargy indicate the onset of life-threatening status asthmaticus and respiratory failure.

History may reveal a family history of allergies and asthma as well as patterns, such as seasonal or episodic occurrence, occurrence outdoors or with exercise, frequency, impact on daily activities, such trigger factors as pets and exercise, previous treatments and effectiveness of each, and family dynamics. It may also reveal associated conditions, including sinusitis, rhinitis, allergies, atopic dermatitis, nasal polyposis, gastroesophageal reflux

disease and, usually, a respiratory infection immediately preceding symptom onset.

In 1997, the National Asthma and Education Prevention Program (NAEPP) of the National Heart, Lung and Blood Institute identified four levels of asthma severity based on the frequency of symptoms and exacerbations, effects on activity level, and lung function study results: mild intermittent, mild persistent, moderate persistent, and severe persistent. (See *Classifying asthma severity*.)

Examination focuses on severity of respiratory distress first, then differentials.

▶ *General:* level of distress
▶ *Skin:* diaphoresis or cyanotic, "allergic shiners" (dark smudges under the eyes)
▶ *Head, eyes, ears, nose, and throat:* nasal flaring or discharge, frontal and maxillary tenderness, postnasal discharge, pharyngeal cobblestone appearance, unilateral purulent nasal discharge, which suggests presence of a foreign body
▶ *Chest:* accessory muscle usage, retractions, adventitious breath sounds, prolonged expirations, unilateral wheeze, which suggests an aspirated foreign body

Differential diagnosis

▶ Chronic bronchitis
▶ Foreign body aspiration
▶ Heart failure
▶ Pneumonia
▶ Tuberculosis
▶ Viral respiratory infection
▶ Vocal cord dysfunction

Diagnostic tests

▶ *Arterial blood gas analysis* provides the best indications of an attack's severity. In acutely severe asthma, partial pressure of arterial oxygen is less than 60 mm Hg, partial pressure of arterial carbon diox-

CLASSIFYING ASTHMA SEVERITY

Clinical features before treatment*

	Symptoms**	Nighttime symptoms	Lung function
Step 4 Severe persistent	▸ Continual symptoms ▸ Limited physical activity ▸ Frequent exacerbations	Frequent	▸ FEV_1 or PEF ≤ 60% predicted ▸ PEF variability > 30%
Step 3 Moderate persistent	▸ Daily symptoms ▸ Daily use of inhaled short-acting beta$_2$-agonist ▸ Exacerbations affect activity ▸ Exacerbations ≥ 2 times per week; may last days	> 1 time per week	▸ FEV_1 or PEF > 60% to < 80% predicted ▸ PEF variability > 30%
Step 2 Mild persistent	▸ Symptoms > 2 times per week but < 1 time per day ▸ Exacerbations may affect activity	> 2 times per month	▸ FEV_1 or PEF ≥ 80% predicted ▸ PEF variability 20% to 30%
Step 1 Mild intermittent	▸ Symptoms ≤ 2 times per week ▸ Asymptomatic and normal peak expiratory flow between exacerbations ▸ Exacerbations brief (from a few hours to a few days); intensity may vary	≤ 2 times per month	▸ FEV_1 or PEF ≥ 80% predicted ▸ PEF variability < 20%

*   The presence of one feature of severity is sufficient to place a patient in that category. An individual should be assigned to the most severe grade in which a feature occurs. The characteristics noted in this figure are general and may overlap because asthma is highly variable. Furthermore, an individual's classification may change over time.

** Patients at any level of severity can have mild, moderate, or severe exacerbations. Some patients with intermittent asthma experience severe and life-threatening exacerbations separated by long periods of normal lung function and no symptoms.

ide ($Paco_2$) is 40 mm Hg or more, and pH is usually decreased.
▸ *Complete blood count* with differential reveals increased eosinophil count.
▸ *Immunoglobulins screening* indicates immunodeficiency and allergic bronchopulmonary aspergillosis.

▸ *Peak expiratory flow* (PEF) rate less than 70% of patient's baseline is an indication for treatment.
▸ *Pulmonary function tests* reveal signs of airway obstruction (decreased PEF rates and forced expiratory volume in 1 second), low-normal or decreased vital capacity,

and increased total lung and residual capacity. However, pulmonary function studies may be normal between attacks.

▶ *Pulse oximetry* may reveal decreased arterial oxygen saturation.

▶ *Chest X-rays* may show hyperinflation with areas of focal atelectasis, or they may be normal.

Management
Acute

●●● **RED FLAG** *PEF less than 60% of*
●●● *patient's baseline indicates the need for emergency care. Acute attacks that don't respond to self-treatment may require hospital care, beta$_2$-adrenergic agonists by inhalation or subcutaneous injection, and oxygen for hypoxemia. If the patient responds poorly, call for emergency medical transport to a medical treatment facility.*

Status asthmaticus is a life-threatening situation resulting from an acute asthma attack. It begins with impaired gas exchange and without rapid intervention may lead to respiratory failure and, eventually, death. The patient is monitored closely for respiratory failure. Management includes oxygen, bronchodilators, epinephrine, corticosteroids, and nebulizer therapy. The patient may require endotracheal intubation and mechanical ventilation if Paco$_2$ increases or if respiratory arrest occurs.

General
The NAEPP created a step-wise method to treat asthma based on the patient's asthma category. These guidelines were updated in 2002. (See *Stepwise approach to managing asthma.*) Dosing of medication as well as adding medications depends on which step the patient falls into at the time of examination. In the patient with asthma, the approach of treating aggressively and then tapering down ther-

apy is widely practiced. Based on patient symptomology, assign the appropriate step of therapy. As the patient gains control of symptoms, "step down" the treatment plan to the preceding step if possible. Medications are grouped as either quick-relief or long-term control agents.

✳ **LIFE SPAN** *Medications used to treat asthma may aggravate an existing medical condition in an elderly patient such as the use of corticosteroids in a patient with osteoporosis. Adjustments may be necessary.*

Medications
Quick-relief agents, such as inhaled short-acting beta$_2$-adrenergic agonists, anticholinergic drugs, and systemic corticosteroids, are geared to abort bronchoconstriction and airflow obstruction. All patients diagnosed with asthma, regardless of classification, should keep a quick-relief inhaler within reach at all times. Nebulized forms of these medications are available for infants or those who can't use a metered dose inhaler.

▶ *Beta$_2$-adrenergic agonists,* such as albuterol and terbutaline, stimulate the sympathetic nervous system to produce smooth-muscle relaxation.

▶ *Anticholinergics,* such as ipratropium, inhibit bronchoconstriction and may increase the benefits of beta$_2$-adrenergic agonists during severe exacerbations. They may also be used as an alternative bronchodilator if the patient can't tolerate beta$_2$-adrenergic agonists.

▶ *Oral corticosteroids* are also considered a quick-relief medication, but they may take approximately 6 hours before clinical improvement is realized.

◐ **CLINICAL PEARL** *Corticosteroids, which are needed to arrest the inflammatory process, shouldn't be withheld. Significant adverse effects*

STEPWISE APPROACH TO MANAGING ASTHMA

This chart, updated by the National Asthma Education and Prevention Program in 2002, may be useful in managing asthma in adults and children older than age 5.

Daily medications required to maintain long-term control

Step 4 Severe persistent	▸ Preferred treatment: –high-dose inhaled corticosteroid AND –long-acting inhaled beta$_2$-adrenergic agonists AND, if needed –Corticosteroid tablets or syrup long term (Make repeat attempts to reduce systemic corticosteroids and maintain control with high-dose inhaled corticosteroids.)
Step 3 Moderate persistent	▸ Preferred treatment: –low-dose inhaled corticosteroids and long-acting inhaled beta$_2$-adrenergic agonists OR –medium-dose inhaled corticosteroids ▸ Alternative treatment: –low-dose inhaled corticosteroids and either leukotriene receptor antagonist or theophylline If needed (particularly in patients with recurring severe exacerbations): ▸ Preferred treatment: –medium-dose inhaled corticosteroids and long-acting beta$_2$-adrenergic agonists ▸ Alternative treatment: –medium-dose inhaled corticosteroids and either leukotriene receptor antagonist or theophylline
Step 2 Mild persistent	▸ Preferred treatment: –low-dose inhaled corticosteroids (with nebulizer or metered dose inhaler [MDI] with holding chamber with or without face mask or dry power inhaler) ▸ Alternative treatment: –cromolyn (nebulizer is preferred or MDI with holding chamber) OR –leukotriene receptor antagonist
Step 1 Mild intermittent	▸ No daily medication needed Bronchodilators as needed for symptoms. Intensity of treatment will depend on severity of exacerbation. ▸ Preferred treatment: –short-acting inhaled beta$_2$-adrenergic agonists by nebulizer or face mask and space/holding chamber ▸ Alternative treatment: –oral beta$_2$-adrenergic agonist

(continued)

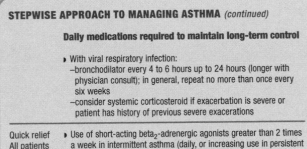

STEPWISE APPROACH TO MANAGING ASTHMA *(continued)*

Daily medications required to maintain long-term control

▸ With viral respiratory infection:
  –bronchodilator every 4 to 6 hours up to 24 hours (longer with physician consult); in general, repeat no more than once every six weeks
  –consider systemic corticosteroid if exacerbation is severe or patient has history of previous severe exacerbations

| Quick relief All patients | ▸ Use of short-acting beta₂-adrenergic agonists greater than 2 times a week in intermittent asthma (daily, or increasing use in persistent asthma) may indicate the need to initiate (increase) long term control therapy. |

Step down
Review treatment every 1 to 6 months; a gradual stepwise reduction in treatment may be possible.

Step up
If control isn't maintained, consider step up. First, review patient medication technique, adherence, and environmental control (avoidance of allergens or other factors that contribute to asthma severity).

NOTE:
▸ The stepwise approach presents general guidelines to assist clinical decision making; it isn't intended to be a specific prescription. Asthma is highly variable; clinicians should tailor specific medication plans to the needs and circumstances of individual patients.
▸ There are very few studies on asthma therapy for infants.
▸ Gain control as quickly as possible (a course of short systemic corticosteroids may be required); then decrease treatment to the least medication necessary to maintain control.
▸ Minimize use of short-acting inhaled beta₂-adrenergic agonists. Overreliance on short-acting inhaled beta₂-adrenergic agonists (their use every day, increasing use or lack of expected effect, or use of approximately one canister a month even if not using it every day) indicates inadequate control of asthma and the need to initiate or intensify long-term control therapy.
▸ Provide patient education on asthma management and controlling environmental factors that make asthma worse, such as allergies and irritants.
▸ Consultation with an asthma specialist is recommended for patients with moderate or severe asthma. Consider consultation for patients with mild persistent asthma.

of short-term corticosteroid use are generally minimal, and their beneficial effects clearly outweigh risks.

Long-term control medications

Long-term control medications, such as inhaled corticosteroids, leukotriene modifiers, methylxanthines, mast-cell stabilizers, long-acting beta₂-adrenergic agonists, and IgE therapy, are indicated for persistent asthma.

Inhaled corticosteroids are the gold standard of long-term asthma control. They're generally well-tolerated and appear to be safe at recommended doses. Benefits of inhaled corticosteroids include decreased inflammation, decreased risk of airway remodeling, decreased bronchial hyperresponsiveness, improvement in lung function, and decreased need for health care intervention.

Data show that inhaled corticosteroids are underused in treatment of asthmatic patients. Patient fears, poor compliance, and underprescribing because of fears about adverse effects might be part of the explanation; however, inhaled corticosteroids have clearly demonstrated a tremendous safety advantage when compared to oral corticosteroids.

CLINICAL PEARL *After asthma is well controlled and spirometry results are optimal, inhaled corticosteroids can be reduced by 25% every 2 to 3 months in an attempt to achieve optimal results using the smallest amount of medication possible.*

Leukotriene modifiers and leukotriene receptor antagonists (LTRAs) inhibit the effects of cysteinyl leukotrienes, including bronchoconstriction, mucus secretion, and vascular permeability of the airway. These medications are effective in reducing the allergen-induced inflammatory response and are also used in exercise-induced and aspirin-sensitive asthma. They can be used as first-line maintenance therapy in the patient with mild persistent asthma, especially if concurrent allergic rhinitis is present. LTRAs can be used as adjunctive therapy to avoid high-dose inhaled corticosteroids.

Although leukotriene modifiers and LTRAs don't replace inhaled corticosteroids as first-line anti-inflammatory treatments, they can be used successfully in patients who experience poor compliance with inhaled corticosteroids.

Methylxanthines, such as theophylline, produce bronchodilation of airway smooth muscle and may have anti-inflammatory properties, although their mechanism of action is still poorly understood. They can be used in tandem with lower doses of inhaled corticosteroids to help lessen the adverse effects that may accompany higher doses of inhaled corticosteroid use. However, methylxanthines are no longer considered first-line agents due to their adverse effect profile, narrow therapeutic window, and serum testing requirements.

Mast cell stabilizers, such as cromolyn and nedocromil, are inhaled agents that help prevent mast cell degranulation and release of inflammatory mediators. These agents are useful for patients who experience exercise-induced asthma or for long-term control in children who suffer from mild persistent asthma. They're also useful in extrinsic, or atopic, asthma when an allergen can't be avoided. Like methylxanthines, mast cell stabilizers may be used in conjunction with lower doses of inhaled corticosteroids to help lessen the adverse effects that may accompany higher doses of inhaled corticosteroid use.

Long-acting beta$_2$-adrenergic agonists, such as salmeterol and sustained-release albuterol, are most useful when inhaled corticosteroids haven't achieved inflammatory control. Be sure to remind the patient that long-acting beta$_2$-adrenergic agonist inhalers aren't quick-relief inhalers due to their slower onset of action.

Omalizumab, an anti-IgE monoclonal antibody, has recently been approved for adults and adolescents with moderate to severe persistent perennial allergic asthma. Human recombinant murine monoclonal antibodies have been thought to attach to IgE antibodies released after allergen exposure. IgE is prevented from attaching to the mast cell, thereby decreasing the overall inflammatory response. This creates the need for a higher level of antigen exposure to invoke the inflammatory cascade leading to asthma. However, omalizumab is ineffective with intrinsic asthma because IgE isn't produced in that category.

Collaborative practice

Consider referring the patient to an allergist or pulmonologist when:

● the diagnosis isn't established and more extensive pulmonary testing is required

● a patient requires step-4 therapy or has had more than two courses of oral steroids in 1 year

● allergy testing or immunotherapy is needed

● the patient has severe persistent asthma or has had a life-threatening emergency department or hospital visit

● the patient is younger than age 3 and requires step-3 or step-4 therapy.

Follow-up

After the patient achieves a stable clinical picture, see him weekly for 2 weeks, then every other week for the next two visits, and then once every 3 months.

Complications

● Acute exacerbations
● Adverse effects of medications
● Atelectasis
● Pneumonia
● Pneumothorax

Patient teaching

● Use a written asthma management plan to help patients obtain a better understanding of the disease. The plan should encompass:

● prevention steps for long-term control, including avoidance strategies, long-term maintenance medications, and peak flow monitoring

● action steps incorporating symptoms of an impending asthma attack, such as chest tightness, wheezing, cough, increase in rescue mediation use, and peak flows below the established personal best

● appropriate uses of quick-relief and long-term medications, including their differences

● use of Diskus or metered dose inhaler and extender or space device

● oral care to prevent candidal infection that may occur with inhaled steroid use

● warning signs that indicate the patient should seek medical attention, such as peak flows below a preestablished value or increased shortness of breath, especially when talking or not exerting himself.

● **CLINICAL PEARL** *A peak flow meter may be one of the most important tools to objectively quantify the severity of asthma in the home, especially in the patient with moderate to severe asthma. After asthma is optimally controlled, a personal best peak flow should be established.*

Resources

● American Academy of Allergy Asthma and Immunology: 1-800-822-2762; *www.aaaai.org*

● American Lung Association: 1-800-LUNG-USA; *www.lungusa.com*

● BREAST CANCER

ICD-9-CM 174.9, carcinoma in situ 233.0

Breast cancer is the most common cancer affecting women, who have a 1-in-8 lifetime risk of developing the disease. Breast cancer also occurs in men, but rarely.

❋ **LIFE SPAN** *Breast cancer is the number two killer (after lung cancer) of women ages 35 to 54. It* *may develop any time after puberty, but is most predominant between the ages of 30 and 80, with peak occurrence between ages 45 and 65.*

The 5-year survival rate for localized breast cancer has improved from the 1940s because of earlier diagnosis and the variety of treatments now available. According to the most recent data, mortality rates continue to decline in white women and, for the first time, are also declining in younger black women. Lymph node involvement is the most valuable prognostic predictor. With adjuvant therapy, a majority of women with negative nodes will survive 10 years.

Causes

The cause of breast cancer isn't known, but its high incidence in women implicates estrogen.

Certain predisposing factors are clear: Women at high risk include those who have a family history of breast cancer, particularly first-degree relatives (mother, sister). Other women at high risk include those who:
▶ began menses early or menopause late
▶ have never been pregnant
▶ were first pregnant after age 30
▶ have had unilateral breast cancer
▶ have had ovarian cancer, particularly at a young age
▶ were exposed to low-level ionizing radiation.

Inconclusive risk factors include exogenous estrogen, high-density fat, or high alcohol use.

CLINICAL PEARL *The discovery of the BRCA-1 and BRCA-2 genes have made genetic predisposition testing an option for women at high risk for breast cancer.*

Women at lower risk include those who:
▶ were pregnant before age 20
▶ have had multiple pregnancies

▶ are Native American or Asian
▶ are breast-feeding or using hormonal contraceptives (possibly).

Breast cancer occurs more commonly in the left breast than the right and more commonly in the outer upper quadrant. Growth rates vary. Theoretically, slow-growing breast cancer may take up to 8 years to become palpable at $^3/_8''$ (1 cm) in size. It spreads by way of the lymphatic system and the bloodstream to the other breast, the chest wall, liver, bone, and brain. Approximately 50% of carcinomas of the breast occur in the upper outer quadrant.

Many refer to the estimated growth rate of breast cancer as "doubling time," or the time it takes the malignant cells to double in number. Survival time for breast cancer is based on tumor size and spread; the number of involved nodes is the single most important factor in predicting survival time.

Breast cancer is classified by histologic appearance and location of the lesion, as follows:
▶ *adenocarcinoma* — arising from the epithelium
▶ *intraductal* — developing within the ducts (includes Paget's disease)
▶ *infiltrating* — occurring in parenchyma of the breast
▶ *inflammatory (rare)* — reflecting rapid tumor growth, in which the overlying skin becomes edematous, inflamed, and indurated
▶ *lobular carcinoma in situ* — reflecting tumor growth involving lobes of glandular tissue
▶ *medullary or circumscribed* — reflecting large tumor with rapid growth rate.

These histologic classifications should be coupled with a staging or nodal status classification system for a clearer understanding of the extent of the cancer.

Clinical presentation

Warning signals of possible breast cancer include:

◗ a lump (usually painless) or mass in the breast (if hard and stony, usually malignant)
◗ change in symmetry or size of the breast (usually enlargement)
◗ change in skin: thickening, scaly skin around the nipple; dimpling; edema (peau d'orange); or ulceration
◗ change in skin temperature (a warm, hot, or pink area; suspect cancer in a non-breast-feeding woman past childbearing age until proved otherwise)
◗ unusual drainage or discharge

RED FLAG *Spontaneous discharge in a non-breast-feeding woman or discharge produced by breast manipulation (greenish black, white, creamy, serous, or bloody) warrants investigation.*

◗ change in the nipple, such as itching, burning, erosion, or retraction
◗ pain (not usually a symptom of breast cancer unless the tumor is advanced, but should be investigated)
◗ bone metastasis, pathologic bone fractures, and hypercalcemia
◗ edema of the arm
◗ axillary node enlargement.

Differential diagnosis
◗ Abscess
◗ Fibroadenoma
◗ Hyperplasia (ductal and lobular)
◗ Lymphoma
◗ Metastatic disease to the breast
◗ Sarcoma

Diagnostic tests

CLINICAL PEARL *Women in their 20s and 30s should have a clinical breast examination (CBE) as part of a regular examination by a health expert evey 3 years. After age 40, women should have a CBE every year.*

◗ *Mammography* is indicated for any woman whose examination suggests an abnormality. However, the value of mammography is questionable for women younger than age 35 (because of the density of the breasts), except those who are strongly suspected of having breast cancer. False-negative results can occur in as many as 30% of all tests. Consequently, with a suspicious mass, a negative mammogram should be disregarded, and a fine-needle aspiration or surgical biopsy should be done.

LIFE SPAN *Women age 40 and older should have annual mammograms.*

◗ *Ultrasonography,* which can distinguish a fluid-filled cyst from a tumor, can be used instead of an invasive surgical biopsy.
◗ *Bone scan, computed tomography scan, measurement of alkaline phosphatase levels, liver function studies,* and *liver biopsy* can detect distant metastasis.
◗ A *hormonal receptor assay* done on the tumor can determine if the tumor is estrogen- or progesterone-dependent. (This test guides decisions to use therapy that blocks the action of the estrogen hormone supporting tumor growth.)

Management

General
Much controversy exists over breast cancer treatments. In choosing therapy, the stage of the disease, the woman's age and menopausal status, and the disfiguring effects of the surgery must be taken into consideration. Treatment of breast cancer may include a combination of methods.

◗ *Peripheral stem cell therapy* may be used for advanced breast cancer.
◗ *Primary radiation therapy* before or after tumor removal is effective

for small tumors in early stages with no evidence of distant metastasis; it's also used to prevent or treat local recurrence. Presurgical radiation to the breast in inflammatory breast cancer helps make tumors more surgically manageable.

Surgery

Surgery involves either mastectomy or lumpectomy. A lumpectomy may be done on an outpatient basis and may be the only surgery needed, especially if the tumor is small and there's no evidence of axillary node involvement. In many cases, radiation therapy is combined with this surgery.

A two-stage surgical procedure, in which the surgeon removes the lump and confirms that it's malignant and then discusses treatment options with the patient, is desirable because it allows the patient to participate in her plan of treatment. Sometimes, if the tumor is diagnosed as clinically malignant, such planning can be done before surgery. In lumpectomy and dissection of the axillary lymph nodes, the tumor and the axillary lymph nodes are removed, leaving the breast intact. A simple mastectomy removes the breast but not the lymph nodes or pectoral muscles. Modified radical mastectomy removes the breast and the axillary lymph nodes. Radical mastectomy, the performance of which has declined, removes the breast, pectoralis major and minor, and the axillary lymph nodes.

Postmastectomy, reconstructive surgery can create a breast mound if the patient desires and doesn't have evidence of advanced disease.

Medication

Chemotherapy, involving various cytotoxic drug combinations, is used as adjuvant or primary therapy, depending on several factors, including staging and estrogen receptor status. Commonly used antineoplastic drugs include cyclophosphamide, fluorouracil, methotrexate, doxorubicin, and vinblastine.

Adjuvant treatment of choice for postmenopausal patients with positive estrogen receptor status is tamoxifen; it has also been found to reduce the risk of breast cancer in high-risk women.

Collaborative practice

▶ Refer the patient to a surgeon and an oncologist.
▶ The patient may need to be referred to a plastic surgeon for reconstructive surgery.
▶ Refer the patient to the American Cancer Society Reach for Recovery for prosthetic information and support.

Follow-up

The patient should be seen as directed by the specialist.

Complications

▶ Infection
▶ Lymphedema
▶ Metastasis
▶ Psychological problems

Patient teaching

▶ Teach the patient about diagnosis and treatment options, including surgery, chemotherapy, and radiation therapy.
▶ Provide psychological and emotional support. Many patients fear cancer, possible disfigurement, and loss of sexual function.
▶ Stress the importance of CBE and mammography following the American Cancer Society guidelines.
▶ Help the patient who has had axillary lymph node dissection prevent lymphedema by instructing her to regularly exercise her hand and arm and to avoid activities that might cause infection or impairment in this hand or arm, which in-

creases the chance of developing lymphedema. Remind her not to let anyone draw blood, start an I.V., give an injection, or take a blood pressure on the affected side because these activities will also increase the chances of developing lymphedema.

Resources

● American Cancer Society: 1-800-ACS-2345; *www.cancer.org*
● National Alliance of Breast Cancer Organizations: 1-888-80-NABCO; *www.nabco.org*
● The Susan G. Komen Breast Cancer Foundation: 1-800-IM-AWARE; *www.komen.org*
● Y-Me National Breast Cancer Organization: 1-800-221-2141; *www.y-me.org*
● Association of Cancer Online Resources: (212) 226-5525; *www.acor.org*

BRONCHITIS, ACUTE

ICD-9-CM 466.0
Bronchitis is an inflammation limited to the tracheobronchial tree, involving the trachea, bronchi, and bronchioles.

Causes

Bronchitis is caused by a number of infections, including viral (adenovirus, influenza, or respiratory syncytial virus), bacterial (*Mycoplasma, Streptococcus pneumoniae, Moraxella catarrhalis,* or *Mycobacterium tuberculosis*) and, rarely, fungal infection. Inflammation of the bronchial tree produces thick secretions that destroy epithelium and inhibit mucociliary function. Other causes of bronchitis include cigarette smoking and exposure to chemicals or smoke.

Clinical presentation

Bronchitis frequently follows a respiratory tract infection, such as a cold and influenza, and is one of the most common diagnoses in the ambulatory care setting. Cough, especially at night, is the primary symptom. A nonproductive cough progresses to produce purulent mucus. The patient may also complain of fever, coughing, mucus with traces of blood after coughing spasms, chest pain, dyspnea, and wheezing. History may reveal close contacts who are sick, a smoking habit, or a chronic respiratory disorder.

Examination findings can be nonspecific for bronchitis, but they have some typical patterns.
● *General:* fever, lymphadenopathy
● *Head, eyes, ears, nose, and throat:* signs of infection
● *Chest:* chest pain, resonance on percussion, and scattered, coarse crackles (in early inspiration and expiration), wheezes, or rhonchi on auscultation

Differential diagnosis

● Asthma
● Bronchogenic tumor
● Heart failure
● Pneumonia
● Reflux esophagitis
● Tuberculosis
● Upper respiratory tract infection

Diagnostic tests

● *Complete blood count* may reveal leukocytosis.
● *Sputum culture and sensitivity testing* and *Gram stain* can detect bacterial causes and sensitivities.
● *Arterial blood gas analysis* detects hypoxemia.
● *Viral titers* (*Mycoplasma* titer less than 1:64) suggest mycoplasma pneumonia; a fourfold rise in titer is diagnostic for the disease.

▶ *Purified protein derivative* may detect tuberculosis.

▶ *Chest X-ray* may reveal pneumonia.

Management
General
Treatment goals are to treat the infection and relieve symptoms. More aggressive treatment and closer monitoring are recommended for patients who are very young (younger than age 4 months), elderly, smokers, immunocompromised, have chronic lung disorders, or have severe symptoms (persistent fever higher than 101° F [38.3° C] in adults or 102.5° F [39.2° C] in children and purulent discharge).
Medication
▶ If bacterial etiology is suspected or there's a need to prevent secondary infection in high-risk patients, *antibiotics* (erythromycin, amoxicillin) may help. Culture and sensitivity results will guide drug choice; for example, macrolides (clarithromycin, azithromycin) treat mycoplasma, and tetracyclines (doxycycline) treat chlamydia as well as mycoplasma.

▶ *Cough suppressants and expectorants* can help with an ineffective cough by decreasing cough frequency while making mucus less viscous and tenacious. Cough suppressants are contraindicated for patients with chronic obstructive pulmonary disease.

▶ *Antipyretic analgesics,* such as nonsteroidal anti-inflammatory drugs and acetaminophen, are recommended for fever and myalgia.

▶ *Bronchodilator and steroid inhalers* are indicated for patients with chronic lung problems and for those who develop hyperreactive airways after infection and mucus production have resolved.

Collaborative practice
Refer the patient to a physician if his condition doesn't improve within 7 days, and refer him to a physician or pulmonologist if bronchitis frequently recurs.
Follow-up
Contact the patient in 2 days to check on fever and response to drugs. See the patient in 1 week to evaluate. If there's no improvement or his condition worsens, refer or consult.

Patients who don't improve after 6 weeks need further evaluation, particularly to determine the cause of persistent cough.

Complications
▶ Acute respiratory failure
▶ Adult-onset asthma
▶ Bronchopneumonia
▶ Secondary infection

Patient teaching
▶ Advise the patient to drink 4 qt (4 L) of noncaffeinated fluid per day, eat a balanced diet, avoid stress, and rest as much as possible to help his body fight infection.

▶ Instruct the patient to use a vaporizer or humidifier or take long, steamy showers to help loosen and thin secretions. (Tell him to breathe in through the nose if it's affected.)

▶ Suggest antipyretic analgesics to relieve body aches for up to 7 days.

▶ Recommend that the patient gargle with salt water(1/4 tsp salt in 8 oz of warm water). For a stuffy nose, the patient may instill saline nose drops (Ocean), leave in for 1 minute, and then blow out, repeating as needed. This may be effective in combination with a hot shower immediately before going to sleep.

▶ Teach smokers how chemicals in cigarette smoke damage ciliary hairs, decreasing the effectiveness of the ciliary escalator. Viral respiratory infection may last 10 to 14 days versus 7 to 10 days for non-smokers. Discuss smoking cessation treatment options, and refer the patient to a smoking cessation program.

▶ To prevent disease transmission, teach the patient to wash his hands with mild soap and water thoroughly and frequently; avoid sharing utensils, toothbrushes, or beverages; and use disposable tissues.

●●● **RED FLAG** *Tell the patient to call*
●●● *and report new signs and symptoms, including the following signs of secondary infection: fever higher than 102.5° F (39.2° C); mucus color changing to dark yellow, green, or brown; inability to swallow liquids; and new onset of severe ear, throat, or sinus pain. Also tell him to call if drug intolerance develops or if a new rash appears after starting the drug or in the event of severe shortness of breath or difficulty breathing.*

Resources

▶ American Academy of Family Physicians: 1-800-274-2237; *www.aafp.org*

CARPAL TUNNEL SYNDROME

ICD-9-CM 354.0

Carpal tunnel syndrome, a form of repetitive stress injury, is the most common of the nerve entrapment syndromes. It results from compression of the median nerve at the wrist, within the carpal tunnel. This compression neuropathy causes sensory and motor changes in the median distribution of the hand. (See *The carpal tunnel.*)

✳ **LIFE SPAN** *Carpal tunnel injury usually occurs in women ages 30 to 60 and poses a serious occupational health problem.*

Assembly-line workers and packers, typists, and people who repeat-

edly use poorly designed tools are most likely to develop this disorder. Strenuous use of the hands — sustained grasping, twisting, or flexing — aggravates this condition.

Causes

The carpal tunnel is formed by the carpal bones and the transverse carpal ligament. Inflammation or fibrosis of the tendon sheaths that pass through the carpal tunnel commonly cause edema and compression of the median nerve. Many conditions can cause the contents or structure of the carpal tunnel to swell and press the median nerve against the transverse carpal ligament. Such conditions include rheumatoid arthritis, flexor tenosynovitis (commonly associated with rheumatic disease), nerve compression, renal failure, menopause, diabetes mellitus, acromegaly, edema following Colles' fracture, hypothyroidism, amyloidosis, myxedema, benign tumors, tuberculosis, and other granulomatous diseases. Another source of damage to the median nerve is dislocation or acute sprain of the wrist. The condition may occur during pregnancy and eventually completely resolve after delivery.

Clinical presentation

▶ Weakness, pain, burning, numbness, or tingling in one or both hands
▶ Paresthesia that affects the thumb, forefinger, middle finger, and half of the fourth finger
▶ Inability to clench hand into a fist
▶ Atrophic nails
▶ Dry and shiny skin

● **CLINICAL PEARL** *Because of vasodilation and venous stasis, symptoms are typically worse at night and in the morning. The pain may spread to the forearm and, in severe cases, as far as the shoulder.*

The patient can usually relieve pain by shaking the hands vigorously or dangling the arm at his side. During the physical examination, ask the patient if pain is relieved with the above maneuver.

Differential diagnosis

▶ Brachial plexus lesion
▶ Generalized peripheral neuropathy

Diagnostic tests

▶ *Physical examination* reveals:
– decreased sensation to light touch or pinpricks in the affected fingers
– thenar muscle atrophy (usually a late sign that occurs in about half of all cases of carpal tunnel syndrome)
– Tinel's sign (tingling over the median nerve on light percussion)
– positive response to Phalen's maneuver. (Holding the forearms vertically and allowing both hands to drop into complete flexion at the wrists for 1 minute reproduces symptoms of carpal tunnel syndrome.)
▶ A *compression test* supports this diagnosis; a blood pressure cuff inflated above systolic pressure on the forearm for 1 to 2 minutes provokes pain and paresthesia along the distribution of the median nerve.
▶ *Electromyography* detects a median nerve motor conduction delay of more than 5 milliseconds.
▶ Other laboratory tests may identify underlying disease.

Management
General

Conservative treatment should be tried first, including resting the hands by splinting the wrist in neutral extension for 1 to 2 weeks and at night for an additional 3 weeks. If a definite link has been established between the patient's occupation and the development of repetitive stress injury, he may have to seek other work. Effective treat-

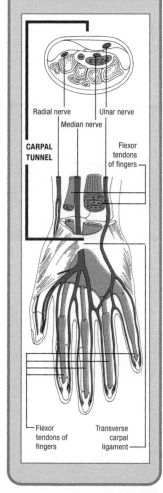

THE CARPAL TUNNEL

The carpal tunnel is clearly visible in this palmar view and cross section of a right hand. Note the median nerve, flexor tendons of fingers, and blood vessels passing through the tunnel on their way from the forearm to the hand.

Radial nerve

Ulnar nerve

Median nerve

CARPAL TUNNEL

Flexor tendons of fingers

Flexor tendons of fingers

Transverse carpal ligament

ment may also require correction of an underlying disorder.

Medication

▶ *Nonsteroidal anti-inflammatory agents,* such as ibuprofen, may provide symptomatic relief.

▶ Injections of *hydrocortisone* into the carpal tunnel every 2 to 3 weeks may provide significant but temporary relief.

Surgery

When conservative treatment fails, the only alternative is surgical decompression of the nerve by resecting the entire transverse carpal tunnel ligament or by using endoscopic surgical techniques. Neurolysis (freeing of the nerve fibers) may also be necessary.

Collaborative practice

▶ Refer the patient to an orthopedic surgeon or neurosurgeon if conservative treatment fails.

▶ Suggest occupational counseling for the patient who has to change jobs because of repetitive stress injury.

Follow-up

The effectiveness of treatment should be monitored initially every 2 weeks, then monthly. For those patients who must remain in their current occupations, suggest ergonomic assessment of the work environment.

Complications

▶ Neural ischemia
▶ Permanent damage with loss of movement and sensation, which may lead to permanent disability
▶ Postoperative infection
▶ Tendon inflammation

Patient teaching

▶ Teach the patient how to apply a splint. Tell him not to make it too tight. Show him how to remove the splint to perform gentle range-of-motion exercises, which should be performed daily.

▶ Advise the patient after surgery to occasionally exercise his hands in warm water. If the arm is in a sling, tell him to remove the sling several times per day to do exercises for his elbow and shoulder.

Resources

▶ American Society for Surgery of the Hand: (847) 384-8300; *www.assh.org*

▶ American Academy of Orthopaedic Surgeons: (847) 823-7186; *www.aaos.org*

● CERVICAL CANCER

ICD-9-CM 180.0

The third most common cancer of the female reproductive system, cervical cancer is classified as either preinvasive or invasive. Cervical carcinoma ranges from minimal cervical dysplasia, in which the lower third of the epithelium contains abnormal cells (75% to 90% cure rate), to carcinoma in situ, in which the full thickness of epithelium contains abnormal cells.

Causes

The human papilloma virus (HPV) is accepted as the cause of virtually all cervical dysplasias and cervical cancers; certain strains of the HPV (16, 18, 31) are associated with an increased risk of cervical cancer.

These predisposing factors have been related to the development of cervical cancer:

▶ intercourse at a young age (before age 16)
▶ multiple sexual partners
▶ herpesvirus 2 and other bacterial or sexually transmitted infections.

Clinical presentation

Cervical dysplasia produces no symptoms or other clinically apparent changes. Early invasive cervical cancer can cause postcoital spotting, dyspareunia, irregular vaginal bleeding, and malodorous vaginal discharge. In advanced stages, it causes pelvic pain, vaginal leakage of urine and feces from a fistula, hematuria, rectal bleeding, anorexia, weight loss, and anemia.

Differential diagnosis
▶ Carcinoma of the endometrium
▶ Cervical polyps
▶ Corpus luteum cyst
▶ Myoma
▶ Severe cervicitis

Diagnostic tests
▶ A *culture* for sexually transmitted illnesses is done as history indicates.
▶ A *cytologic examination (Papanicolaou [Pap] test)* can detect cervical cancer before symptoms appear. Abnormal Pap test specimens must be carefully evaluated. The Bethesda System of Cervical Cytology uses diagnostic terminology to indicate the adequacy of Pap test specimens for diagnosis. It can be used to make follow-up recommendations.
▶ *Colposcopy* is indicated for abnormal Pap tests. Consider endocervical sampling in patients older than age 40 with possible chronic anovulation and in patients younger than age 40 with signs or symptoms of hyperplasia or neoplasia. This test can detect the presence and extent of preclinical lesions.
▶ *Cervical cone biopsy* is done with colposcopic examination to confirm the diagnosis and determine the extent of invasion. This procedure frequently leads to a cure if the carcinoma is detected early.
▶ Laboratory studies include *complete blood count* (anemia due to blood loss), *creatinine* (ureteral obstruction), *liver function tests* (metastases), *prolactin*, and *thyroid panel* (may reveal anovulation).
▶ *Computed tomography scan, magnetic resonance imaging,* and *bone scan* can detect metastases.

Management
General
Appropriate treatment depends on accurate clinical staging. Preinvasive lesions may be treated with total excisional biopsy, cryosurgery, laser destruction, and conization. Frequent Pap test follow-up is recommended.

Surgery
Therapy for invasive squamous cell carcinoma may include radical hysterectomy and radiation therapy (internal, external, or both).

Medication
Pharmaceutical treatment includes chemotherapy (fluorouracil, carboplatin) and antiemetics (ondansetron, metoclopramide) to deal with adverse effects of chemotherapy.

Collaborative practice
Refer the patient to a gynecologist or gynecologic oncologist for colposcopy, counseling, or treatment.

Follow-up
The patient should be seen as directed by the gynecologist.

Complications
▶ Hemorrhage
▶ Loss of ovarian function
▶ Metastatic cancer
▶ Pelvic infection
▶ Ureteral fistula

Patient teaching
▶ Teach the patient about the diagnosis and treatment options.
▶ Teach the patient the importance of a regular Pap test. (Schedule depends on age and risk factors.)
▶ Before a biopsy, explain to the patient that she may feel pressure, minor abdominal cramps, or a pinch from the punch forceps. Reassure her that pain is minimal because the cervix has few nerve endings.
▶ Before cryosurgery, explain to the patient that she may experience abdominal cramps, headache, and sweating, but reassure her that

she'll feel little pain. Cryosurgery will cause a *large* amount of watery discharge for up to 10 days.

▶ Before laser therapy, explain to the patient that the procedure takes approximately 30 minutes and may cause abdominal cramps.

▶ After these procedures, tell the patient to expect a discharge or spotting for about 1 week; also tell her not to douche, use tampons, or engage in sexual intercourse during this time. Tell her to watch for and report signs of infection. Stress the need for a follow-up Pap test and a pelvic examination in 3 months.

▶ Before radiation therapy, teach the patient to watch for and report discomfort that persists and seems to stay in one area. Radiation may increase susceptibility to infection by lowering the white blood cell count; therefore, the patient should avoid persons with obvious infections during therapy.

▶ Teach the patient to use a vaginal dilator to prevent vaginal stenosis and to facilitate vaginal examinations and sexual intercourse.

▶ Reassure the patient that this disease and its treatment shouldn't radically alter her lifestyle or prohibit sexual intimacy.

▶ Use resources to get educational information (for example, on chemotherapy, support services, and cancer's effect on sexuality).

●●● **RED FLAG** *Tell the patient to call her primary care provider to report new signs and symptoms, including postmenopausal bleeding.*

Resources

▶ American Cancer Society: 1-800-ACS-2345; *www.cancer.org*
▶ Cancer Information Service: 1–800-4-CANCER; *http://cis.nci.nih.gov*
▶ Association of Cancer Online Resources: (212) 226-5525; *www. acor.org*

CHRONIC OBSTRUCTIVE PULMONARY DISEASE

ICD-9-CM COPD 496, emphysema 492.8, chronic bronchitis 491
Chronic obstructive pulmonary disease (COPD) — also called *chronic obstructive lung disease* — is a chronic airway obstruction that results from emphysema, chronic bronchitis, asthma, or a combination of these disorders. Usually, more than one of these underlying conditions coexist; most typically, bronchitis and emphysema occur together.

The most common chronic lung disease, COPD affects an estimated 17 million Americans, and its incidence is rising. It affects men more commonly than women probably because, until recently, men were more likely to smoke heavily. It doesn't always produce symptoms, and it causes only minimal disability in many patients; however, COPD tends to worsen with time.

Causes

Predisposing factors include cigarette smoking, recurrent or chronic respiratory infections, air pollution, and allergies. Familial and hereditary factors (for example, deficiency of alpha$_1$-antitrypsin) paired with cigarette smoking may be responsible for emphysema.

Smoking is by far the most important of these factors; it impairs ciliary action and macrophage function and causes inflammation in airways, increased mucus production, destruction of alveolar septae, and peribronchiolar fibrosis. Early inflammatory changes may reverse if the patient stops smoking before lung destruction is extensive.

Clinical presentation

The typical patient, a long-term cigarette smoker, has no symptoms until middle-age, when his ability to exercise or do strenuous work gradually starts to decline and he begins to develop progressive exertional dyspnea and a productive cough. While subtle at first, these signs become more pronounced as the patient gets older and the disease progresses.

The patient eventually develops dyspnea on minimal exertion, frequent respiratory infections, and intermittent or continuous hypoxemia. Emphysema and bronchitis are both present to varying degrees. In its advanced form, COPD may cause thoracic deformities, overwhelming disability, cor pulmonale, severe respiratory failure, and death.

History may reveal fatigue, weight loss, and decreased libido. Examination may reveal tachypnea, accessory muscle usage, increased anteroposterior diameter, hyperresonance on percussion, decreased heart and lung sounds, and prolonged expirations.

Differential diagnosis

▸ Acute bronchitis
▸ Asthma
▸ Heart failure
▸ Malignancy
▸ Sleep apnea

Diagnostic tests

▸ *Complete blood count* may detect polycythemia caused by chronic hypoxemia indicating chronic bronchitis or emphysema.
▸ *Arterial blood gas analysis* may detect hypercapnia and moderate to severe hypoxemia.
▸ *Pulmonary function testing* shows increased residual volume with decreased vital capacity and forced expiratory volume.

▸ *Chest X-ray* is typically normal in the course of COPD; however, it's useful in differentiating chronic bronchitis from emphysema. Increased bronchovascular markings and cardiomegaly revealed on X-ray indicate chronic bronchitis, whereas a small heart, hyperinflation, flat diaphragms, and bullous changes suggest emphysema.

Management
Acute

The patient must be hospitalized for respiratory failure, exacerbation, and infection; treatment dependents on the clinical picture.

General

The main goal of treatment is to relieve symptoms and prevent complications. Effective coughing, postural drainage, and chest physiotherapy can help mobilize secretions.

For patients using metered-dose inhalers, consider using a spacer device to facilitate proper administration. If the patient reports a strong taste in his mouth, he's usually getting the dose in his mouth instead of his lungs, with decreased effectiveness.

Tell the patient to avoid using antihistamines, cough suppressants, sedatives, tranquilizers, and opioids because of their effects on the respiratory system.

Encourage the patient to participate in local support groups and rehabilitation programs (physical and pulmonary).

Surgery

Lung volume reduction surgery is a procedure for carefully selected patients with emphysema. Nonfunctional parts of the lung (diseased tissue that provides little ventilation or perfusion) are surgically removed. Removal allows more functional lung tissue to expand and the diaphragm to return to its normally elevated position.

Medication

▶ *Bronchodilators* can be given by metered-dose inhalers (beta-adrenergic bronchodilators [albuterol, terbutaline]), by mouth (theophylline), or by nebulizer or nasal spray (anticholinergic bronchodilator [ipratropium]), to help alleviate bronchospasm and enhance mucociliary clearance of secretions.

▶ *Corticosteroids* (prednisone) are useful as anti-inflammatory agents, with the greatest results noted in early stages when lung tissue reversibility is greatest.

▶ *Pneumococcal vaccination* and *annual influenza vaccinations* are important preventive measures. This is particularly important as more antibiotic-resistant organisms emerge.

▶ *Antivirals* (amantadine) are used after exposure to influenza A, for high-risk populations during flu season, and during acute influenza infection.

▶ *Antibiotics* are used as needed to treat secondary respiratory infections.

▶ Low concentrations of *oxygen* help relieve symptoms.

▶ In rare cases of alpha$_1$-antitrypsin deficiency, it can be replaced by a weekly I.V. injection of human alpha$_1$ proteinase inhibitor (Prolastin).

Collaborative practice

The patient should be referred to a pulmonologist or physician if nonresponsive or if his response is unsatisfactory, if the clinical picture is deteriorating rapidly, or if cor pulmonale is present.

Refer the patient to a local pulmonary and physical therapy rehabilitation program to build endurance and strength after he's cleared medically.

Follow-up

The patient should be seen initially every 2 weeks for evaluation of treatment. Thereafter, monitor according to severity of the disorder.

Complications

▶ Cor pulmonale
▶ Hypoxemia
▶ Infection
▶ Left ventricular heart failure
▶ Malnutrition
▶ Pulmonary hypertension
▶ Respiratory acidosis
▶ Respiratory failure
▶ Secondary polycythemia

Patient teaching

▶ Because most patients with COPD receive outpatient treatment, provide comprehensive patient teaching to help them comply with therapy and understand the nature of this chronic, progressive disease.

▶ Encourage the patient to enroll in available pulmonary rehabilitation programs.

▶ Encourage regular, consistent aerobic exercise, particularly upper extremity and diaphragmatic exercises and pursed-lip breathing.

▶ Urge the patient to stop smoking. Evaluate his progress with smoking cessation at each follow-up visit.

▶ Encourage the patient to avoid respiratory irritants, install an air conditioner with an air filter in the home, and regularly change air filters.

▶ Review the use and adverse effects of drugs.

▶ Review the signs of infection, and warn the patient to avoid contact with persons who have respiratory infections. Encourage good oral hygiene to help prevent infection.

▶ Review deep breathing, coughing, and chest physiotherapy.

▶ Encourage noncaffeinated fluids and the use of a humidifier to correct dehydration or to thin and loosen thick secretions.

▸ Emphasize the importance of a balanced diet and small frequent meals (4 to 6 per day) to avoid fatigue and to decrease diaphragmatic elevation caused by gastric distention.

▸ If ordering oxygen therapy at home, teach the patient the importance of using equipment correctly. Because the patient may tire easily while eating, teach the importance of using nasal oxygen while eating.

▸ Discuss with the patient and his family ways to adjust their lifestyles to accommodate the limitations imposed by this debilitating chronic disease. Instruct the patient to exercise daily and allow for daily rest periods.

●●● RED FLAG *Tell the patient to call*
●●● *the primary care provider to report new or persistent signs and symptoms, including fever higher than 101° F (38.3° C) or a cough producing green, brown, or dark yellow mucus; difficulty eating because of shortness of breath; increasing shortness of breath or increasing orthopnea (requiring use of extra pillows to elevate the head in order to sleep); breathing that becomes rapid or increasingly difficult; or unusual drowsiness.*

●●● RED FLAG *If the patient won't*
●●● *respond, his lips become dusky or blue, or his respirations become very irregular, activate emergency medical services.*

Resources

▸ American Lung Association: 1-800-LUNG-USA; *www.lungusa.org*
▸ National Heart, Lung and Blood Institute: (301) 592-8573; *www.nhlbi.nih.gov*

COLORECTAL CANCER

ICD-9-CM primary 154.0, secondary 197.5, in situ 230.4, benign 211.4, uncertain 235.2

In the United States and Europe, colorectal cancer is the second leading visceral neoplasm. Incidence is equally distributed between men and women, mostly those older than age 50, except in familial polyposis. Colorectal malignant tumors are almost always adenocarcinomas. About half of these are sessile lesions (flat-based) of the rectosigmoid area; the rest are pedunculated (stalked) lesions. Sessile lesions are more likely to become malignant.

Colorectal cancer tends to progress slowly and remains localized for a long time. Consequently, it's potentially curable in 75% of patients if an early diagnosis allows resection before nodal involvement. With early diagnosis, the overall 5-year survival rate is nearly 50%. The larger the lesion, the greater the incidence of invasive cancer. (See *TNM staging*, page 196.)

Causes

While most colorectal cancers arise from adenomas, the exact cause of colorectal cancer is unknown. There are known risk factors. Dietary risk factors include low-fiber and high-fat intake. Other risk factors include a history of inflammatory bowel disease, familial polyposis, a first-degree relative with a history of colon cancer, or adenomatous polyps.

Clinical presentation

Adenomas are precursors for most colorectal cancers. These polyps are treatable lesions but usually produce no symptoms until they're very large. Bleeding from polyps is

TNM STAGING

The TNM (tumor, node, and metastasis) system developed by the American Joint Committee on Cancer provides a consistent method for classifying malignant tumors based on the extent of the disease. It also offers a convenient structure to standardize diagnostic and treatment protocols. Differences in classification may occur, depending on the primary cancer site.

T for primary tumor
The anatomic extent of the primary tumor depends on its size, depth of invasion, and surface spread. Tumor stages progress from TX to T4 as follows:

TX — Primary tumor can't be assessed
T0 — No evidence of primary tumor
Tis — Carcinoma in situ
T1, T2, T3, T4 — Increasing size or local extent (or both) of primary tumor

N for nodal involvement
Nodal involvement reflects the tumor's spread to the lymph nodes as follows:

NX — Regional lymph nodes can't be assessed
N0 — No evidence of regional lymph node metastasis
N1, N2, N3 — Increasing involvement of regional lymph nodes

M for distant metastasis
Metastasis denotes the extent (or spread) of disease. Levels range from MX to M4 as follows:

MX — Distant metastasis can't be assessed
M0 — No evidence of distant metastasis
M1 — Single, solitary distant metastasis
M2, M3, M4 — Multiple foci or multiple organ metastasis

---

usually scanty and intermittent. Manifestations of colorectal cancer result from local obstruction and, in later stages, from direct extension to adjacent organs (bladder, prostate, ureters, vagina, sacrum) and distant metastasis (usually to the liver).

In early stages, signs and symptoms are typically vague and depend on the anatomic location and function of the affected bowel segment. Later, they generally include pallor, cachexia, ascites, hepatomegaly, lymphangiectasis (dilation of the lymphatic vessels), fatigue, weakness, iron deficiency anemia, constipation or diarrhea, tenesmus, urgency, and hematochezia.

Cancer on the right side
On the right side of the colon, which absorbs water and electrolytes, early tumor growth causes no signs of obstruction because the tumor tends to grow along the bowel rather than surround the lumen, and the fecal content in this area is normally liquid. It may, however, cause black, tarry stools; anemia; and abdominal aching, pressure, or dull cramps.

As the disease progresses, the patient develops weakness, fatigue, exertional dyspnea, vertigo and, eventually, diarrhea, obstipation (extreme, persistent constipation), anorexia, weight loss, vomiting, and other signs and symptoms of intestinal obstruction. In addition, a tumor on the right side may be palpable.

Cancer on the left side
On the left side, a tumor causes signs and symptoms of an obstruc-

tion even in early stages because, in this area, stool is of a formed consistency. A tumor commonly causes rectal bleeding (typically ascribed to hemorrhoids), intermittent abdominal fullness or cramping, and rectal pressure.

As the disease progresses, the patient develops obstipation, diarrhea, or "ribbon" (pencil-shaped) stool. Typically, he notices that passage of stool or flatus relieves the pain. At this stage, bleeding from the colon becomes obvious, with dark or bright red blood in the stool and mucus in or on the stool.

Rectal tumor signs

With a rectal tumor, the first symptom is a change in bowel habits, commonly beginning with an urgent need to defecate on arising ("morning diarrhea") or obstipation alternating with diarrhea. Other indications include blood or mucus in stool and a sense of incomplete evacuation. Late in the disease, pain begins as a feeling of rectal fullness that later progresses into a dull, and sometimes constant, ache confined to the rectum or sacral region.

Differential diagnosis

- Benign adenomas
- Colitis
- Hemorrhoids or rectal polyps
- Infection
- Irritable bowel syndrome
- Neoplasm from other primary site

RED FLAG *A patient with a GI complaint whose examination reveals an abdominal mass, severe abdominal tenderness, fever, weight loss, or acute onset without obvious cause requires aggressive evaluation. Other red flags include nocturnal wakening due to GI complaints, family history of malignancy, positive fecal occult blood test, and abnormal blood counts (decreased hemoglobin and hematocrit).*

Diagnostic tests

Only a tumor biopsy can verify colorectal cancer, but the following tests help detect it.

- *Digital rectal examination* discovers almost 15% of colorectal cancers by detecting a rectal mass.
- A *fecal occult blood test* can detect blood in stool but has low specificity for colorectal cancer. Sensitivity is improved with serial testing (three to six specimens).
- *Complete blood count* detects anemia, which may indicate an occult hemorrhage.
- *Carcinoembryonic antigen (CEA),* although not specific or sensitive enough for an early diagnosis, is helpful in monitoring patients before and after treatment to detect metastasis or recurrence.
- *Urinary 5-hydroxyindoleacetic acid levels* may be high in colorectal cancer.
- *Proctoscopy* or *sigmoidoscopy* can detect up to 66% of colorectal cancers.
- *Colonoscopy* permits visual inspection (and photographs) of the colon up to the ileocecal valve and gives access for polypectomies and biopsies of suspected lesions. It's a useful screening tool for high-risk patients.
- *Computed tomography scan* helps to detect extent of metastasis.
- *Barium X-ray,* using a dual contrast with air, can locate lesions that are undetectable manually or visually. Barium examination should follow endoscopy or excretory urography because the barium sulfate interferes with these tests.

Management

Acute

The most effective treatment for colorectal cancer is surgery to remove the malignant tumor and adjacent tissues as well as lymph nodes that may contain cancer cells.

Before surgery

▶ Order diet modifications, laxatives, enemas, and antibiotics to clean the bowel and to decrease abdominal and perineal cavity contamination during surgery.

▶ If the patient is having a colostomy, teach him and his family about the procedure. Refer the patient to the wound, ostomy, continence nurse for stoma siting, patient education, and postoperative follow-up.

After surgery

▶ Explain to the patient's family members the importance of their positive reactions to the patient's adjustment.

▶ Encourage the patient to look at the stoma and participate in its care as soon as possible. Emphasize importance of good hygiene and skin care.

▶ If indicated, instruct the patient with a sigmoid colostomy to do his own irrigation as soon as he can after surgery.

Physical activity

▶ Inform the patient that a structured, gradually progressive exercise program to strengthen abdominal muscles may be instituted under medical supervision.

▶ Before achieving bowel control, the patient can resume physical activities, including sports.

▶ Avoid injury to the stoma or surrounding abdominal muscles.

▶ Instruct the patient to avoid heavy lifting because herniation or prolapse may occur through weakened muscles in the abdominal wall.

Medication

▶ *Chemotherapy* is indicated for patients with metastasis, residual disease, or a recurrent inoperable tumor. Drugs used in such treatment commonly include fluorouracil with levamisole, leucovorin, methotrex-

ate, or streptozocin. Patients whose tumor has extended to regional lymph nodes may receive fluorouracil and levamisole for 1 year postoperatively.

▶ *Radiation therapy* induces tumor regression and may be used before or after surgery or combined with chemotherapy, especially fluorouracil.

Collaborative practice

Refer the patient to a gastroenterologist or other physician for colonoscopy, to a gastroenterologic surgeon and oncologist for evaluation and treatment as indicated, and to a home health agency for follow-up care as needed. The patient should see the wound, ostomy, continence nurse to set up a colostomy care regimen.

Sexual counseling is important for men because most are impotent after an abdominoperineal resection. Refer the patient to a psychologist or psychiatrist for coping mechanisms to deal with changes in body image.

Follow-up

The patient should be seen as directed by the specialist. After resection, monitor CEA levels quarterly. Every 6 months the patient needs serial fecal occult blood tests, physical examination, chest X-ray, and liver function tests. Colonoscopy is needed yearly for 2 years. If all findings are negative, progress to colonoscopy every 2 to 3 years. If an adenomatous polyp is detected, refer for removal and follow up with colonoscopy in 6 months.

Complications

▶ Anastomotic problems
▶ Diarrhea
▶ Pneumonia
▶ Stomatitis
▶ Temporary alopecia
▶ Urinary tract infection
▶ Wound infection

Patient teaching

▶ Teach the patient about the disease process, treatment options, and colostomy care.

▶ Teach the patient about risk factors (family history of polyposis or colorectal cancer), and reinforce the need for colorectal cancer screening, especially if he's a member of a high-risk group. Recommend a specific screening protocol based on his risk factors.

● ● ● **RED FLAG** *Tell the patient to call his primary care provider to report any new or persistent signs and symptoms, including signs of infection in the postoperative period (fever higher than 101° F [38.3° C] or increasing pain, swelling, drainage, odor, and wound size), change in bowel habits or appearance of stool (diarrhea, constipation, blood in stool), palpable mass in abdomen or rectal area, rectal bleeding, and increasing or persistent abdominal pain.*

Resources

▶ American Cancer Society: 1-800-ACS-2345; *www.cancer.org*
▶ Cancer Information Service: 1-800-4-CANCER; *http://cis.nci.nih.gov*
▶ Cancer Care: 1-800-813-HOPE; *www.cancercare.org*
▶ United Ostomy Association: 1-800-826-0826; *www.uoa.org*
▶ Wound, Ostomy, and Continence Nurse Society: 1-800-826-0826; *www.wocn.org*
▶ Association of Cancer Online Resources: (212) 226-5525; *www.acor.org*

DEPRESSION, MAJOR

ICD-9-CM major depressive disorder 296.2, recurrent episode 296.3
Depression is the fourth most common reason patients visit the primary care provider. Depression manifests in many ways, but it occurs when a patient experiences more stress and negative emotions than he can handle. About 50% of all depressed patients experience a single episode and recover completely. Major depression can profoundly alter a person's ability to function. Suicide is the most serious complication of major depression. Nearly twice as many women as men attempt suicide, but men are far more likely to succeed.

Causes

The exact cause of depression isn't known. Current theory states that each individual is able to handle a certain amount of negative (or positive) stress. The body compensates by altering the rate of uptake of neurotransmitters by synaptic receptors. When an individual experiences a major stressor (such as the death of a spouse) or a series of smaller stresses (car accident, job insecurity, major expenses, pregnancy), the synapses reset to a lower mood (similar to adjusting a home thermostat). After synapses are reset, removing the original stress doesn't necessarily reverse the mood.

Depression commonly occurs secondary to many medical disorders such as cancer. The existence of a reason for the patient's depression doesn't stop the diagnosis and shouldn't delay treatment.

Many commonly abused substances (such as alcohol) as well as drugs prescribed for medical and psychiatric conditions can also cause depression. Examples include antihypertensives, psychotropics, opioid and nonopioid analgesics, antiparkinsonian drugs, cardiovascular drugs, oral antidiabetics, antimicrobials, steroids, chemotherapeutic agents, and cimetidine.

Clinical presentation

The primary features of major depression are a predominantly sad mood, a loss of interest or pleasure in daily activities (anhedonia), a significant change in appetite, a sleep disorder (insomnia or hypersomnia), fatigue or loss of energy nearly every day, restlessness, irritability, social withdrawal, perpetual feelings of unworthiness or inappropriate guilt, an inability to concentrate or make decisions, and suicidal ideation. *Dysthymic disorder* is a milder, chronic form of depression.

The patient may report an increase or a decrease in appetite, sleep disturbance, a lack of interest in sexual activity, constipation, or diarrhea. When taking the patient's history, it's important to note affect and inattentiveness. Examination focuses on ruling out suspected causes but frequently reveals other signs, including agitation (such as hand wringing or restlessness) and reduced psychomotor activity (such as slowed speech).

Take special note of high-risk factors for suicide. These include certain age-groups (teenagers and the elderly); recurrent depressive episodes; previous suicide attempt; history of substance abuse (particularly alcohol); thought process disorder (such as hearing a dead relative calling him); lack of a social support system; lack of a significant other; presence of a chronic or disabling or painful disorder; a specific suicidal plan; giving away personal belongings; suddenly feeling happy or energetic without cause; or having a family member or friend who has committed suicide. The more risk factors, the more closely the patient should be monitored.

Failure to detect suicidal thoughts early may encourage the patient to attempt suicide. The risk of suicide increases as the depression starts to lift, and the patient regains the energy to carry out plans.

If you're uncomfortable asking about suicidal ideation, practice this approach. After reaching the diagnosis of depression, say, "There's another symptom that you haven't mentioned, but more than 90% of patients with dysthymia have it. Do you ever get the feeling that you and just about everybody else would be better off if you weren't around?" If the patient denies it vehemently or states that their religious convictions are too strong to permit thoughts of suicide, be more concerned than if they state they have the occasional suicidal thoughts. If you're confident the patient isn't actively suicidal, understands the diagnosis and treatment plan, and knows he can contact you anytime he feels bad, you can follow up in the office.

Differential diagnosis

- Anxiety disorder
- Bipolar depression
- Dementia
- Dysthymic disorder
- Medical conditions, such as thyroid or endocrine disorders
- Schizophrenic disorder

Diagnostic tests

The diagnosis is made on clinical grounds but is supported by psychological tests.

- *The Beck Depression Inventory* or *Children's Depression Inventory* may help determine the onset, severity, duration, and progression of depressive symptoms.
- A *toxicology screening* may suggest drug-induced depression.
- *Thyroid-stimulating hormone levels* will indicate hypothyroidism.

Management

Acute

If the patient is a danger to himself or others, have someone else activate emergency medical services or get help while you engage the patient in conversation. State that you understand how he feels, and express your certainty that this feeling will pass and that there's help and hope.

General

Because of slowed responses, give the patient extra time to answer questions, ask questions, and express feelings. If you act rushed or fail to make eye contact, you may discourage him from confiding in you.

Pharmacologic therapy is usually an adjunct to psychotherapy. Antidepressants may mask deep-rooted problems. Never remove a patient's coping mechanism without giving him an acceptable replacement.

Teach carefully about diagnosis and drugs.

▶ Patient education increases compliance with management regimen, including pharmacologic and nonpharmacologic measures.

▶ Dysthymia isn't thoroughly understood, but current theory is that a chemical imbalance develops. Replacing that chemical helps the patient reset the synapses and relieves symptoms.

▶ Results take 2 to 8 weeks, depending on the drug, and are gradual.

▶ The patient may not receive the most effective drug the first time, but with the right drug and the right dose, the patient will feel better.

▶ The primary care provider will work with the patient until the right drug is found.

You must be willing to work with the patient until he feels better and must be available at all times during an acute episode.

Medication

In depression, drug therapy includes selective serotonin reuptake inhibitors (SSRIs), tricyclic antidepressants (TCAs), monoamine oxidase (MAO) inhibitors, and bupropion.

▶ *SSRIs,* including fluoxetine, trazodone, paroxetine, and sertraline, are increasingly becoming the drugs of choice. They're effective and produce fewer adverse effects than TCAs; however, they're associated with sleep and GI problems and alterations in sexual desire and function.

▶ *TCAs,* such as amitriptyline, clomipramine, and desipramine, prevent the reuptake of norepinephrine, serotonin, or both into the presynaptic nerve endings, resulting in increased synaptic concentrations of these neurotransmitters. They also cause a gradual loss in the number of beta-adrenergic receptors.

▶ *MAO inhibitors,* such as phenelzine, selegiline, and tranylcypromine, block the enzymatic degradation of norepinephrine and serotonin. These agents are usually prescribed for patients with atypical depression (for example, depression marked by an increased appetite and need for sleep, rather than anorexia and insomnia) and for some patients who fail to respond to TCAs.

MAO inhibitors are associated with a high risk of toxicity; patients treated with one of them must be able to comply with the necessary dietary restrictions. Conservative doses of an MAO inhibitor may be combined with a TCA for patients refractory to either drug alone.

▶ The mechanism of action of *bupropion* is unknown.

After resolution of the acute episode, patients commonly remain on antidepressants for 6 months to 2 years. If depression recurs, the patient may be maintained on low doses of antidepressants.

Collaborative practice

If appropriate, refer the patient to a psychiatrist or psychologist. An appointment is urgent for patients who are in their teens or younger; for those over age 64; for those who are pregnant or sexually active without contraceptive measures; for those who are unable to function, have comorbidities, and are nonresponsive to two trials of antidepressant drugs; and for those who are suicidal or having a recurrence of depression.

A counselor can provide the patient with alternatives that others have tried successfully in the past, so the patient won't be limited to coping mechanisms that are already familiar. Support groups specific to the patient's profile (Incest Survivors, Narcotics Anonymous) are useful.

Follow-up

Follow-up should be weekly until improvement is noted (if no improvement in 6 to 8 weeks, consider another drug), then monthly for 3 months, and then quarterly. Focus on the adverse effects, dosage, and effectiveness of the drug regimen.

Complications

▶ Nonresponsiveness to therapy
▶ Recurrence
▶ Suicidal ideations

Patient teaching

▶ Teach the patient that it normally takes 6 to 8 weeks for effects to show. Effects are gradual, not dramatic.
▶ Help the patient to develop a structured routine, including noncompetitive activities, to build his self-confidence and encourage interaction with others. Urge him to join group activities and to socialize.
▶ Inform the patient that he can help ease depression by expressing his feelings, participating in pleasurable activities, and improving grooming and hygiene.
▶ Help the patient to recognize distorted perceptions that may contribute to his depression. When he learns to recognize depressive thought patterns, he can consciously begin to substitute self-affirming thoughts.
▶ Teach the patient about prescribed medications. Stress the need to comply with the drug regimen and to report adverse effects. For drugs with anticholinergic effects, such as amitriptyline and amoxapine, suggest sugarless gum or hard candy to relieve dry mouth.
▶ Many antidepressants are sedating (for example, amitriptyline and trazodone); warn the patient taking these drugs to avoid activities that require alertness, including driving and operating mechanical equipment, until the central nervous system (CNS) effects of the drug are known.
▶ Caution the patient taking a TCA to avoid drinking alcoholic beverages or taking other CNS depressants during therapy.
▶ If the patient is taking a MAO inhibitor, emphasize that he must avoid foods that contain tyramine, caffeine, or tryptophan. The ingestion of tyramine can cause a hypertensive crisis. Examples of foods that contain these substances are cheese, sour cream, pickled herring, liver, canned figs, raisins, bananas, avocados, chocolate, soy sauce, fava beans, yeast extracts, meat tenderizers, coffee, colas, beer, Chianti wine, and sherry.
●●● **RED FLAG** *Tell the patient to call*
●●● *the primary care provider to*

report new or persistent signs and symptoms, including inability to perform daily activities, weight loss, and increasing feelings of frustration, anger, or hopelessness.

Resources

▶ Depression and Bipolar Support Alliance: 1-800-826-3632; *www. dbsalliance.org*

▶ National Foundation for Depressive Illness: 1-800-239-1265; *www.depression.org*

▶ National Mental Health Association: (703) 684-7722; *www.nmha. org*

DIABETES MELLITUS

ICD-9-CM 250.0, with nephropathy 250.4, with ophthalmopathy 250.5, with neuropathy 250.6

A chronic disease of absolute or relative insulin deficiency or resistance, diabetes mellitus is characterized by disturbances in carbohydrate, protein, and fat metabolism.

This disorder occurs in two forms: type 1 and the more prevalent type 2. Type 1 usually occurs before age 30 (although it may occur at any age); the patient is usually thin and requires exogenous insulin and dietary management to achieve control. Conversely, type 2 used to be called "adult-onset diabetes" because it occurred mostly in obese adults after age 40. However, changing dietary patterns, sedentary lifestyles, and increasing rates of obesity are causing type 2 diabetes to develop in younger people, even children. Type 2 diabetes is most commonly treated with diet, exercise, and antidiabetic drugs, but treatment may include insulin therapy.

CULTURAL KEY *High-risk groups for type 2 diabetes include Blacks, Asians, Hispanics, and Native Americans. The incidence of* type 2 diabetes has dramatically increased in obese children, particularly among minority populations in North America. Currently, 30% of patients with newly diagnosed diabetes are in their second decade of life.

A leading cause of death from disease in the United States, diabetes contributes to about 50% of myocardial infarctions and about 75% of strokes as well as to renal failure and peripheral vascular disease. Diabetes is also the leading cause of new blindness in the United States.

Causes

The effects of diabetes mellitus result from insulin deficiency. Insulin transports glucose into the cells for use as energy and storage as glycogen. It also stimulates protein synthesis and free fatty acid storage in the fat deposits. Insulin deficiency compromises the body tissues' access to essential nutrients for fuel and storage.

The cause of type 1 diabetes is thought to be an autoimmune process that's triggered by a virus or environmental factor; however, the cause of the idiopathic form of type 1 diabetes isn't known. Patients with this form exhibit no evidence of an autoimmune process.

The cause of type 2 diabetes is thought to be beta cell exhaustion due to lifestyle habits and hereditary factors. Risk factors thought to contribute to the development of type 2 diabetes include obesity, family history, ethnic background, and history of gestational diabetes during pregnancy.

Other risk factors for diabetes include the following:

▶ Physiologic or emotional stress can cause prolonged elevation of stress hormone levels (cortisol, epinephrine, glucagon, and growth hormone). This raises blood glucose levels, placing an increased demand on the pancreas.

▸ Pregnancy causes weight gain and increases hormonal levels (estrogen, progesterone, prolactin, and human placental lactogen), which cause insulin resistance.

▸ Some medications can antagonize the effects of insulin, including thiazide diuretics, adrenal corticosteroids, and hormonal contraceptives.

The patient history should focus on symptoms associated with hyperglycemia and hypoglycemia, reviewing the patient's glucose testing diary, and complications of diabetes. Elicit dietary habits, ideal-weight maintenance attempts, exercise (frequency and duration), and drug treatment and compliance. If the patient is noncompliant due to an inability to pay for medications or supplies, refer him to social services or suggest resources. Assess cardiac risk factors: obesity, hypertension, smoking, high triglycerides, high low-density lipoproteins, low high-density lipoproteins (HDLs), and stress.

Clinical presentation

In type 1 diabetes, symptomatology may be insidious or dramatic, as with ketoacidosis. The most common symptom is fatigue from energy deficiency and a catabolic state.

Insulin deficiency causes the three P's of diabetes: polyphagia, polydipsia, and polyuria. Hyperglycemia pulls fluid from body tissues, causing osmotic diuresis, polyuria, dehydration, polydipsia, dry mucous membranes, and poor skin turgor. In ketoacidosis and hyperosmolar hyperglycemic nonketotic syndrome (HHNS), dehydration may cause hypovolemia and shock. Wasting of glucose in the urine usually produces weight loss and hunger in type 1 diabetes, even with polyphagia.

● **CLINICAL PEARL** *Glucosuria without hyperglycemia is present in benign renal glucosuria and renal tubular disease. Polyuria and polydipsia without hyperglycemia occur in diabetes insipidus. Hyperglycemia and glucosuria are seen in pheochromocytoma, Cushing's syndrome, and acromegaly. Hyperglycemia occurs in acute periods of severe stress from infection, trauma, and burns.*

Long-term effects

In diabetes, long-term effects may include cardiovascular problems, retinopathy, nephropathy, atherosclerosis, peripheral and autonomic neuropathy, and an increased susceptibility to infection.

●●● **RED FLAG** *Macrovascular complications are the major cause of death in patients with diabetes. Additional risk factors exacerbate the problem. These include smoking tobacco, obesity, sedentary lifestyle, hypertension, and dyslipidemia.*

A condition known as *metabolic syndrome,* which is related to insulin resistance, occurs if a patient has all of the following risk factors: obesity, high blood pressure, high triglyceride levels, and low HDL levels (each of which is an independent risk factor for heart disease). Metabolic syndrome is associated with a high risk of developing type 2 diabetes and coronary artery disease. The components (risk factors) of this syndrome are associated with high insulin levels that result from peripheral insulin resistance. Eliminating or reducing individual components will decrease the overall risk; however, most measures that affect one component will affect the others as well, providing additional risk reduction.

Retinopathy can progress to blindness, nephropathy to kidney failure, and atherosclerosis to cardiovascular events.

Peripheral neuropathy usually affects the hands and feet and may cause numbness or pain. Autonomic neuropathy may manifest itself in several ways, including gastroparesis (leading to delayed gastric emptying and a feeling of nausea and fullness after meals), nocturnal diarrhea, impotence, and orthostatic hypotension.

Because hyperglycemia impairs the patient's resistance to infection, diabetes may result in skin and urinary tract infections (UTIs) and vaginitis. The glucose content of the epidermis and urine encourages bacterial growth.

Differential diagnosis

▶ Benign renal glucosuria
▶ Gestational diabetes mellitus
▶ Secondary diabetes (results from endocrine, metabolic, or genetic disorders or may be drug-induced)

Other conditions need to be considered before reaching a diagnosis of diabetes. Glucosuria without hyperglycemia can occur in benign renal glucosuria or in renal tubular disease. Diabetes insipidus presents with polyuria and polydipsia but not hyperglycemia. Secondary diabetes may result from endocrine or metabolic disorders that cause hyperglycemia and glucosuria, such as Cushing's syndrome, pheochromocytoma, and acromegaly. Transient hyperglycemia can also occur in severe stress from trauma, burns, or infection.

Diagnostic tests

In nonpregnant adults, one of the following findings confirms diabetes mellitus:

▶ typical symptoms of uncontrolled diabetes and a *random blood glucose level* equal to or above 200 mg/dl (SI, 11.1 mmol/L)

▶ a *fasting plasma glucose level* equal to or greater than 126 mg/dl (SI, 7 mmol/L) on at least two occasions

▶ if the fasting glucose test is normal, a *blood glucose level* above 200 mg/dl (SI, 11.1 mmol/L) during a glucose tolerance test with 75-g glucose load.

An *ophthalmologic examination* may show diabetic retinopathy. *Glycosylated hemoglobin* (Hb A_{1c}) reflects glucose control during the previous 3 months; this isn't diagnostic but is useful in long-term management.

Management
General
Types 1 and 2

Effective treatment for both types of diabetes normalizes blood glucose and decreases complications. Therefore, review applicable information about diabetes, self-monitoring, foot care, physical activity, and diet management at each visit.

Treatment of both types of diabetes requires a diet designed to meet nutritional needs, control blood glucose levels, and reach and maintain appropriate body weight. For the obese patient with type 2 diabetes, weight reduction is a goal. In type 1, the calorie allotment may be high, depending on growth stage and activity level. For success, the diet must be followed consistently and meals eaten at regular times.

Support groups and classes certified by the American Diabetes Association can help with education, motivation, and compliance.

Researchers are also making progress in gene therapy. Genes have been developed that regulate and produce insulin, but the genes need to be placed in a permanent spot in the deoxyribonucleic acid chain so the effect doesn't die along with the individual cell.

Surgery

Treatment of long-term diabetic complications may include transplantation or dialysis for renal failure, photocoagulation for retinopathy, and vascular surgery for peripheral arterial disease. Pancreas transplantation may be indicated for a patient with type 1 diabetes who's also experiencing end-stage pancreatic disease.

Medication

Type 1 diabetes

In type 1 diabetes mellitus, treatment includes insulin replacement. Current forms of insulin replacement include single-dose, mixed-dose, split–mixed dose, and multiple-dose regimens. The multiple-dose regimens may use an insulin pump. Insulin inhalers and insulin patches are being studied.

Insulin may be rapid-acting, short-acting, intermediate-acting, long-acting, or a combination of rapid-acting and intermediate-acting; it may be standard or purified, and it may be derived from beef, pork, or human sources. Purified human insulin is used commonly today.

Type 2 diabetes

Exercise and dietary changes are first-line therapy in many patients with new-onset type 2 diabetes. The success rate of diet and exercise alone is 3% to 5%. Therefore, type 2 diabetes may require oral antidiabetic drugs to stimulate endogenous insulin production, increase insulin sensitivity at the cellular level, delay carbohydrate absorption from the GI tract, and suppress hepatic gluconeogenesis.

Medications for type 2 diabetes include sulfonylureas (glipizide, glyburide), which stimulate insulin production; biguanides (metformin), which inhibit hepatic glucose production and increase peripheral insulin sensitivity without increasing insulin levels; alpha-glucosidase inhibitors (acarbose), which decrease the rate of absorption of carbohydrates and so decrease postprandial peaks of blood glucose; and thiazolidinediones (pioglitazone, rosiglitazone), which reduce peripheral insulin resistance. Combination therapy is becoming more common and achieving better control with fewer episodes of hypoglycemia.

Insulin can be added to or temporarily replace oral antidiabetics when maximum dosage or combinations of oral drugs aren't controlling hyperglycemia, during times of major stress or infection, and during pregnancy.

Collaborative practice

The patient should see an endocrinologist for new or poorly controlled diabetes, an ophthalmologist (yearly) for a dilated-eye examination to check for retinopathy, a podiatrist for early intervention with foot disorders, and a dietitian for diet management.

He should be referred to an endocrinologist or another physician if he has ketosis or uncontrolled blood glucose levels, fails to respond to conventional regimens, switches from oral antidiabetics to insulin, or experiences chest pain, painful neuropathy, mental confusion, or skin ulcers. Genetic counseling may be considered for young adult diabetics who are planning families.

Follow-up

When the drug regimen is changed, see the patient weekly until his glucose level is controlled and then every 2 to 4 months if Hb A_{1c} testing reflects control. Visit frequency is influenced by compliance, metabolic control, and signs of end-organ damage. At each visit, review symptoms, blood glucose record, laboratory results, funduscopy, cardiac status (especially blood pressure), and foot status (examine for skin integrity, blood supply, and neuropathy). After 3 years, schedule an annual dilated-eye examination for retinopathy.

Other follow-up includes routine urinalysis for proteinuria and creatinine to detect renal insufficiency, an annual random urine specimen for albumin-to-creatinine ratio, or 24-hour urine collection. (If urinalysis indicates decreased kidney function, repeat twice; if two out of three tests suggest decreased kidney function, the patient should begin taking an angiotensin-converting enzyme inhibitor such as captopril.) Consider scheduling the patient for a periodic lipid panel because diabetics are at high risk for atherosclerosis and cardiac events.

Complications

Treatment of long-term diabetic complications may include transplantation or dialysis for renal failure, photocoagulation for retinopathy, drugs for hypertension and lipid abnormalities, and vascular surgery for large-vessel disease. Tight glucose control is essential in minimizing all of these complications, probably due to decreasing the arterial changes caused by hyperglycemia. Other complications include HHNS, gangrene, glaucoma, cataracts, skin ulceration, and Charcot joints.

The Diabetes Control and Complications Trial findings demonstrated that intensive drug therapy that focuses on keeping glucose at near-normal levels for 5 years or more reduces the onset and progression of retinopathy (by up to 63%), nephropathy (by up to 54%), and neuropathy (by up to 60%).

Patient teaching

●●● **RED FLAG** *Stress to the patient*
●●● *that compliance with the prescribed program is essential. Emphasize the effects of strict blood glucose control on long-term health (delaying or preventing blindness, impotence, stroke, heart attack, and amputation). Teach him to check blood glucose levels and medicate per individualized parameters. If levels exceed the highest range of the personal treatment plan, tell him to notify his primary care provider.*

●●● **RED FLAG** *Instruct the patient to*
●●● *watch for acute complications of diabetic therapy, especially hyperglycemia and hypoglycemia (lethargy, dizziness, weakness, pallor, diaphoresis). Check blood glucose levels; if they're low, immediately give carbohydrates in the form of 6 oz fruit juice or one piece of hard candy.*

▶ Teach the patient how to manage his diabetes when he has a minor illness, such as a cold, the flu, or an upset stomach.

▶ Have the patient monitor diabetic control by testing and recording blood glucose levels. Tell him to bring the record and glucometer to the office with each visit; have him demonstrate proper technique and correct as needed.

▶ Teach the effects of diabetes on the blood vessels, eyes, kidneys, peripheral nervous system, and autonomic nervous system. Reinforce that the best treatment is prevention with close control of blood glucose levels.

▶ Treat all injuries, cuts, and blisters (particularly on the legs or feet) meticulously.

▶ Be alert for signs of UTI and renal disease (decreased, concentrated, dark, or cloudy urine with or without discomfort).

▶ Remind the patient of the need for yearly ophthalmologic examinations to detect diabetic retinopathy.

▶ Teach the patient the signs of diabetic neuropathy (numbness or pain in the hands and feet, footdrop, impotence, neurogenic bladder). Stress the need for personal safety precautions; explain that decreased sensation can mask injuries.

▶ Teach the patient to care for his feet by washing them daily, drying carefully between the toes, and inspecting for corns, calluses, redness, swelling, bruises, and breaks in the skin. Encourage him to avoid over-the-counter products for corn and callus removal, and follow up with the primary care provider for problems. Advise him to wear nonconstricting shoes and to avoid walking barefoot.

▶ To delay the clinical onset of diabetes, teach persons at high risk to avoid risk factors.

●●● **RED FLAG** *Tell the patient to call*
●●● *the primary care provider to report new or persistent signs and symptoms, including signs of infection, signs of cardiac distress (chest pain, palpitations, dyspnea, confusion), changes in vision, peripheral numbness or tingling, constipation, anorexia, and blisters or skin openings, particularly on the feet.*

Resources

▶ American Association of Diabetes Educators: 1-800-338-3633; *www.aadenet.org*
▶ American Diabetes Association: 1-800-DIABETES; *www.diabetes.org*
▶ Juvenile Diabetes Research Foundation International: 1-800-533-CURE; *www.jdf.org*
▶ The Neuropathy Association: (212) 692-0662; *www.neuropathy.org*

DIVERTICULAR DISEASE

ICD-9-CM diverticulosis 562.10, diverticulitis 562.11

In diverticular disease, bulging pouches (diverticula) in the GI wall push the mucosal lining through the surrounding muscle. The most common site for diverticula is in the sigmoid colon, but they may develop anywhere, from the proximal end of the pharynx to the anus.

Other typical sites are the duodenum, near the pancreatic border (the ampulla of Vater), and the jejunum. Diverticular disease of the stomach is rare and is commonly a precursor of peptic or neoplastic disease. Diverticular disease of the ileum (Meckel's diverticulum) is the most common congenital anomaly of the GI tract but is rarely symptomatic after age 5.

Diverticular disease has two clinical forms. In *diverticulosis*, diverticula are present but don't cause symptoms. In *diverticulitis*, diverticula are inflamed and may cause potentially fatal obstruction, infection, or hemorrhage.

Causes

Diverticular disease is most prevalent after age 60 and is rare before age 40. Diverticula probably result from high intraluminal pressure on areas of weakness in the GI wall, where blood vessels enter.

Diet may also be a contributing factor because lack of roughage reduces fecal residue, narrows the bowel lumen, and leads to higher intra-abdominal pressure during defecation. The fact that diverticulosis is most prevalent in Western industrialized nations, where processing removes much of the roughage from foods, supports this theory. Diverticulosis is less common in nations where the diet contains more natural bulk and fiber.

In diverticulitis, retained undigested food mixed with bacteria accumulates in the diverticular sac, forming a hard mass (fecalith). This substance cuts off the blood supply to the thin walls of the sac, making them more susceptible to attack by colonic bacteria. Inflammation follows, possibly leading to perforation, abscess, peritonitis, obstruction, or hemorrhage. Occasionally, the inflamed colon segment may form a fistula by adhering to the bladder or other organs.

Clinical presentation

The two forms of diverticular disease produce different clinical effects.

Diverticulosis

Although diverticulosis usually produces no symptoms, the patient may complain of recurrent left lower quadrant pain. Such pain, typically accompanied by alternating constipation and diarrhea, is relieved by defecation or the passage of flatus. Symptoms resemble irritable bowel syndrome and suggest that both disorders may coexist.

In older patients, a rare complication of diverticulosis (without diverticulitis) is hemorrhage from colonic diverticula, usually in the right colon. Such hemorrhage is usually mild to moderate and easily controlled, but it may occasionally be massive and life-threatening.

Diverticulitis

Mild diverticulitis produces moderate left lower quadrant pain, gas, and irregular bowel habits. Additionally, the patient may complain of mild nausea, low-grade fever, and leukocytosis.

In severe diverticulitis, the diverticula can rupture and produce abscesses or peritonitis. Rupture occurs in up to 20% of such patients;

its symptoms include abdominal rigidity and left lower quadrant pain.

Peritonitis follows the release of fecal material from the rupture site and causes signs of sepsis and shock (high fever, chills, hypotension). Rupture of the diverticulum near a vessel may cause microscopic or massive hemorrhage, depending on the vessel's size.

Chronic diverticulitis may cause fibrosis and adhesions that narrow the bowel's lumen and lead to bowel obstruction. Signs and symptoms of incomplete obstruction include constipation, ribbonlike stools, intermittent diarrhea, and abdominal distention. Signs and symptoms of increasing obstruction include abdominal rigidity and pain, diminishing or absent bowel sounds, nausea, and vomiting.

Differential diagnosis

▶ Angiodysplasia (with rectal bleeding)
▶ Appendicitis
▶ Colon cancer
▶ Crohn's disease
▶ Gastroenteritis
▶ Irritable bowel syndrome
▶ Ulcerative colitis

●●● **RED FLAG** *A patient with a GI*
●●● *complaint whose examination reveals an abdominal mass, severe abdominal tenderness, fever, weight loss, or acute onset without obvious cause requires aggressive evaluation. Other red flags include nocturnal wakening due to GI complaints, family history of malignancy, positive fecal occult blood test, and abnormal blood counts.*

Diagnostic tests

▶ *White blood cell* (WBC) elevation with immature polymorphs indicates diverticulitis.
▶ A low *hemoglobin* reading indicates bleeding.

▶ *Erythrocyte sedimentation rate* elevation indicates diverticulitis.

▶ *Urinalysis* showing WBCs, red blood cells, or pus cells suggests possible fistula formation.

▶ *Urine culture* of persistent infection suggests colovesical fistula.

▶ *Blood culture*, if positive, indicates diverticulitis with generalized peritonitis.

▶ An *upper GI series* confirms or rules out diverticulosis of the esophagus and upper bowel.

▶ In nonacute diverticular disease, *flexible sigmoidoscopy* or *colonoscopy* rules out or confirms diverticulosis.

▶ *Barium enema* confirms or rules out diverticulosis of the lower bowel. Barium-filled diverticula can be single, multiple, or clustered like grapes and may have a wide or narrow mouth. Barium outlines, but doesn't fill, diverticula blocked by impacted feces. In patients with acute diverticulitis, a barium enema may rupture the bowel, so this procedure requires caution.

▶ *Abdominal X-rays* may detect peritonitis, perforation, free air and, if irritable bowel syndrome accompanies diverticular disease, colonic spasm.

▶ *Computed tomography (CT) scan* of the abdomen and pelvis with or without contrast is diagnostic for abscess, fistula, and measuring an inflammatory mass.

▶ *Angiography* is diagnostic and therapeutic for diverticular bleeding.

▶ *Spiral CT scan* with bolus of I.V. contrast may detect bleeding.

▶ *Colonoscopy* and *flexible sigmoidoscopy* may detect cancer and ulcerative or ischemic colitis.

▶ *Cystoscopy* is indicated if colovesical fistula is suspected.

▶ A *biopsy* rules out cancer; however, a colonoscopic biopsy isn't recommended during acute diverticu-

lar disease because of the strenuous bowel preparation it requires.

Management

The two forms of the disease call for different treatment regimens.

Diverticulosis

Asymptomatic diverticulosis generally doesn't require treatment. Intestinal diverticulosis with pain, mild GI distress, constipation, or difficult defecation generally responds to a liquid or bland diet, stool softeners, and occasional doses of mineral oil. These measures relieve symptoms, minimize irritation, and lessen the risk of progression to diverticulitis. After pain subsides, patients also benefit from a high-residue diet and bulk laxatives such as psyllium.

Diverticulitis

Treatment of mild diverticulitis without signs of perforation aims to prevent constipation and combat infection. It may include bed rest, a liquid diet, a broad-spectrum antibiotic (ciprofloxacin), stool softeners, an opioid pain reliever (such as meperidine) to control pain and relax smooth muscle, and an antispasmodic (such as hyoscyamine or propantheline) to control muscle spasms.

Surgery

Diverticulitis that doesn't respond to medical treatment requires a colon resection to remove the involved segment. Perforation, peritonitis, obstruction, or a fistula that accompanies diverticulitis may require a temporary colostomy to drain abscesses and rest the colon, followed by later anastomosis.

Patients who hemorrhage need blood replacement and careful monitoring of fluid and electrolyte balance. Such bleeding usually stops spontaneously. If bleeding continues, angiography may be performed to guide catheter placement for infusing vasopressin into the bleeding vessel.

Collaborative practice

Refer the patient to a gastroenterologist for evaluation and colonoscopy as needed and to a physician if the condition is nonresponsive in 2 to 3 days. Hospitalization may be needed for toxicity, septicemia, or peritonitis. The patient should see a wound, ostomy, and continence nurse if an ostomy is placed.

Follow-up

See the patient in 2 to 3 days to evaluate response. If the patient is being treated with antibiotics, see him in 1 week. If the patient is stable, see him yearly.

Complications

▶ Abscess
▶ Bowel obstruction
▶ Fistula
▶ Hemorrhage
▶ Perforation
▶ Peritonitis
▶ Septicemia
▶ Toxicity

Patient teaching

If the patient has diverticulosis, include the following points in your teaching:

▶ Explain what diverticula are and how they form.
▶ Make sure the patient understands the importance of dietary roughage and the harmful effects of constipation and straining during defecation. Encourage increased intake of foods high in indigestible fiber, including fresh fruits and vegetables, whole-grain bread, and wheat or bran cereals. Warn that a high-fiber diet may temporarily cause flatulence and discomfort.
▶ Advise the patient to relieve constipation with stool softeners or bulk-forming cathartics. Caution against taking bulk-forming cathartics without plenty of water; if

swallowed dry, they may absorb enough moisture in the mouth and throat to swell and obstruct the esophagus or trachea.

●●● **RED FLAG** *Tell the patient to call*
●●● *the primary care provider to report new or persistent signs and symptoms, including abdominal pain that worsens or is nonresponsive to treatment; fever above 101° F (38.3° C); signs of dehydration (light-headedness, voiding small amounts of dark concentrated urine, excessive thirst); vomiting blood or coffee-ground material; bright red, black, tarry, or maroon-colored stools; yellow skin or eyes; or no bowel movement for 5 days.*

Resources

▶ Wound, Ostomy and Continence Nurses Society: 1-888-224-WOCN; *www.wocn.org*
▶ For patient information on irritable bowel syndrome: *www.medscape.com*

HEADACHE

ICD-9-CM headache 784, classic migraine 346.0, unspecified migraine 346.9, tension headache 307.81, cluster headache 346.2
Headache is the most common complaint in primary care. The three most common types are migraine, tension-type, and cluster.

Causes

Most chronic headaches result from tension — muscle contraction — which may be caused by emotional stress, fatigue, menstruation, or environmental stimuli (noise, crowds, bright lights). The cause of migraine headaches isn't known, but one proposed mechanism is neuronal dysfunction, possibly of the trigeminal nerve pathway with secondary constriction and dilation of cranial arteries, indicating a process that causes neurogenic inflammation. One theory stating that disruption of neurotransmitters (serotonin and norepinephrine) occurs during migraines is supported by research findings that antidepressant drugs that regulate neurotransmitters are effective against migraine in some cases.

More than 80% of migraine patients have a family history of migraines, and a chromosomal abnormality has been found in at least one type of migraine. Research suggests that classic migraine, common migraine, and chronic tension-type headache (present more than 15 days a month) are actually variants of the same disorder. This, in turn, is supported by another theory, which states that chronic headaches are caused by a biochemical condition similar to depression.

Other causes of headache include glaucoma; inflammation of the eyes or mucosa of the nasal or paranasal sinuses; diseases of the scalp, teeth, extracranial arteries, and external or middle ear; and muscle spasms of the face, neck, or shoulders.

Headaches may also be secondary to drugs such as vasodilators (nitrates, alcohol, histamine), systemic disease, hypoxia, hypertension, head trauma and tumor, intracranial bleeding, abscess, or aneurysm.

Clinical presentation

The three common categories of headache can be differentiated by presentation.

Migraine headaches

For diagnosis of migraine, two of the following characteristics must be present: pulsatile, throbbing pain; unilateral location aggravated by normal physical activity; nausea and vomiting; photophobia; or phonophobia. History may reveal that the migraine was preceded by scintillating scotoma (visual aura), hemianopsia, unilateral paresthesia,

or speech disorders; aura typically occurs 20 minutes before migraine onset. The patient may experience irritability and anorexia and may be bedridden. Possible association exists with neck muscle contraction and pain, cervical osteoarthritis, vasodilation, epilepsy, and low plasma serotonin levels. Common migraine is the same as classic migraine but without an aura.

Tension-type headaches

Tension-type headaches produce a dull, persistent ache, tender spots on the head and neck, and a feeling of tightness around the head, with a characteristic "hatband" distribution. The pressure or tightness is bilateral with mild to moderate pain that isn't aggravated by activity. Examination may reveal associated neck muscle contraction and pain, cervical osteoarthritis, vasodilation, epilepsy, or low plasma serotonin levels.

Cluster headaches

Cluster headaches typically develop within 2 hours of falling asleep. The pain is so excruciating that patients can't sit still. Many patients who use alcohol and tobacco, which trigger these headaches, abstain during attacks. Pain is unilateral during an episode but may switch sides from cycle to cycle. The eye on the affected side is commonly erythematous and edematous. These headaches typically occur in clusters of up to four times per day for 1 to 4 months, disappear completely for 6 months to 2 years, and then the cycle repeats. The patient presents with at least one of the following: conjunctival injection, lacrimation, nasal congestion, rhinorrhea, miosis, ptosis, or eyelid edema.

An accurate diagnosis requires a history of recurrent headaches and physical examination of the head and neck that includes percussion, auscultation for bruits, inspection for signs of infection, and palpation for defects (hardened, nonpulsatile temporal arteries), crepitus, or tender spots (especially after trauma). A firm diagnosis also requires a complete neurologic examination and assessment for other systemic diseases (such as hypertension) and depression.

Differential diagnosis

▶ Aneurysm
▶ Brain tumor
▶ Caffeine dependence
▶ Cervical spondylosis
▶ Chronic sinusitis
▶ Hemorrhage
▶ Hypertension
▶ Meningitis
▶ Temporal arteritis
▶ Temporomandibular joint syndrome

●●● RED FLAG *Warning signs that* **●●●** *suggest a serious underlying cause needing prompt consultation or referral include patient complaints of a cluster, migraine, or chronic tension-type headache for the first time in his life; increasingly frequent and severe headaches or new onset of severe headaches after age 50; changes in cognition; syncope; seizures; being wakened by a headache; vomiting without nausea; history of recent head injury; tender nonpulsatile temporal arteries; or nuchal rigidity and high fever. More aggressive evaluation is needed if papilledema is observed during funduscopy, if the patient has symptoms suggesting another systemic illness (such as weight loss), or if his headaches fail to respond to treatment.*

Diagnostic tests

▶ *Elevated sedimentation rate* in patients over age 50 may indicate temporal arteritis.

▶ *Complete blood count* is done if anemia or polycythemia is suspected.

▶ *Electrolyte* and *thyroid studies* detect metabolic and endocrine disorders.

▶ *X-rays of the cervical spine and sinuses* detect arthritis and chronic sinus infection.

▶ *Computed tomography, magnetic resonance imaging,* and *magnetic resonance angiography* are performed for a new onset or change in the headache pattern, or if neurologic abnormalities are found on examination. These tests can detect hemorrhage and tumors.

▶ *Lumbar puncture* can reveal infection.

Management

Treatment depends on the length and severity of the headaches. Other measures include identification and elimination of trigger factors and, possibly, psychotherapy if emotional stress is a trigger.

Migraine headaches
Acute

The patient may require hospitalization for severe pain, concurrent medical problems such as dehydration, or medication-withdrawal problems. Urgently institute abortive drug therapy because early intervention assists in management.

General

Explain the diagnosis clearly, and validate the patient's pain. Evaluate the impact of the migraine headaches on the patient's quality of life. A tool, such as the migraine disability assessment scale, is helpful in determining the illness' impact on the patient's lifestyle. Discuss with the patient how to develop a plan to manage the headaches effectively and provide a quality lifestyle. Teach the patient biofeedback techniques so that he can gain conscious control over various auto-

214 • Disease management

nomic functions with the help of electronic monitors. By observing the fluctuations of a particular bodily function, such as heart rate or blood pressure, on the monitor, he'll eventually learn to adjust his thinking to control that function. For instance, electromyelographic (measuring muscle tension) biofeedback is used to treat muscle contraction headaches.

Massage, gentle exercise, and a balanced diet may help by decreasing overall muscle tension and improving subclinical health problems, such as plaque buildup in arteries and decreasing insulin sensitivity.

Medication
Migraine headaches
🔵 **CLINICAL PEARL** *The most effective management of a migraine headache is to treat it early. Instruct the patient to treat the migraine as soon as there's throbbing pain aggravated by movement.*

▶ *Migraine medication* may be *abortive* (such as medications taken after a headache has begun) or *preventive* (such as daily medications used to reduce frequency of attacks).

▶ Abortive drugs include 5HT$_1$-receptor agonists (sumatriptan), dihydroergotamine, and nonsteroidal anti-inflammatory drugs (NSAIDs). If nausea and vomiting make oral administration impossible, some drugs can be given by alternative routes, such as subcutaneous injection and nasal spray. Antiemetics (metoclopramide) are a helpful adjunct to other therapies; corticosteroids (prednisone) reduce neurogenic inflammation.

▶ Preventive drugs include propranolol, atenolol, clonidine, and amitriptyline.
Chronic tension-type headaches
▶ *Prophylactic antidepressants* (sertraline) are useful.

▶ For exacerbations, *NSAIDs* (naproxen) and *muscle relaxants* (methocarbamol) may be used.
Cluster headaches
▶ *Prophylactic drugs* include calcium channel blockers (verapamil), corticosteroids (prednisone, tapered over 1 month), and ergotamine vasoconstrictors (dihydroergotamine, ergotamine).

▶ *Abortive drugs* include oxygen (7 to 10 L by face mask), 5-HT$_1$-receptor agonists (subcutaneous sumatriptan), ergotamine vasoconstrictors (sublingual ergotamine), or local anesthetics (intranasal lidocaine).

Collaborative practice
Refer the patient to a specialist (neurologist, ophthalmologist), as indicated by the findings. A psychologist or psychiatrist can assist with biofeedback and pain management. Refer to a primary care provider if you're unsure of diagnosis, for concurrent medical conditions, for drug-seeking behavior, or if the condition is nonresponsive to therapy.

Follow-up
Focus on documenting frequency of attacks, pain behaviors, and medication usage; also stress avoiding triggers through behavior modification.

Complications
▶ Adverse effects of medications
▶ Cerebral ischemia
▶ Disruption of lifestyle
▶ Drug dependence
▶ Unremitting migraine

Patient teaching
▶ Explain to the patient that migraine is a hereditary disorder that's treatable but not curable. Drug therapy can decrease the severity and length of migraines, and avoiding trigger factors can reduce their frequency.

▶ Trigger factors consist of changes in routine: sleep changes, weather changes, a change in caffeine intake (from diet or over-the-counter [OTC] analgesics), hormonal changes, letdown after stress, and missing meals. If food is a trigger, it will have an effect within 30 minutes to 12 hours after ingestion.

▶ Encourage the patient to keep a headache diary to help pinpoint individual triggers and most effective therapies. Record the duration and location of the headache, the time of day it usually begins, the nature of the pain, concurrent symptoms such as blurred vision, and precipitating factors, such as tension, menstruation or menopause, loud noises, use of alcohol, use of medications such as hormonal contraceptives, and prolonged fasting.

▶ Provide information about the rationale for drug classes, drug actions, and limitations, including rebound headaches that may occur with over use of OTC analgesics such as acetaminophen.

▶ Advise the patient to lie down in a dark, quiet room during an attack and to place ice packs on his forehead or a cold cloth over his eyes.

▶ Instruct him to take medication at the onset of migraine symptoms.

▶ Stress that drinking plenty of fluids is important because dehydration is common.

●●● RED FLAG *Tell the patient to call*
●●● *the primary care provider to report new or persistent signs and symptoms, including headache lasting more than 24 hours despite therapy, difficulty moving extremities, slurred speech, confusion, difficulty walking normally, blurred or double vision, vomiting without nausea, increasing severity or frequency, headaches present on waking (if the patient had a head injury), and fever higher than 101° F (38.3° C) for adults and 102.5° F (39.2° C)*

for children ages 4 months to 17 years with a stiff neck.

Resources

▶ American Council for Headache Education: (856) 423-0258; *www. achenet.org*

▶ National Headache Foundation: 1-888-NHF-5552; *www.headaches.org*

▶ New England Center for Headache: (203) 968-1799; *www. headachenech.com*

▶ Patient information on headaches: *www.medscape.com*

HEART FAILURE

ICD-9-CM congestive heart failure 428.0

A syndrome characterized by myocardial dysfunction, heart failure leads to impaired pump performance (reduced cardiac output) or to frank heart failure and abnormal circulatory congestion. Congestion of systemic venous circulation may result in peripheral edema or hepatomegaly; congestion of pulmonary circulation may cause pulmonary edema, which is an acute, life-threatening emergency. (See *Classifying heart failure,* page 216.)

Pump failure usually occurs in a damaged left ventricle (left-sided heart failure) but may occur in the right ventricle (right-sided heart failure) either as a primary disorder or secondary to left-sided heart failure. Sometimes left- and right-sided heart failure develop simultaneously.

Although heart failure may be acute (as a direct result of myocardial infarction [MI]), it's generally a chronic disorder associated with retention of sodium and water by the kidneys. Advances in diagnostic and therapeutic techniques have greatly improved the outlook for patients with heart failure, but the prognosis still depends on the underlying cause and its response to treatment.

CLASSIFYING HEART FAILURE

The New York Heart Association classification is a universal gauge of heart failure severity based on physical limitations.

Class I: Minimal
▸ No limitations
▸ Ordinary physical activity doesn't cause undue fatigue, dyspnea, palpitations, or angina

Class II: Mild
▸ Slightly limited physical activity
▸ Comfortable at rest
▸ Ordinary physical activity results in fatigue, palpitations, dyspnea, or angina

Class III: Moderate
▸ Markedly limited physical activity
▸ Comfortable at rest
▸ Less than ordinary activity produces symptoms

Class IV: Severe
▸ Can't perform physical activity without discomfort
▸ Angina or symptoms of cardiac insufficiency may develop at rest

Causes

Heart failure may result from a primary abnormality of the heart muscle (such as an infarction), inadequate myocardial perfusion due to coronary artery disease, or cardiomyopathy. Other causes include mechanical disturbances in ventricular filling during diastole when there's too little blood for the ventricle to pump, as in mitral stenosis secondary to rheumatic heart disease or constrictive pericarditis, atrial fibrillation, myocarditis, endocarditis, and other arrhythmias. Systolic hemodynamic disturbances — such as excessive cardiac workload due to volume overloading or pressure overload — that limit the heart's pumping ability, can also cause heart failure. Other precipitating causes include infection, anemia, thyrotoxicosis, and pregnancy. These disturbances can result in mitral or aortic insufficiency, which causes volume overloading, and aortic stenosis or systemic hypertension, which results in increased resistance to ventricular emptying.

Reduced cardiac output triggers three compensatory mechanisms — cardiac dilation, ventricular hypertrophy, and increased sympathetic activity. These mechanisms improve cardiac output at the expense of increased ventricular work.

In *cardiac dilation,* an increase in end-diastolic ventricular volume (preload) causes increased stroke work and stroke volume during contraction, stretching cardiac muscle fibers beyond optimal limits and producing pulmonary congestion and pulmonary hypertension, which lead in turn to right-sided heart failure.

In *ventricular hypertrophy,* an increase in muscle mass or the diameter of the left ventricle allows the heart to pump against increased resistance (impedance) to the outflow of blood; however, the increase in ventricular diastolic pressure needed to fill the enlarged ventricle may compromise diastolic coronary blood flow, limiting oxygen supply to the ventricle and causing ischemia and impaired myocardial contractility.

As a response to decreased cardiac output and blood pressure, *increased sympathetic activity* enhances peripheral vascular resistance, contractility, heart rate, and venous return.

Signs of increased sympathetic activity, such as cool extremities and clamminess, may indicate impending heart failure. Increased sympathetic activity also restricts blood flow to the kidneys, which respond by reducing the glomerular filtration rate and increasing tubular reabsorption of sodium and water, in turn expanding the circulating blood volume. This renal mechanism, if unchecked, can aggravate congestion and produce overt edema.

Chronic heart failure may worsen as a result of respiratory tract infections, pulmonary embolism, stress, increased sodium or water intake, and failure to comply with the prescribed treatment regimen.

Clinical presentation

Left-sided heart failure primarily produces pulmonary signs and symptoms; right-sided heart failure primarily produces systemic signs and symptoms. Heart failure commonly affects both sides of the heart.

Left-sided heart failure

Clinical signs of left-sided heart failure include dyspnea, orthopnea, paroxysmal nocturnal dyspnea, Cheyne-Stokes respirations, crackles, wheezing, hypoxia, respiratory acidosis, cough, cyanosis or pallor, palpitations, arrhythmias, elevated blood pressure, S_3 and S_4 heart sounds, and pulsus alternans.

Right-sided heart failure

Clinical signs of right-sided heart failure include dependent peripheral edema, hepatomegaly, splenomegaly, jugular vein distention (JVD), ascites, slow weight gain, arrhythmias, hepatojugular reflex, abdominal distention, nausea, vomiting, anorexia, jaundice, weakness, fatigue, dizziness, and syncope.

The patient history should elicit previous heart problems, difficulty

breathing, cardiac risk factors (smoking, diabetes, hypertension, dyslipidemia), family history of cardiac disorders, drug and alternative therapies tried, and patient response.

Examination focuses on perfusion.

▶ *General:* level of distress, blood pressure, weight
▶ *Head, eyes, ears, nose, and throat:* funduscopy, enlarged thyroid, JVD, or hepatojugular reflux
▶ *Skin:* color, diaphoresis, turgor
▶ *Chest:* tachycardia, tachypnea, crackles, extra heart sounds, murmurs, point of maximal impulse shifted left and down
▶ *Abdomen:* hepatomegaly, ascites
▶ *Extremities:* clubbing, cyanosis, edema

Differential diagnosis

▶ Asthma
▶ Chronic obstructive pulmonary disease
▶ Cirrhosis
▶ Hypertrophic cardiomyopathy
▶ MI
▶ Nephrotic syndrome or acute glomerulonephritis
▶ Pulmonary embolism
▶ Valvular disease
▶ Venous insufficiency

Diagnostic tests

▶ *Echocardiography* shows the size and function of ventricles, atria, pericardial effusion, valve deformities, shunts, and wall motions. It may, for instance, reveal left ventricular dysfunction with a reduced ejection fraction.
▶ *Electrocardiography* reflects heart strain, enlargement, and ischemia. It may also reveal left ventricular enlargement, tachycardia, and extrasystole.
▶ *Chest X-ray* shows increased pulmonary vascular markings, interstitial edema, pleural effusion, and cardiomegaly.

● *Pulmonary artery monitoring* typically demonstrates elevated pulmonary artery wedge pressures, left ventricular end-diastolic pressure in left-sided heart failure, and elevated right atrial pressure or central venous pressure in right-sided heart failure.

● *Urinalysis, blood urea nitrogen levels,* and *serum creatinine levels* reveal renal impairment.

● *Cardiac enzymes* detect MI.

● *Liver function tests* detect liver impairment.

● *Chemistry panel* reveals electrolyte imbalance (commonly due to drugs).

● *Thyroid-stimulating hormone levels* reveal thyroid dysfunction.

Management

General

The goal of therapy is to improve pump function by reversing the compensatory mechanisms that are producing the symptoms. Nonpharmacologic therapy consists of checking daily weights, restricting sodium (less than 2 g/day), and restricting fluids. Immunizations against influenza and pneumococcal pneumonia are strongly encouraged, as are lifestyle modifications to reduce symptoms of heart failure, such as weight loss if obese, smoking cessation, stress reduction, and an exercise program.

Surgery

Surgical options include cardiac transplantation for end-stage heart failure and ventricular surgery. A ventricular assist device (VAD) is commonly used while a patient waits for a heart transplant or for patients with end-stage heart failure. (See *VAD: Help for a failing heart.*)

Medication

● *Diuretics* (hydrochlorothiazide) reduce total blood volume in venous return and preload.

● *Angiotensin-converting enzyme inhibitors* for patients with left ventricular dysfunction reduce production of angiotensin II, resulting in preload and afterload reduction.

● *Cardiac glycosides* (digoxin) strengthen myocardial contractility.

● *Beta-adrenergic blockers* are used in patients with mild to moderate heart failure caused by left ventricular systolic dysfunction.

● *Diuretics, nitrates, morphine,* and *oxygen* treat pulmonary edema.

Collaborative practice

After diagnosis, refer the patient to a primary care provider or cardiologist for initial treatment, exacerbations, and also if he develops ischemic heart disease, arrhythmias, renal insufficiency, liver impairment, or anemia.

●●● **RED FLAG** *Refer the patient to a* ●●● *physician and medical treatment facility at once for suspected cardiogenic shock (severe hypotension, oliguria, change in mental status) or pulmonary edema with crackles and hypoxia.*

Follow-up

If treatment is initiated in the hospital, see the patient in 1 week. If the patient is treated in the office, contact him 1 day after an exacerbation; if his condition hasn't improved, consult a physician. If his condition has improved, see him every 1 to 2 weeks, depending on the clinical picture, until his symptoms have resolved and his weight goal has been met; afterward, see him monthly for 3 months and then quarterly.

Complications

● Arrhythmias
● Cerebral insufficiency
● Digoxin toxicity
● Pulmonary edema
● Renal insufficiency with severe electrolyte imbalance

▶ Venostasis with a predisposition to thromboembolism (associated primarily with prolonged bed rest)

Patient teaching

▶ Explain the rationale for checking daily weights, monitoring intake and output, and checking for peripheral edema.

▶ Advise the patient to schedule activities to allow adequate rest periods.

▶ Advise the patient to avoid foods high in sodium, such as canned or commercially prepared foods and dairy products, to curb fluid overload.

▶ Explain to the patient that the potassium he loses through diuretic therapy must be replaced by taking a prescribed potassium supplement and eating potassium-rich foods, such as bananas, apricots, and orange juice.

▶ Stress the need for regular follow-up care.

▶ Emphasize the importance of taking digoxin exactly as prescribed. Tell the patient to watch for and immediately report signs of toxicity, such as anorexia, vomiting, and yellow vision.

▶ Explain to the patient how supplemental oxygen and high Fowler's position will help him breathe more easily.

⦿⦿⦿ **RED FLAG** *Tell the patient to call the primary care provider to report pulse irregularities, dizziness, blurred vision, shortness of breath, persistent dry cough, palpitations, increased fatigue, paroxysmal nocturnal dyspnea, swollen ankles, decreased urine output, and rapid weight gain (more than 5 lb [2.3 kg] in a week).*

Resources

▶ American Heart Association: 1-800-AHA-USA-1; *www.americanheart.org*

VAD: HELP FOR A FAILING HEART

The ventricular assist device (VAD) functions somewhat like an artificial heart. The major difference is that the VAD assists the heart, whereas the artificial heart replaces it. The VAD is designed to aid one or both ventricles. The pumping chambers themselves aren't usually implanted in the patient.

The permanent VAD is implanted in the patient's chest cavity. Although a VAD usually provides only temporary support, in November 2002 the Food and Drug Administration approved the use of a left VAD as a permanent implant for terminally ill patients with end-stage heart failure who aren't eligible for a heart transplant. The device receives power through the skin by a belt of electrical transformer coils (worn externally as a portable battery pack). It can also operate off an implanted, rechargeable battery for up to 1 hour at a time.

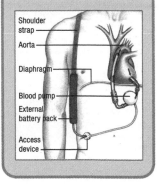

Shoulder strap
Aorta
Diaphragm
Blood pump
External battery pack
Access device

▶ National Heart, Lung, and Blood Institute: (301) 592-8573; *www.nhlbi.nih.gov*

COMPARING TYPES OF HEPATITIS

This chart compares the features of each type of viral hepatitis characterized to date.

Feature	Hepatitis A	Hepatitis B	Hepatitis C
Incubation	15 to 45 days	30 to 180 days	15 to 160 days
Onset	Acute	Insidious	Insidious
Age-group most affected	Children, young adults	Any age	More common in adults
Transmission	Fecal-oral, sexual (especially oral-anal contact), non-percutaneous (sexual, maternal-neonatal), percutaneous (rare)	Blood-borne; parenteral route, sexual, maternal-neonatal; virus is shed in all body fluids	Blood-borne; parenteral route
Severity	Mild	Commonly severe	Moderate
Prognosis	Generally good	Worsens with age and debility	Moderate
Progression to chronicity	None	Occasional	10% to 50% of cases

● For providers — Drug affordability: *www.needymeds.com* (contains information about many drug company programs that provide financial assistance to patients who need their drugs)

HEPATITIS, VIRAL

ICD-9-CM 070.9, type A 070.1, type B acute 070.30, type B chronic 070.32, type B with D 070.31, type C acute 070.51, type C chronic 070.54, type E 070.53, type E prophylaxis V05.3

A fairly common systemic disease, viral hepatitis is marked by hepatic cell destruction, necrosis, and autolysis, leading to anorexia, jaundice, and hepatomegaly. Hepatitis A (HAV) causes no chronic liver disease, and hepatitis E (HEV) is rare. Hepatitis B, C, and D (HBV, HCV, HDV, respectively) cause more severe symptoms plus an increased likelihood of persistent hepatitis and chronic disease, such as cirrho-

Hepatitis D	Hepatitis E	Hepatitis G
14 to 64 days	14 to 60 days	2 to 6 weeks
Acute	Acute	Presumed insidious
Any age	Ages 20 to 40	Any age, primarily adults
Parenteral route; most people infected with hepatitis D are also infected with hepatitis B	Primarily fecal-oral	Blood-borne; similar to Hepatitis B and C
Can be severe and lead to fulminant hepatitis	Highly virulent with common progression to fulminant hepatitis and hepatic failure, especially in pregnant patients	Moderate
Fair, worsens in chronic cases; can lead to chronic hepatitis D and chronic liver disease	Good unless pregnant	Generally good; no current treatment recommendations
Occasional	None	Not known; no association with chronic liver disease

sis and hepatocellular carcinoma. Advanced age and serious underlying disorders, such as human immunodeficiency virus, make complications more likely. The prognosis is poor if edema and hepatic encephalopathy develop.

Causes

The six major forms of viral hepatitis result from infection with the causative viruses: A, B, C, D, E, and G. (See *Comparing types of hepatitis*.)

Type A hepatitis

One third of all Americans have antibodies to HAV. This disease is highly contagious and is rising among those with immunosuppression related to human immunodeficiency virus infection. It's usually transmitted by the fecal-oral route. Rarely, it's transmitted parenterally. HAV usually results from ingestion of contaminated food, milk, or water. Outbreaks of HAV are usually traced to ingestion of seafood from polluted water.

Type B hepatitis

Chronic HBV affects about 1 million people in North America. Formerly thought to be transmitted only by direct exchange of contaminated blood or through sexual contact, HBV is now known to be transmitted by body secretions and feces. As a result, nurses, physicians, laboratory technicians, and dentists are frequently exposed to HBV, usually as a result of wearing defective gloves. Routine screening of donor blood for the hepatitis B surface antigen (HBsAg) has reduced the incidence of posttransfusion cases, but transmission by needles shared by drug abusers remains a major problem.

CLINICAL PEARL *Hepatitis B is considered a sexually transmitted disease because of its high incidence and ratio of transmission by this route.*

Type C hepatitis

Chronic HCV affects about 4 million people in North America — 20% of all hepatitis cases. Although the hepatitis C virus has been isolated, few patients have tested positive for it, perhaps reflecting the test's poor specificity. HCV is most commonly transmitted via transfused blood from asymptomatic donors. In up to 40% of patients, the mode of transmission is unknown.

CLINICAL PEARL *Most patients with HCV are asymptomatic. HCV is associated with a high rate of chronic liver disease (chronic hepatitis, cirrhosis, and an increased risk of hepatocellular carcinoma), which develops in 50% to 80% of those infected. People who have chronic HCV are considered infectious.*

Type D hepatitis

HDV occurs in 1% of patients with HBV but infects 50% of all who develop fulminant hepatitis, which is associated with a very high mortality. HDV is found only in patients with an acute or chronic episode of HBV and requires the presence of HBsAg. HDV depends on the double-shelled type B virus to replicate. For this reason, HDV infection requires prior infection with HBV. Thus, immunization against HBV also protects the patient from HDV. HDV is rare in the United States except in I.V. drug abusers.

Type E hepatitis

HEV is transmitted enterically, much like HAV. Because this virus is inconsistently shed in feces, detection is difficult.

CULTURAL KEY *HEV (formerly grouped with type C under the name non-A, non-B hepatitis) is uncommon in North America, occurring primarily in people who have recently returned from an endemic area, such as India, Africa, Asia, or Central America. It's more common in young adults and more severe in pregnant women.*

Type G hepatitis

Hepatitis G (HGV) appears to be transmitted much like HCV and frequently appears as a coinfection with HCV. Not much is known about HGV, but it appears to play a minor role in both acute and chronic hepatitis.

Clinical presentation

Assessment findings are similar for the different types of hepatitis. Typically, signs and symptoms progress in three stages: prodromal (preicteric), clinical (icteric), and recovery (posticteric).

Prodromal stage

In the prodromal stage, the patient typically complains of easy fatigue and anorexia (possibly with mild weight loss), generalized malaise, depression, headache, weakness, arthralgia, myalgia, photophobia, and nausea with vomiting. He may also describe changes in his senses of taste and smell.

Assessment of vital signs may reveal a fever of 100° to 102° F (37.8° to 38.9° C). As the prodromal stage draws to a close, usually 1 to 5 days before the onset of the clinical jaundice stage, inspection of urine and stool specimens may reveal dark-colored urine and clay-colored stools. The patient is most infectious in the 2 weeks prior to the appearance of jaundice.

Clinical stage

If the patient has progressed to the clinical jaundice stage, he may report pruritus, abdominal pain or tenderness, and indigestion. Early in this stage, he may complain of anorexia; later, his appetite may return. Inspection of the sclerae, mucous membranes, and skin may reveal jaundice, which can last for 1 to 2 weeks. Jaundice indicates that the damaged liver is unable to remove bilirubin from the blood; however, its presence doesn't indicate the severity of the disease. Jaundice typically appears shortly after the most acute phase passes. Occasionally, hepatitis occurs without jaundice.

During the clinical jaundice stage, inspection of the skin may detect rashes, erythematous patches, or urticaria, especially if the patient has HBV or HCV. Palpation may disclose abdominal tenderness in the right upper quadrant, an enlarged and tender liver and, sometimes, splenomegaly and cervical adenopathy.

Recovery stage

During the recovery stage, most of the patient's symptoms decrease or subside. On palpation, a decrease in liver enlargement may be noted. The recovery phase commonly lasts from 2 to 12 weeks, although sometimes this phase lasts longer in patients with HBV, HCV, or HEV.

Differential diagnosis

▸ Cytomegalovirus infection
▸ Drug- or alcohol-induced hepatitis
▸ Infectious mononucleosis
▸ Primary or secondary hepatic malignancy

Diagnostic tests

In suspected viral hepatitis, a hepatitis profile is routinely performed. This study identifies antibodies specific to the causative virus, establishing the type of hepatitis as follows:

▸ *Type A:* Detection of an antibody to HAV confirms the diagnosis (anti-HAV immunoglobulin [Ig] M [acute case] or IgG [previous exposure])

▸ *Type B:* The presence of HBsAg and HBV antibodies confirms the diagnosis. Anti-hepatitis B surface antigen (anti-HBsAg) and anti-hepatitis B core antigen (anti-HBcAg) IgM reveal the acute stage. IgG and anti-HBcAg reveal a chronic state.

▸ *Type C:* The diagnosis depends on serologic testing for the specific antibody (anti-HCV on enzyme-linked immunosorbent assay) 1 or more months after the onset of acute hepatitis. Until then, the diagnosis is established primarily by obtaining negative test results for HAV, HBV, and HDV. HCV ribonucleic acid (RNA) on polymerase chain reaction (PCR) is the most sensitive test for early stages but is revealed only intermittently in the chronic state.

▸ *Type D:* The detection of intrahepatic delta antigens or IgM antidelta antigens in acute disease (or IgM and IgG in chronic disease) establishes the diagnosis.

▸ *Type E:* IgM anti-HEV and IgG anti-HEV may be detected, but levels rapidly fall after acute infection resolves. These tests aren't routinely done.

▸ *Type G:* HGV RNA on PCR may be detected.

The following additional findings from liver function studies support the diagnosis.

▶ *Serum aspartate aminotransferase (AST)* and *serum alanine aminotransferase (ALT) levels* are increased in the prodromal stage of acute viral hepatitis.

▶ *Serum alkaline phosphatase levels* are slightly increased.

▶ *Serum bilirubin levels* are elevated. Levels may continue to be high late in the disease, especially in severe cases.

▶ *Prothrombin time* is prolonged. (More than 3 seconds longer than normal indicates severe liver damage.)

▶ *White blood cell counts* commonly reveal transient neutropenia and lymphopenia followed by lymphocytosis.

▶ *Urinalysis* may reveal protein, bilirubin, or both.

▶ *Liver biopsy* is performed if chronic hepatitis is suspected (diagnostic for type and reveals extent of liver damage, also required before starting interferon).

▶ *Ultrasound* may detect ascites or obstruction.

Management
Acute

▶ Report all newly diagnosed cases to the local health authorities.

▶ Correct coagulation defects, fluid and electrolyte imbalances, acid-base imbalance, hypoglycemia, and impaired renal function.

▶ Administer supplemental vitamins and commercial feedings. If symptoms are severe and the patient can't tolerate oral intake, provide I.V. therapy and parenteral nutrition.

▶ Record the patient's weight daily, and keep intake and output records. Note changes in stool color, consistency, and amount as well as frequency of bowel movements.

▶ Watch for signs of fluid shift, such as weight gain and orthostasis.

▶ Watch for signs of hepatic coma, dehydration, pneumonia, vascular problems, and pressure ulcers.

▶ In fulminant hepatitis, maintain electrolyte balance and a patent airway, prevent infections, and control bleeding. Correct hypoglycemia and other complications while awaiting liver regeneration and repair.

▶ Protein intake should be reduced if signs of precoma — lethargy, confusion, and mental changes — develop. Large meals are usually better tolerated in the morning because many patients experience nausea late in the day.

▶ In acute viral hepatitis, hospitalization usually is required only for patients with severe symptoms or complications. Parenteral nutrition may be required if the patient experiences persistent vomiting and is unable to maintain oral intake.

Medications

No specific drug therapy has been developed for hepatitis, with the exception of HBV and HCV, which have been treated somewhat successfully with interferon alfa. Instead, the patient is advised to rest in the early stages of the illness and to combat anorexia by eating small, high-calorie, high-protein meals.

Antiemetics may be given one half-hour before meals to relieve nausea and prevent vomiting; phenothiazines have a cholestatic effect and should be avoided. For severe pruritus, the resin cholestyramine may be given.

Collaborative practice

Refer patients with a positive diagnosis as well as all cases of acute hepatitis, to a gastroenterologist or another physician for evaluation and treatment.

Follow-up

See the patient regularly (exact frequency depends on the clinical picture) and monitor diagnostic tests (serial measurements of serum AST and ALT; serum viral markers as indicated; chemistry panel to detect metabolic complications; complete blood count [platelets if taking interferon]; and liver biopsy). In HCV, HCV-RNA levels monitor the patient's response to treatment; if results are negative after 3 months, an elevated sustained response is likely. In HBV, HBeAg levels indicate increased viral replication and thus an increased viral load. High HBeAg levels are also associated with an increased risk of transmission.

Complications

▶ Hepatic failure
▶ Hepatitis (chronic active or chronic)
▶ Hepatocellular malignancy (HBV, HCV)
▶ Necrosis (acute or subacute)

Patient teaching

▶ Use enteric precautions when caring for patients with HAV or HEV hepatitis. Practice standard precautions for all patients.
▶ Inform the patient and his family about isolation precautions.
▶ Instruct the patient to allow rest periods throughout the day. He can gradually add activities to his schedule as he begins to recover.
▶ Encourage the patient to eat small, frequent, balanced meals, and encourage plenty of calories and foods high in vitamin K (green, leafy vegetables).
▶ Encourage fluids (at least 4,000 ml daily). Encourage the anorectic patient to drink fruit juices. Chipped ice and effervescent soft drinks can hydrate without inducing vomiting.
▶ Explain the disease process, symptoms, treatment, pros and cons of drugs, and how to prevent

transmission. Strongly recommend abstaining from alcohol and medications metabolized by the liver, such as acetaminophen and ibuprofen. Explain to female patients that, because hormonal contraceptives tend to increase bilirubin levels, they should consider an alternative form of contraception.

●●● RED FLAG *Tell the patient to call*
●●● *the primary care provider to report new or persistent signs and symptoms, including personality changes (disorientation, forgetfulness, slurred speech), slight tremor, lethargy, and abnormal movements of wrists and fingers (asterixis).*

Resources

▶ American Liver Foundation (Hepatitis): 1-888-443-7872; *www.liverfoundation.org*
▶ Hepatitis Foundation International: 1-800-891-0707; *www.hepfi.org*
▶ Hepatitis B Foundation: (215) 489-4900; *www.hepb.org*

HUMAN IMMUNODEFICIENCY VIRUS

ICD-9-CM HIV or AIDS 042, HIV-2 079.53

Currently one of the most widely publicized diseases, acquired immunodeficiency syndrome (AIDS) is marked by progressive failure of the immune system. Although it's characterized by gradual destruction of cell-mediated (T-cell) immunity, it also affects humoral immunity and even autoimmunity because of the central role of the CD4$^+$ T lymphocyte in immune reactions. The resultant immunodeficiency makes the patient susceptible to opportunistic infections, unusual cancers, and other abnormalities that define AIDS.

This syndrome was first described by the Centers for Disease Control and Prevention (CDC) in 1981.

Since then, the CDC has declared a case surveillance definition for AIDS and has modified it several times in recent years.

A retrovirus — the human immunodeficiency virus (HIV) type I — is the primary etiologic agent. Transmission of HIV occurs by contact with infected blood or body fluids and is associated with identifiable high-risk behaviors. It's therefore disproportionately represented in homosexual and bisexual men, I.V. drug users, neonates of HIV-infected women, recipients of contaminated blood or blood products (dramatically decreased since the mid-1980s), and heterosexual partners of persons in the former groups. Because of similar routes of transmission, AIDS shares epidemiologic patterns with hepatitis B and sexually transmitted diseases (STDs).

The natural history of AIDS infection begins with infection by the HIV retrovirus, which is detectable only by laboratory tests, and ends with the severely immunocompromised, terminal stage of this disease. Depending on individual variations and the presence of cofactors that influence progression, the time elapsed from acute HIV infection to the appearance of symptoms (mild to severe) to the diagnosis of AIDS and, eventually, to death varies greatly.

❋ **LIFE SPAN** *HIV is predominantly found in young people, with most cases involving those between ages 17 and 55; however, it has also been reported in elderly men and women. In the United States, AIDS is the fifth leading cause of death among people ages 25 to 44 and is the leading cause of death for black men in this age group.*

Causes

AIDS results from infection with HIV, which strikes cells bearing the CD4+ antigen; the latter (normally a receptor for major histocompatibility complex molecules) serves as a receptor for the retrovirus and lets it enter the cell. HIV prefers to infect the CD4+ lymphocyte or macrophage but may also infect other CD4+ antigen-bearing cells of the GI tract, uterine cervical cells, and neuroglial cells. The virus gains access by binding to the CD4+ molecule on the cell surface along with a coreceptor (thought to be the chemokine receptor CCR5).

After invading a cell, HIV replicates, leading to cell death, or becomes latent. HIV infection leads to profound pathology, either directly — through destruction of CD4+ cells, other immune cells, and neuroglial cells — or indirectly — through the secondary effects of CD4+ T-cell dysfunction and resultant immunosuppression.

The infection process takes three forms:

▶ *immunodeficiency*: opportunistic infections and unusual cancers

▶ *autoimmunity*: lymphoid interstitial pneumonitis, arthritis, hypergammaglobulinemia, and production of autoimmune antibodies

▶ *neurologic dysfunction:* AIDS dementia complex, HIV encephalopathy, and peripheral neuropathies.

HIV is transmitted by direct inoculation during intimate sexual contact, especially associated with the mucosal trauma of receptive rectal intercourse; transfusion of contaminated blood or blood products (a risk diminished by routine testing of all blood products); sharing of contaminated needles; or transplacental or postpartum transmission from infected mother to fetus (by cervical or blood contact at delivery and in breast milk).

Accumulating evidence suggests that HIV isn't transmitted by casual household or social contact. The average time between exposure to the virus and diagnosis of AIDS is 8 to 10 years, but shorter and longer incubation times have also been recorded.

Clinical presentation

HIV infection manifests itself in many ways. After a high-risk exposure and inoculation, the infected person usually experiences a mononucleosis-like syndrome, which may be attributed to a flu or other virus and then may remain asymptomatic for years. In this latent stage, the only sign of HIV infection is laboratory evidence of seroconversion.

When symptoms appear, they may take many forms.

▶ Persistent generalized adenopathy
▶ Nonspecific symptoms (weight loss, fatigue, night sweats, fevers)
▶ Neurologic symptoms resulting from HIV encephalopathy
▶ Opportunistic infection or cancer

❈ **LIFE SPAN** *The clinical course varies slightly in children with AIDS. Their incubation time is apparently shorter, with a mean of 17 months. Signs and symptoms resemble those of adults, except for findings related to STDs. Children show virtually all of the opportunistic infections observed in adults, with a higher incidence of bacterial infections: otitis media, sepsis, chronic salivary gland enlargement, lymphoid interstitial pneumonia,* Mycobacterium avium *complex function, and pneumonias, including* Pneumocystis carinii.

The patient history may reveal fevers, night sweats, diarrhea, weight loss, lymphadenopathy, frequent candidal infections, difficulty swallowing, mental status changes, visual changes, and severe headaches. Find out the patient's reason for being tested, current high-risk behaviors, past diagnosis

of and treatment for tuberculosis (TB) and hepatitis, and immunization history.

Examination focuses on signs of infection, malignancy, and neurologic involvement.

▶ *General:* fever, lymphadenopathy
▶ *Abdomen:* hepatomegaly, splenomegaly
▶ *Anogenital:* STDs, neoplasia (high risk for cervical carcinoma)
▶ *Chest:* pneumonia, cardiomyopathy
▶ *Central nervous system (CNS):* mental status changes, other CNS involvement
▶ *Head, eyes, ears, nose, and throat:* retinopathy, oral lesions
▶ *Skin:* lesions, including infectious types such as herpes, autoimmune types such as psoriasis, and neoplastic types such as Kaposi's sarcoma

Differential diagnosis

▶ Prolonged illness without ready explanation
▶ Dependent on the stage of HIV infection

Diagnostic tests

The CDC defines AIDS as an illness characterized by one or more "indicator" diseases coexisting with laboratory evidence of HIV infection and other possible causes of immunosuppression. The CDC's current AIDS surveillance case definition requires laboratory confirmation of HIV infection in people who have a $CD4^+$ T-cell count of 200 cells/µl or who have an associated clinical condition or disease.

▶ The most commonly performed tests, antibody tests, indicate HIV infection indirectly by revealing HIV antibodies. The recommended protocol requires initial screening of individuals and blood products with an enzyme-linked immunosorbent assay (ELISA). A positive ELISA test should be repeated and then confirmed by an alternate method, usually the Western blot or an immunofluorescence assay; however, antibody testing isn't always reliable. Because the body takes a variable amount of time to produce a detectable level of antibodies, a "window" varying from a few weeks to as long as 35 months (in one documented case) allows an HIV-infected person to test negative for HIV antibodies.

▶ Antibody tests are also unreliable in neonates because transferred maternal antibodies persist for 6 to 10 months. To overcome these problems, direct testing is performed to detect HIV. Direct tests include antigen tests (p24 antigen), HIV cultures, nucleic acid probes of peripheral blood lymphocytes with determination of HIV-1 ribonucleic acid levels, and the polymerase chain reaction (PCR).

▶ Additional tests to support the diagnosis and help evaluate the severity of immunosuppression include CD4$^+$ and CD8$^+$ T-cell subset counts, erythrocyte sedimentation rate, complete blood cell count, serum beta$_2$-microglobulin, p24 antigen, neopterin levels, and anergy testing. Because many opportunistic infections in AIDS patients are reactivations of previous infections, patients are also tested for syphilis, hepatitis B, tuberculosis, toxoplasmosis and, in some areas, histoplasmosis. When diagnosed with HIV, other needed screening tests include cytomegalovirus (CMV) titer, Papanicolaou (Pap) test, and chest X-ray to detect cancer.

Management
Acute
Treat new interstitial pneumonitis, severe vomiting, or diarrhea with dehydration. Neurologic manifestations require intensive supportive treatment.

General
Be aware that a diagnosis of AIDS is profoundly distressing because of the disease's social impact and the discouraging prognosis. The patient may lose his job and financial security as well as the support of his family and friends. Coping with an altered body image, the emotional burden of serious illness, and the threat of death may overwhelm the patient.

Patients engaging in unprotected sex need family counseling as well as transmission counseling. Zidovudine (AZT) taken by the mother during pregnancy has decreased vertical transmission but not completely. The probability of a child losing a parent early in life is also an issue.

Medication
No cure has yet been found for AIDS; however, primary therapy for HIV infection includes three types of antiretroviral agents:

▶ *protease inhibitors (PIs)*, such as ritonavir, indinavir, nelfinavir, and saquinavir

▶ *nucleoside reverse transcriptase inhibitors (NRTIs)*, such as zidovudine, didanosine, zalcitabine, lamivudine, and stavudine

▶ *nonnucleoside reverse transcriptase inhibitors (NNRTIs)*, such as nevirapine and delavirdine.

HIV treatment is undergoing change so rapidly that new drugs and new information may substantially alter treatment guidelines; however, the founding principles that guide treatment will probably still be applicable. The antiretrovirals, used in various combinations, are designed to inhibit HIV viral replication. Other potential therapies include immunomodulatory agents designed to boost the weakened immune system and anti-infective and antineoplastic agents to combat opportunistic infections and associated cancers. Some of these drugs are used prophylactically to help patients resist opportunistic infections.

Current treatment protocols combine two or more agents in an effort to gain the maximum benefit with the fewest adverse reactions. Such regimens typically include one PI plus two NRTIs or one NNRTI plus two NRTIs for persons unable to tolerate a PI or who develop lipodystrophy (abnormal fat distribution). Many variations and drug interactions are being studied. Combination therapy helps inhibit the production of resistant, mutant strains. The drug regimen is changed when the patient develops drug toxicity or intolerable adverse effects, or when treatment fails (as indicated by development of opportunistic infections, increasing viral load, or decreasing T-cell count). To prevent cross-resistance, all drugs must be stopped simultaneously when resistance develops to one drug.

Supportive treatments help maintain nutritional status as well as relieve pain and other distressing physical and psychological symptoms. Many pathogens in AIDS respond to anti-infective drugs but tend to recur after treatment ends. For this reason, most patients need continuous anti-infective treatment, presumably for life or until the drug is no longer tolerated or effective.

Recommended immunizations are pneumonia vaccine, influenza vaccine, tuberculosis booster, and hepatitis B vaccine.

✿ **LIFE SPAN** *Administer inactivated polio virus to children.*

✿ **LIFE SPAN** *AZT is commonly combined with other agents such as lamivudine, but it has also been used as a single agent for pregnant HIV-positive women.*

Collaborative practice

Refer the patient to an infectious disease or HIV/AIDS specialist after diagnosis for evaluation and initial treatment plan as well as for signs of drug failure (opportunistic infection, increasing viral load, decreasing T-cell count). The patient may need to see a neurologist or neurosurgeon for intracranial lesions, a gastroenterologist for intractable diarrhea or painful swallowing not responsive to antifungal drugs, a pulmonologist for interstitial pneumonitis, social services for financial and home care needs, and a psychologist or psychiatrist for counseling and developing coping mechanisms.

Follow-up

See the patient initially every 3 months for viral load and CD4$^+$ count. At each visit, check for shortness of breath, dyspnea on exertion (*Pneumocystis carinii* pneumonia), diarrhea, fever, night sweats (TB), odynophagia (oral cavity or esophageal candidiasis), neurologic manifestations (infection, cancer, or dementia), and visual changes (retinitis due to CMV). Increase frequency as indicated by clinical picture. Women need a pelvic examination and Pap test every 6 months due to the high risk of cervical carcinoma. Patients on AZT need a complete blood count and liver function tests every 3 months as well.

Complications

The many possible complications include opportunistic infections and cancers, meningoencephalitis, neuropsychiatric manifestations, thrombocytopenia, wasting syndrome, and premature death. (See *Opportunistic infections in AIDS*, page 230.)

OPPORTUNISTIC INFECTIONS IN AIDS

This chart shows the complicating infections that may occur in acquired immunodeficiency syndrome (AIDS).

Microbiological agent	Organism	Condition
Protozoa	*Pneumocystis carinii* *Cryptosporidium* *Toxoplasma gondii* *Histoplasma*	Pneumocystosis Cryptosporidiosis Toxoplasmosis Histoplasmosis
Fungi	*Candida albicans* *Cryptococcus neoformans*	Candidiasis Cryptococcosis
Viruses	Herpes Cytomegalovirus (CMV)	Herpes simplex 1 and 2 CMV retinitis
Bacteria	*Mycobacterium tuberculosis* *Mycobacterium avium*	Tuberculosis *M. avium* complex

Note: Other opportunistic conditions include Kaposi's sarcoma, wasting syndrome, and AIDS dementia complex.

Patient teaching

● Emphasize that combination antiretroviral therapy aims for maximum suppression of HIV replication, thereby improving survival. Poor drug compliance leads to drug resistance and treatment failure. Patients must understand that medication regimens must be followed closely and may be required for many years, if not throughout life.
● Stress the importance of notifying those who may have been infected.
● Encourage safer sex practices.
● Emphasize that needles must not be shared.
● Stress the importance of good nutrition, vitamin supplements, and regular exercise in maintaining health.
● Advise the patient never to eat raw or possibly contaminated food.
● Inform the patient of national and local support groups and services.

● Explain treatment options, including how drugs work, expected adverse effects, dosage scheduling, and monitoring needed.

●●● RED FLAG *Tell the patient to call the primary care provider to report signs and symptoms of infection or cancer (fever higher than 101° F [38.3° C], cloudy or colored discharge, nonhealing wound, chills, weight loss, increasing fatigue, enlarged lymph nodes, mouth sores or painful swallowing, cough, dyspnea, visual changes, headaches, increasing congestion [particularly with purulent drainage], or rash); vomiting or diarrhea with signs of dehydration (fewer than three voidings in 24 hours; dark, concentrated, urine with strong odor; constant thirst; skin tenting); change in mental status or depression; intolerable drug adverse effects; and possible pregnancy.*

Resources

▶ National AIDS Hotline: 1-800-342-2437; Spanish: 1-800-344-7432

▶ For consumers and providers (site sponsored by the Food and Drug Administration) — Texas AIDS Health Fraud Information Network: 1-800-758-5152; *www.tahfin.org*

▶ For providers — Drug affordability: *www.needymeds.com* (contains information regarding many drug company programs that provide financial assistance for their drugs)

▶ National Nonoccupational HIV Postexposure Prophylaxis (PEP) Registry (collects data [without use of identifying data] about type of exposure, decision to use or not use PEP, drugs taken, risk-reduction referrals made, and results of HIV testing): 1-877-448-1737; *www. hivpepregistry.org*

HYPERTENSION

ICD-9-CM essential 401.1
An intermittent or sustained elevation in diastolic or systolic blood pressure, hypertension affects more than 20% of adults in the United States. If untreated, it carries a high mortality.

Hypertension is a major cause of stroke, cardiac disease, and renal failure; however, the prognosis is good if this disorder is detected early and if treatment begins before complications develop.

Causes

Hypertension occurs as two major types: essential (primary) and secondary. The cause of essential hypertension is unknown but commonly accompanies the risk factors for cardiovascular disease. (See *Cardiovascular disease risk factors.*)

Causes of secondary hypertension include coarctation of the aorta; renal artery stenosis and parenchymal disease; brain tumor; pheochromo-

---

CARDIOVASCULAR DISEASE RISK FACTORS

Major risk factors

▶ Hypertension
▶ Cigarette smoking
▶ Obesity (body mass index ≥ 30)
▶ Physical inactivity
▶ Dyslipidemia
▶ Diabetes mellitus
▶ Microalbuminuria
▶ Age (younger than age 55 for men, younger than age 65 for women)
▶ Family history of cardiovascular disease

Target organ damage or clinical cardiovascular disease

▶ Heart diseases
 – Left ventricular hypertrophy
 – Angina or prior myocardial infarction
 – Prior coronary revascularization
 – Heart failure
▶ Stroke or transient ischemic attack
▶ Nephropathy
▶ Peripheral arterial disease
▶ Retinopathy

Adapted from the National Heart, Lung, and Blood Institute. *The Seventh Report of the Joint National Committee on Prevention, Detection, Evaluation and Treatment of High Blood Pressure (JNC 7).* Bethesda, Md.: National Institutes of Health, 2003. Pub. #03-5231.

---

cytoma; Cushing's syndrome; thyroid, pituitary or parathyroid dysfunction; and primary aldosteronism.

CULTURAL KEY *Hypertension is most common in blacks.*

Blood pressure regulation
Increased blood volume, cardiac rate, and stroke volume as well as

arteriolar vasoconstriction can raise blood pressure. The link to sustained hypertension, however, is unclear. Hypertension may also result from the failure of the following intrinsic regulatory mechanisms.

▶ *Renal hypoperfusion* causes the release of renin, which is converted by angiotensinogen, a liver enzyme, to angiotensin I. Angiotensin I is converted to angiotensin II, a powerful vasoconstrictor. The resulting vasoconstriction increases afterload.

▶ *Angiotensin II* stimulates adrenal secretion of aldosterone, which increases sodium reabsorption. Hypertonic-stimulated release of anti-diuretic hormone from the pituitary gland follows, increasing water reabsorption, plasma volume, cardiac output, and blood pressure.

▶ *Autoregulation* changes the diameter of an artery to maintain perfusion despite fluctuations in systemic blood pressure. The intrinsic mechanisms that are responsible include stress relaxation, in which vessels gradually dilate when blood pressure rises to reduce peripheral resistance and capillary fluid shift, in which plasma moves between vessels and extravascular spaces to maintain intravascular volume.

▶ When the blood pressure drops, *baroreceptors* in the aortic arch and carotid sinuses decrease their inhibition of the medulla's vasomotor center, which increases sympathetic stimulation of the heart by norepinephrine. This, in turn, increases cardiac output by strengthening the contractile force, increasing the heart rate, and augmenting peripheral resistance by vasoconstriction.

▶ *Stress* can also stimulate the sympathetic hormones, which increases cardiac output and peripheral vascular resistance.

Clinical presentation

Serial blood pressure measurements greater than 140/90 mm Hg confirm hypertension. In those with a high cardiac risk profile, serial readings greater than 135/80 mm Hg confirm hypertension. (See *Classifying blood pressure readings*.) Auscultation may reveal bruits over the abdominal aorta and the carotid, renal, and femoral arteries; ophthalmoscopy reveals arteriovenous nicking and, in hypertensive encephalopathy, papilledema.

Hypertension is known as the "silent killer" because it usually produces no symptoms until significant damage has occurred. Highly elevated blood pressure damages the intima of small vessels, resulting in fibrin accumulation in the vessels, local edema and, possibly, intravascular clotting.

Symptoms produced by this process depend on the location of the damaged vessels or the target organ.

▶ *Brain:* stroke, transient ischemic attack
▶ *Retina:* blindness
▶ *Heart:* myocardial infarction (MI)
▶ *Kidneys:* proteinuria, edema and, eventually, renal failure

Hypertension increases the heart's workload, causing left ventricular hypertrophy. Progressive damage causes left- and right-sided heart failure and pulmonary edema.

Differential diagnosis

▶ Coarctation of the aorta
▶ Cushing's syndrome
▶ Drug reaction
▶ Hypertension (primary and secondary)
▶ Hyperthyroidism
▶ Neurologic disorder
▶ Pheochromocytoma
▶ Primary aldosteronism
▶ Renal disease

CLASSIFYING BLOOD PRESSURE READINGS

In 2003, the National Institutes of Health issued *The Seventh Report of the Joint National Committee on Prevention, Detection, Evaluation, and Treatment of High Blood Pressure* (*The JNC 7 Report*). Updates since *The JNC 6* report include a new category, prehypertension, and the combining of stages 2 and 3 hypertension. Categories now are normal, prehypertension, and stages 1 and 2 hypertension.

The revised categories are based on the average of two or more readings taken on separate visits after an initial screening. They apply to adults ages 18 and older. (If the systolic and diastolic pressures fall into different categories, use the higher of the two pressures to classify the reading. For example, a reading of 160/92 mm Hg should be classified as stage 2.)

Normal blood pressure with respect to cardiovascular risk is a systolic reading below 120 mm Hg and a diastolic reading below 80 mm Hg. Patients with prehypertension are at increased risk for developing hypertension and should follow health-promoting lifestyle modifications to prevent cardiovascular disease.

In addition to classifying stages of hypertension based on average blood pressure readings, clinicians should also take note of target organ disease and additional risk factors, such as a patient with diabetes, left ventricular hypertrophy, and chronic renal disease. This additional information is important to obtain a true picture of the patient's cardiovascular health.

Category	Systolic		Diastolic
Normal	< 120 mm Hg	AND	< 80 mm Hg
Prehypertension	120 to 139 mm Hg	OR	80 to 89 mm Hg
Hypertension Stage 1	140 to 159 mm Hg	OR	90 to 99 mm Hg
Stage 2	≥ 160 mm Hg	OR	≥ 100 mm Hg

Diagnostic tests

▶ On *urinalysis,* moderate and higher proteinuria indicates kidney disease.
▶ *Complete blood count* baseline is done for comparison.
▶ *Electrolytes* may indicate adrenal dysfunction.
▶ *Fasting blood glucose* detects diabetes, an additional cardiac risk.
▶ Elevations in *blood urea nitrogen* and *serum creatinine levels* indicate renal disease.
▶ *Lipid panel* detects additional cardiac risk factors.

▶ *Electrocardiography* detects left ventricular hypertrophy or ischemia.
▶ *Chest X-ray* is done if cardiomegaly is suspected.
▶ *Excretory urography* is performed if renal atrophy and unilateral renal disease are suspected.

Management
Acute

●●●
●●● **RED FLAG** *For signs of hypertensive crisis (blood pressure exceeding 180/100 mm Hg), hypertensive encephalopathy, intracranial*

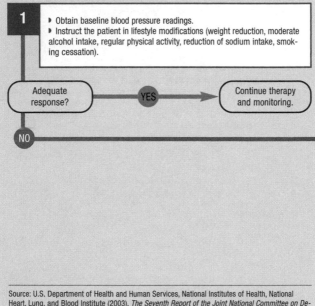

CLINICAL PEARL
MANAGING ANTIHYPERTENSIVE THERAPY

This flowchart is based on the approach to antihypertensive therapy endorsed by the Joint National Committee on the Detection, Evaluation, and Treatment of High Blood Pressure.

Diagnosis of hypertension suspected and confirmed

1
▶ Obtain baseline blood pressure readings.
▶ Instruct the patient in lifestyle modifications (weight reduction, moderate alcohol intake, regular physical activity, reduction of sodium intake, smoking cessation).

Adequate response? — **YES** → Continue therapy and monitoring.

NO

Source: U.S. Department of Health and Human Services, National Institutes of Health, National Heart, Lung, and Blood Institute (2003). *The Seventh Report of the Joint National Committee on Detection, Evaluation, and Treatment of High Blood Pressure (JNC 7).* Bethesda, Md.: National Institutes of Health, 2003. Pub. #03-5231.

hemorrhage, unstable angina, acute MI, acute left ventricular failure with pulmonary edema, dissecting aortic aneurysm, eclampsia, or signs associated with optic disk edema or progressive organ damage, treat blood pressure immediately with parenteral or oral drugs. Typically, hypertensive emergencies require parenteral administration of a vasodilator or an adrenergic inhib-

itor, or oral administration of a selected drug — such as nifedipine, captopril, clonidine, or labetalol — to rapidly reduce blood pressure. Have the patient take the drug in the office, and then recheck in 1 hour. If there's no response, refer him to the emergency department.

General
Encourage the patient diagnosed with hypertension to track and

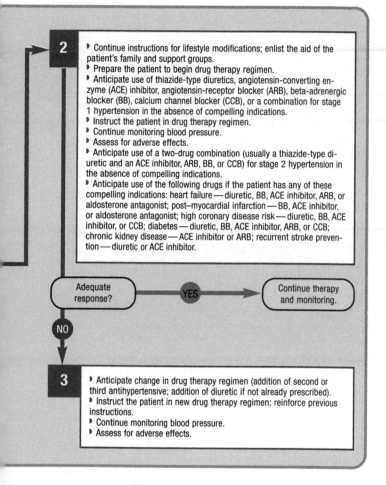

2
- Continue instructions for lifestyle modifications; enlist the aid of the patient's family and support groups.
- Prepare the patient to begin drug therapy regimen.
- Anticipate use of thiazide-type diuretics, angiotensin-converting enzyme (ACE) inhibitor, angiotensin-receptor blocker (ARB), beta-adrenergic blocker (BB), calcium channel blocker (CCB), or a combination for stage 1 hypertension in the absence of compelling indications.
- Instruct the patient in drug therapy regimen.
- Continue monitoring blood pressure.
- Assess for adverse effects.
- Anticipate use of a two-drug combination (usually a thiazide-type diuretic and an ACE inhibitor, ARB, BB, or CCB) for stage 2 hypertension in the absence of compelling indications.
- Anticipate use of the following drugs if the patient has any of these compelling indications: heart failure — diuretic, BB, ACE inhibitor, ARB, or aldosterone antagonist; post–myocardial infarction — BB, ACE inhibitor, or aldosterone antagonist; high coronary disease risk — diuretic, BB, ACE inhibitor, or CCB; diabetes — diuretic, BB, ACE inhibitor, ARB, or CCB; chronic kidney disease — ACE inhibitor or ARB; recurrent stroke prevention — diuretic or ACE inhibitor.

Adequate response? — YES → Continue therapy and monitoring.

NO

3
- Anticipate change in drug therapy regimen (addition of second or third antihypertensive; addition of diuretic if not already prescribed).
- Instruct the patient in new drug therapy regimen; reinforce previous instructions.
- Continue monitoring blood pressure.
- Assess for adverse effects.

record his daily blood pressure at home and to bring the written record to the office on each visit. Home monitoring lets the patient check early morning blood pressure, which is usually the highest, and detects "white-coat hypertension" (readings that are higher in the health care provider's office).

Medication

The National Institutes of Health has developed an algorithm for treatment of hypertension based on *The Seventh Report of the Joint National Committee on Prevention, Detection, Evaluation and Treatment of High Blood Pressure.* (See *Managing antihypertensive therapy.* See also *Compelling indications for in-*

COMPELLING INDICATIONS FOR INDIVIDUAL DRUG CLASSES IN HYPERTENSION TREATMENT

In 2003, the National Institutes of Health issued *The Seventh Report of the Joint National Committee on Prevention, Detection, Evaluation and Treatment of High Blood Pressure.* Patients with hypertension and specific compelling indications may require combination therapy with two or more antihypertensive medications from different drug classes to achieve their blood pressure goal. The addition of another drug from a different class is initiated when blood pressure control isn't achieved with a single agent.

This chart lists compelling indications with their initial therapy options.

Compelling indication	Initial therapy options
Heart failure	Thiazide diuretic, beta-adrenergic blocker, angiotensin-converting enzyme (ACE) inhibitor, angiotensin receptor blocker, aldosterone antagonist
Post–myocardial infarction	Beta-adrenergic blocker, ACE inhibitor, aldosterone antagonist
High cardiovascular disease risk	Thiazide diuretic, beta-adrenergic blocker, ACE inhibitor, calcium channel blocker
Diabetes	Thiazide diuretic, beta-adrenergic blocker, ACE inhibitor, angiotensin receptor blocker, calcium channel blocker
Chronic kidney disease	ACE inhibitor, angiotensin receptor blocker
Recurrent stroke prevention	Thiazide diuretic, ACE inhibitor

Adapted from: U.S. Department of Health and Human Services. National Institutes of Health. *The Seventh Report of the Joint National Committee on Prevention, Detection, Evaluation, and Treatment of High Blood Pressure.* 2003. Pub. #03-5231.

dividual drug classes in hypertension treatment.)

Collaborative practice

Refer the patient to a physician or medical treatment facility if blood pressure is above 180/110 mm Hg to prevent end-organ damage. Refer him to a cardiologist (depending on risk factors) if blood pressure is higher than 160/100 mm Hg and he has cardiac risk factors. Follow up within 3 days. Refer him to a nephrologist or urologist for indications of primary or secondary renal pathology. Refer him to an endocrinologist for endocrine disorders and to another physician for abnormal electrocardiogram.

Follow-up

Follow up every 2 weeks until the patient is stable, then every 3 months for 1 year. If the goal blood pressure is maintained for 1 year, consider reducing or eliminating drugs while continuing lifestyle modifications. Follow up at least every 3 to 6 months, focusing on behavior and drug compliance, adverse reactions, and quality of life issues (impotence, fatigue). Schedule annual urinalysis and creatinine, potassium, and glucose levels to monitor kidney function and detect diabetes.

Complications

▶ Heart failure
▶ Hypertensive heart disease
▶ MI
▶ Renal failure
▶ Stroke

Patient teaching

▶ Help the patient examine and modify his lifestyle, such as by reducing stress and exercising regularly.
▶ To increase compliance, suggest a daily routine for taking drugs.
▶ Warn the patient that uncontrolled hypertension may cause stroke and heart attack. Stress that the goal of treatment is to prevent morbidity and mortality.
▶ Stress the importance of reporting adverse reactions so drugs can be changed or adjusted to minimize the impact on quality of life.
▶ Stress the importance of smoking cessation.
▶ Emphasize the importance of curbing daily alcohol intake (2 oz hard liquor, 24 oz beer, or 10 oz wine).
▶ Encourage progressive aerobic exercise, for example, working up to 45 minutes five times weekly.
▶ Advise the patient to avoid high-sodium antacids and over-the-counter cold and sinus medications, which contain vasoconstrictors.
▶ Tailor diet to the patient's needs — for example, weight reduction or low saturated fat and cholesterol — as indicated. Urge all patients to avoid high-sodium foods (pickles, potato chips, condiments, dried meats, canned soups, cold cuts) and not to add salt to food.

Explain the importance of getting the recommended daily allowance of potassium and magnesium.
▶ Have the patient keep a record of blood pressure measurements and of drugs used in the past, noting their effectiveness, and bring this record to each visit.

●●● RED FLAG *Tell the patient to call* **●●●** *the primary care provider to report new or persistent signs and symptoms, including signs and symptoms of stroke or MI (severe headache, slurred speech, dizziness, weakness on one side of the body, shortness of breath, excessive sweating and chest pain or pressure that may or may not radiate up to the jaw, neck, or arm). Also tell the patient to call the primary care provider if he can't tolerate the adverse effects of the medications.*

Resources

▶ American Heart Association: 1-800-AHA-USA-1; *www.americanheart.org*
▶ National Kidney Foundation: 1-800-622-9010; *www.kidney.org*
▶ For providers — Drug affordability: *www.needymeds.com* (contains information regarding many drug company programs that provide financial assistance for their drugs)

HYPOTHYROIDISM

ICD-9-CM primary 244.9, postsurgical 244.0
Hypothyroidism, a state of low serum thyroid hormone, results from hypothalamic, pituitary, or thyroid insufficiency. The disorder can progress to life-threatening myxedema coma.

Causes

Hypothyroidism results from inadequate production of thyroid hormone, usually from dysfunction of the thyroid gland due to surgery (thyroidectomy), irradiation therapy, inflammation, chronic autoimmune thyroiditis (Hashimoto's disease) or, rarely, such conditions as amyloidosis and sarcoidosis. It may also result from pituitary failure to produce thyroid-stimulating hormone (TSH), hypothalamic failure to produce thyrotropin-releasing hormone, inborn errors of thyroid hormone synthesis, inability to synthesize thyroid hormone because of iodine deficiency (rare in the United States), or the use of antithyroid drugs such as propylthiouracil. In children, it's a congenital, autoimmune disorder or may be caused by the mother taking antithyroid drugs during pregnancy.

In patients with hypothyroidism, infection, exposure to cold, and sedatives may precipitate myxedema coma.

Clinical presentation

Early clinical features are vague — fatigue, forgetfulness, sensitivity to cold, unexplained weight gain, and constipation. As the disorder progresses, characteristic myxedematous signs appear — decreasing mental stability; dry, flaky, inelastic skin; puffy face, hands, and feet; hoarseness; periorbital edema; ptosis (upper eyelid droop); loss of lateral third of eyebrows; dry, sparse hair; and thick, brittle nails.

Cardiovascular involvement leads to decreased cardiac output, slow pulse rate, signs of poor peripheral circulation and, occasionally, cardiomegaly. Other common effects include anorexia, abdominal distention, menorrhagia, decreased libido, infertility, ataxia, intention tremor, and nystagmus. Reflexes show delayed relaxation time, especially the Achilles tendon.

Progression to myxedema coma is usually gradual, but when stress aggravates severe or prolonged hypothyroidism, coma may develop abruptly. Clinical effects include progressive stupor, hypoventilation, hypoglycemia, hyponatremia, hypotension, and hypothermia.

❋ **LIFE SPAN** *Hypothyroidism is characterized in infants by respiratory difficulties, persistent jaundice, and hoarse crying and in older children by stunted growth, bone and muscle dystrophy, and mental deficiency. If left untreated, children may suffer irreversible mental retardation; skeletal abnormalities are reversible with treatment.*

Differential diagnosis

▶ Adrenal disease
▶ Chronic autoimmune thyroiditis
▶ Depression
▶ Liver disease
▶ Nephrotic syndrome
▶ Pituitary tumor

Diagnostic tests

▶ Increased *TSH levels* are diagnostic of primary hypothyroidism; total serum thyroxine (T_4) is low; triiodothyronine (T_3) resin uptake is high; and the free T_4 index is low.
▶ High *antithyroid titers* detect autoimmune thyroiditis. If diagnosis is suspected, test cholesterol, liver enzymes, and electrolytes for baseline (may improve when hypothyroidism is controlled).

Management

Acute

Hypothermia or myxedema coma requires immediate intervention at a medical treatment facility.

Medication

Pharmacologic therapy includes gradual thyroid hormone replacement (levothyroxine, T_4); start low and go slow, particularly in elderly or cardiac patients. Monitor for drug interactions (anticoagulants, hypoglycemics, estrogens, and corticosteroids). Give cathartics and stool softeners as needed.

Collaborative practice

Refer the patient to an endocrinologist if the condition is nonresponsive to treatment and to an endocrinologist or other physician if the diagnosis is suspected in a child.

Follow-up

Follow up monthly to monitor response and draw TSH. When stable, visits can be every 6 months for examination (focus on cardiac system in elderly patients and patients with a known history of heart disease) and to check TSH level.

Complications

▶ Adrenal crisis with rapid increases in thyroid hormone
▶ Bone demineralization (consider hormone replacement therapy and calcium supplements)
▶ Immunocompromised status
▶ Infertility
▶ Hypersensitivity to opiates
▶ Megacolon
▶ Myxedema coma
▶ Organic psychosis
▶ Treatment-induced heart failure (in patients with coronary artery disease)

Patient teaching

▶ Teach the patient about diagnosis and the need for lifelong, uninterrupted therapy, even though symptoms subside.
▶ Encourage the patient to eat a high-bulk, low-calorie diet and to increase activity to combat constipation and promote weight loss.
▶ Notify anyone who prescribes drugs of the underlying hypothyroidism.
●●● **RED FLAG** *Tell the patient to call*
●●● *his primary care provider to report new or persistent signs and symptoms, including infections; signs of hyperthyroidism (restlessness, heat intolerance, weight loss despite increased appetite, sweating, diarrhea, tremor, and palpitations) or hypothyroidism (fatigue, cold*

intolerance, weight gain despite loss of appetite, constipation, and depression); and signs of aggravated cardiovascular disease (chest pain, tachycardia, palpitations, dyspnea).

Resources

▶ Thyroid Foundation of America, Inc.: 1-800-832-8321; *www.tsh.com*

IRON DEFICIENCY ANEMIA

ICD-9-CM 280.9

In iron deficiency anemia, an inadequate supply of iron is available for optimal formation of red blood cells (RBCs). Body stores of iron, including plasma iron, decrease as does transferrin, which binds with and transports iron. Insufficient body stores of iron lead to a depleted RBC mass, which in turn results in a lower hemoglobin concentration (hypochromia) and decreased oxygen-carrying capacity of the blood.

Causes

Iron deficiency anemia may occur because of inadequate dietary intake of iron (less than 2 mg/day), as in prolonged unsupplemented breast- or bottle-feeding, or during periods of stress, such as rapid growth in children and teenagers or poor nutrition in the elderly. Other causes include:

▶ *iron malabsorption,* as in chronic diarrhea, partial or total gastrectomy, and malabsorption syndromes such as celiac disease
▶ *blood loss secondary to drug-induced GI bleeding* (from anticoagulants, aspirin, steroids) or due to heavy menses, hemorrhage from trauma, GI ulcers, cancer, or varices
▶ *pregnancy,* which diverts maternal iron to the fetus for erythropoiesis
▶ *intravascular hemolysis-induced hemoglobinuria* or *paroxysmal nocturnal hemoglobinuria*

● *mechanical erythrocyte trauma* caused by a prosthetic heart valve or vena cava filters.

❋ **LIFE SPAN** *Iron deficiency anemia occurs most commonly in infants (particularly premature or low-birth-weight infants), children, adolescents (especially girls), and premenopausal women.*

Clinical presentation

Because of the gradual progression of iron deficiency anemia, many patients are initially asymptomatic, except for symptoms of an underlying condition. They tend not to seek medical treatment until anemia is severe.

At advanced stages, the patient may develop dyspnea on exertion, fatigue, listlessness, pallor, excessive menstrual flow, inability to concentrate, irritability, headache, and a susceptibility to infection. Decreased oxygen perfusion causes compensatory tachycardia and may cause palpitations.

In chronic iron deficiency anemia, the patient may present with koilonychia (nails become spoon-shaped and brittle), cheilosis (the corners of the mouth crack), and a smooth-textured tongue, and the patient may complain of dysphagia or develop pica. Associated neuromuscular effects include vasomotor disturbances, peripheral paresthesias, and neuralgic pain.

Differential diagnosis

● Anemia of chronic disease
● Conditions that cause acute or chronic blood loss
● Megaloblastic anemias

Diagnostic tests

● *Complete blood count with differential* identifies which type of anemia is present. Indicators of iron deficiency anemia are low RBC count with microcytic, hypochromic cells and decreased mean corpuscu-

lar hemoglobin. (In early stages, RBC count may be normal.)

● *Serum ferritin* may detect iron deficiency anemia.

● A high *total iron-binding capacity (TIBC)* indicates iron deficiency; a low TIBC may indicate chronic disease or malnutrition.

● Low *serum iron* indicates iron deficiency, chronic disease, or pernicious anemia.

● *Serial fecal occult blood test, endoscopy,* or *colonoscopy* detects occult GI bleeding.

● *Bone marrow aspiration* detects depleted or absent iron stores and normoblastic hyperplasia.

Management

Acute

●●● **RED FLAG** *Hemoglobin levels less than 8 g/dl may require transfusion.*

General

Investigate possible sources of bleeding and correct as indicated. Schedule rest periods to conserve the patient's energy, particularly with low cardiac output, angina, or light-headedness. Increase dietary iron and ascorbic acid (vitamin C).

Medication

Give ferrous sulfate by mouth in tablets or capsule or use as an elixir. Parenteral administration is available for patients with malabsorption.

❋ **LIFE SPAN** *In pregnant women, give ferrous sulfate twice per day for 2 weeks, then once daily. If hemoglobin levels don't improve, further testing is indicated.*

Collaborative practice

Refer the patient to a physician if you're unable to identify the cause of the anemia or if the condition doesn't respond to treatment.

Follow-up

See the patient every 2 weeks for 1 month, monthly for 2 months, then quarterly to semiannually to check for recurrences and reinforce preventive measures. See pregnant women who aren't improved at 2 weeks; check total iron, TIBC, folate, and vitamin B_{12}. If B_{12} is deficient, she'll need B_{12} injections.

Complications

▶ Hemorrhage from an identified source
▶ Undetected bleeding malignant tumor

Patient teaching

▶ To increase compliance, advise the patient not to stop therapy, even if he feels better, because replacement of iron stores takes time. Tell the patient to report adverse reactions, such as nausea, vomiting, diarrhea, constipation, fever, and severe stomach pain. Inform him that iron may cause stools to turn black.
▶ Tell the patient to take an iron supplement with meals to help decrease gastric irritation. If an elixir is used, instruct the patient to put it in a glass of orange juice and to sip it through a straw to prevent staining his teeth.
▶ Emphasize the need for high-risk individuals, such as premature infants, children under age 2, and pregnant women, to take prophylactic oral iron as ordered. (Children under age 2 should also receive supplemental cereals and formulas high in iron.)
▶ Tell the patient to avoid dairy products or antacids within 2 hours of taking dietary or supplemental iron because of iron's poor absorption. If GI upset occurs, tell him to take the iron with food. This decreases absorption by 50%, but vitamin C can increase absorption.
▶ Heme iron is easily absorbed from meat, poultry, and fish. To increase absorption of nonheme iron from other sources, such as fortified cereal or bread and leafy green vegetables, teach the patient to include vitamin C in the meal, such as from citrus fruits and strawberries.

■■■ **RED FLAG** *Tell the patient to call*
■■■ *the primary care provider to report new or persistent signs and symptoms, including abnormal bleeding, bruising, increasing fatigue, or inability to perform normal activities.*

Resources

▶ National Heart, Lung, and Blood Institute: (301) 592-8573; *www.nhlbi.nih.gov*

IRRITABLE BOWEL SYNDROME

ICD-9-CM irritable colon 564.1
Also known as *spastic colon* or *functional bowel pain*, irritable bowel syndrome (IBS) is a variable combination of chronic or recurrent GI symptoms with no detectable pathology. The disorder is marked by chronic or periodic diarrhea alternating with constipation and accompanied by gaseousness, straining, and abdominal cramps. The prognosis is good. Supportive treatment or avoidance of a known irritant usually relieves symptoms.

Causes

Mechanisms involved in IBS include visceral hypersensitivity and altered colonic motility. IBS is generally associated with psychological stress, which results in increased colonic contractions. It may also result from physical factors, such as diverticular disease, ingestion of irritants (coffee, raw fruits, or vegetables), or lactose intolerance. Autonomic nervous system abnormalities, genetic and psychosocial factors, and a luminal component (impaired digestion and absorption of certain carbohydrates, such as artificial sweeteners and lactose) may also play a role. Secondary IBS can be caused by abuse of laxatives, food poisoning, or colon cancer.

✱ LIFE SPAN *IBS occurs most frequently in women younger than age 45.*

Clinical presentation

IBS characteristically produces episodes of lower abdominal pain that are usually relieved by bowel movement, or it appears with an alteration in frequency or consistency of stools. Diarrhea is common but typically doesn't disrupt sleep. Stools are usually small and contain visible mucus. Dyspepsia, abdominal distention, and feelings of incomplete evacuation may occur.

Patients present with a combination of symptoms, though many state a predominance of diarrhea, constipation, or abdominal bloating and discomfort. These symptoms alternate with normal bowel function; the presence of symptoms at least 25% of the time without detectable pathology indicates IBS.

Differential diagnosis

▶ Amebiasis
▶ Colon cancer
▶ Crohn's disease
▶ Diverticulitis
▶ Endometriosis
▶ Lactose intolerance
▶ Ulcerative colitis

⣿ RED FLAG *A patient with a GI complaint whose examination reveals an abdominal mass, severe abdominal tenderness, fever, weight loss, or acute onset without obvious cause requires aggressive evaluation. Other red flags include nocturnal wakening due to GI complaints, family history of cancer, positive fecal occult blood test, abnormal blood counts, signs and symptoms of malabsorption, and new onset after age 50.*

Diagnostic tests

Appropriate diagnostic procedures to rule out pathology include erythrocyte sedimentation rate (a check for infection, inflammation, and cancer), complete blood count (to check for infection and blood loss), sigmoidoscopy, colonoscopy, barium enema, rectal biopsy, and stool examination for blood, parasites, and bacteria.

Management

The best treatment is education and reassurance. Explain the natural history of IBS. Emphasize that it isn't a mental disorder, but a biological response to stress or irritants and that it affects the quality of life but not longevity.

Therapy aims to relieve symptoms and includes counseling to help the patient understand the relationship between stress and his illness. Studies have found psychological therapy more beneficial than medical therapy in selected patients. Psychological therapy is more beneficial in patients who are aware of the role of stress in their disorder, don't have constant pain, and have fewer pain sites, shorter duration of symptoms, treatable anxiety or depression, and a realistic goal. Rest and heat applied to the abdomen are helpful, as is biofeedback.

Increased fiber (dietary and or supplemental) may be effective for both constipation and diarrhea. Work with the patient to monitor modifications for effectiveness. Patients do better with frequent, supportive contact from the primary care provider.

If the cause of IBS is chronic laxative abuse, bowel training may help correct the condition.

Medication

▶ *Bulk laxative* (psyllium) helps prevent constipation and diarrhea.

▸ *Antispasmodics* (anticholinergics, including phenobarbital, hyoscyamine, atropine, and hyoscine) relieve spasms.

▸ *Analgesics* (Donnatal) may be used for pain but can be addicting.

▸ *Antidiarrheals* (loperamide or attapulgite) can be used for diarrhea.

▸ *Osmotic laxatives* (magnesium hydroxide) are given for constipation.

▸ *Lactase capsules or tablets* counteract milk intolerance.

▸ *Antidepressants* (tricyclic antidepressants and serotonin reuptake inhibitors) in low doses may improve GI symptoms.

▸ *5-HT$_4$ receptor partial agonist* (Tegaserod) may be used for short-term treatment of women with IBS whose primary symptom is constipation. It also relieves abdominal discomfort and bloating.

▸ *5-HT$_3$ receptor antagonist* (Alosetron) is selective antagonists used for short-term treatment of women with IBS who have severe diarrhea. It's available through a restricted marketing program because of serious GI adverse effects, such as ischemic colitis and serious complications of constipation, including obstruction, perforation, and toxic megacolon. Only practitioners enrolled in the prescribing program can write a prescription for it.

Collaborative practice

Possible referrals include to a nutritionist for diet counseling, to a psychologist or psychiatrist for counseling and coping mechanisms as needed, and to a gastroenterologist or another physician for further workup and management for nonresponsiveness.

Follow-up

See the patient every 2 weeks until condition improves, then every 6 months. If the patient is over age 40, schedule an annual sigmoidoscopy and digital rectal examination because of an increased incidence of diverticulitis and colon cancer.

Complications

▸ Dehydration

▸ Laxative abuse and drug dependence

▸ Malnutrition

Patient teaching

▸ Emphasize the natural history of the disorder; it affects the quality of life but not longevity. This disorder can't be cured, but the patient can control the symptoms to improve his quality of life.

▸ Explain that antidepressants are given for their GI benefits and, in these dosages, generally have no psychotropic effects.

▸ Recommend a symptom diary to establish a record of association between symptoms and specific foods, stress, and emotional state. This will allow the patient to analyze and modify lifestyle, gaining some control as well as relief of symptoms. It's important not to exclude a food until it's correlated with symptoms at least three times (to avoid the risk of an overly limited diet). Questionable foods include poorly absorbed carbohydrates (such as sorbitol and lactose), high-fat foods, and alcohol.

▸ Encourage the patient to decrease stress and develop healthy coping mechanisms. Warn him against dependence on sedatives or antispasmodics.

▸ Encourage regular checkups because IBS is associated with a higher-than-normal incidence of diverticulitis and colon cancer. For patients over age 40, emphasize the need for an annual sigmoidoscopy and rectal examination.

●●● **RED FLAG** *Tell the patient to*
●●● *call the primary care provider to report any persistent, changing,*

worsening, anxiety-producing, or specific signs and symptoms, including fever higher than 101° F (38.3° C), vomiting blood or coffee-ground material, passing tarry black stools or blood, jaundice, and no bowel movements in 5 days.

Resources

▸ Crohn's and Colitis Foundation of America: 1-800-932-2423; *www.ccfa.org*

▸ For patient information on IBS: *www.medscape.com*

LUMBOSACRAL STRAIN

ICD-9-CM intervertebral disk disorders 722, unspecified backache 724.5

Lumbosacral strain refers to the stretching or tearing of muscles, tendons, ligaments, or the back due to trauma or chronic mechanical stress. Pain can be acute, chronic, or recurring in the lumbosacral spine area. Adults ages 20 to 40 are at greatest risk. Twenty percent of Americans complain of lower back pain that's slow to resolve and recurs easily without conscious, daily preventive measures.

Causes

Most acute back pain is caused by muscle strain or spasm of the paraspinal muscles. It can also result from trauma or mechanical causes that tear or physically stress the structures of the back.

Risk factors include chronic occupational strain, obesity, improper body mechanics when lifting, poor posture, weak back and abdominal muscles, and structural abnormalities, such as an abnormal forward pelvic tilt and unequal leg lengths.

Clinical presentation

Pain is the most significant presenting sign. Onset of pain and stiffness occurs 12 to 36 hours after the injury or activity. Pain is usually moderate to severe, located across the lumbosacral area and down through the buttocks and thighs, and unilateral or bilateral. Aggravating factors include movement, particularly standing and back flexion. Pain and spasm will increase on palpation. Relieving factors are rest and reclining. Muscle spasms may be present and can last several days.

The patient may present with gait and posture that are stiff or slow, and decreased range of motion with increased pain on flexion of the back. Point tenderness and muscle spasm are common. Positive straight-leg raises (elevate each leg passively with flexion at hip and extension of knee) reveal radicular pain when the leg is raised more than 60 degrees. Positive crossed-leg raises (when the patient complains of radicular pain in the leg that isn't raised during a straight-leg raise) strongly suggest a vertebral disk injury. Pain on the Patrick's test (the heel is placed on the opposite knee and lateral force is exerted) suggests hip or sacroiliac disease.

Abnormal reflexes may indicate more serious spinal cord involvement. A lack of sensation of the perineum is a warning sign and indicates further evaluation for cauda equina syndrome. To detect complaints of back pain that have secondary reward (attention-getting behavior) as the root of the problem, do something that should cause no back pain and see if the patient overreacts. For instance, applying slight pressure to the top of the head shouldn't produce pain. Distracting the patient while doing passive tests may elicit a different response.

Differential diagnosis

Initially, differentiate between mechanical and nonmechanical causes of back pain. (Mechanical is defined as being related to the motion of the body in daily activities and posture.) Mechanical causes include strains, disk disease, and spinal stenosis.

It's crucial to consider nonmechanical causes of back pain (such as osteomyelitis, metabolic bone disease, neoplasm, spinal cord disease, and abdominal aneurysm), which account for 4% of all cases, because sequelae can be life-threatening.

⦿⦿⦿ RED FLAG *More aggressive evaluation is indicated if you suspect a nonmechanical diagnosis; risk factors include age younger than 20 or older than 55, fever, unrelenting pain, extreme hypertension, and abdominal pain.*

Diagnostic tests

No tests are routinely indicated for initial presentation with lower back pain.

▶ *Complete blood count* with elevated white blood cells and an elevated sedimentation rate suggest infection. Low serum calcium may indicate osteoporosis. Alkaline phosphatase can indicate renal disease. Serum immunoelectrophoresis can reveal inflammatory disorders, malignancies, diffuse bone disease, or renal disease. Urinalysis may reveal a urinary tract infection.

▶ *Radiology studies* have a high false-positive rate and by themselves are insufficient for diagnosis. They should be done for high-risk groups, such as trauma patients and those suspected of having been abused. X-rays detect fracture in trauma cases (substance abusers may deny or not remember trauma) and pathologic fractures from use of steroids, osteoporosis, or metastasis. They may also detect a malig-

nant tumor (suspect in patients over age 50 with fever or a recent weight loss).

▶ *Magnetic resonance imaging* detects nonmusculoskeletal causes, such as disk disease and neoplasms.

▶ *Bone scan* detects malignancy and osteoporosis.

Management

Acute

⦿⦿⦿ RED FLAG *Immediate evaluation is needed for pain extending below the knees, lack of sensation in the perineum, and abnormal findings of motor, sensory, and reflex function in the lower extremities.*

General

Regardless of the treatment plan, 33% of lower back pain cases resolve in 1 week, and 98% resolve within 3 months. Highest patient satisfaction rates result when the patient is provided an explanation and understanding of his back pain.

Initial conservative management of the patient with back pain includes a period of controlled physical activity plus drugs; analgesics should be used only for short periods to avoid risk of drug dependence. Physical therapy must be part of the management plan, including cold and heat treatments to decrease pain and spasm.

Medication

▶ *Nonsteroidal anti-inflammatory drugs (NSAIDs)*, such as ibuprofen and naproxen, can decrease pain and inflammation while the tissues heal. These drugs should be used for a limited time (1 to 2 weeks).

▶ For back spasms, *muscle relaxants* (such as cyclobenzaprine or methocarbamol) are frequently used in conjunction with NSAIDs.

▶ *Opioids* should be prescribed only in severe trauma cases. The patient may resume full activity too soon and cause further injury. There's also a risk of drug dependence because of the chronic nature of the disorder.

Collaborative practice

Refer the patient to an orthopedist if the condition is nonresponsive after 1 week. Refer for physical therapy for back strengthening exercises and proper body mechanics training.

Follow-up

See the patient weekly for evaluation until pain resolves and then at 1 month to reinforce back precautions and exercises.

Complications

● Chronic lower back pain
● Opioid addiction

Patient teaching

● Teach the patient that back pain is slow to ease and can recur with minimal additional stress or injury. It's important to continue back exercises when the pain eases. Most back injuries don't happen suddenly; they're the result of long-term insult (keeping the back in flexion for large amounts of each day for years and poor body mechanics).

● Tell the patient to sleep on a firm mattress.

● For the first 72 hours, the patient should apply ice packs or cold compresses to the area, no more than 20 minutes at a time, four or more times per day. This will decrease swelling, inflammation, spasms, and pain.

● After 72 hours, the patient can apply a heating pad (set at medium) to the area, no more than 20 minutes at a time (to avoid burns), four or more times per day. This will relax the muscles, enhance blood exchange at the site, and ease stiffness and pain. A hot bath or shower with the water aimed at the site has the same effect.

● Advise the patient to start moving slowly but progressively after the first day, to avoid prolonged sitting or standing (longer than 15 minutes without changing positions), to avoid bending or twisting the back, and to bend at the knees and keep the back straight when lifting. Tell him to begin extension exercises, such as walking or swimming, as soon as pain eases as tolerated and to progress as tolerated.

● Teach the patient to place a folded towel or lumbar back roll (available at medical supply houses) in the small of the back when sitting for more than 15 minutes at a time or when riding in a car.

● Have the patient learn and practice daily back extension exercises such as the McKenzie exercises. As ambulation increases, decrease medication doses.

● Instruct the patient to avoid strenuous or high-impact activities and actions, such as lifting and pushing, for 6 weeks because healing is a slow process.

● Have the patient decrease his risk of recurrences by reducing weight (if overweight), increasing daily exercise for overall conditioning, and using good body mechanics at all times.

● For patients who need to return to activity early, consider a back support such as a corset. This may provide support but seems to function more by increasing awareness of the back and its relationship with activity. A back support is of questionable use after 3 months and increases the risk of injury after 6 months; patients may attempt more strenuous activities because they feel "protected," and minimizing extension or flexion over long periods tends to weaken the muscles.

● ● ● **RED FLAG** *Tell the patient to call*
● ● ● *the primary care provider to report new or persistent signs and*

symptoms, including pain lasting
more than 1 week, weakness or
numbness in the legs, bowel or bladder dysfunction, or severe pain
that's worsened by the management
plan.

Resources
▶ Arthritis Foundation: 1-800-283-
7800; *www.arthritis.org*
▶ McKenzie Institute: 1-800-635-
8380; *www.mckenziemdt.org/
index_us.cfm*

OSTEOARTHRITIS

ICD-9-CM 715.9
Osteoarthritis, the most common
form of arthritis, is a chronic disease that causes deterioration of the
joint cartilage and formation of reactive new bone at the margins and
subchondral areas of the joints.
This degeneration results from a
breakdown of chondrocytes, most
commonly in the distal interphalangeal and proximal interphalangeal joints, but also in the hip
and knee joints. Primary osteoarthritis is strongly associated with
aging, which predisposes the patient to cartilage degeneration.

Osteoarthritis is widespread, occurring equally in both sexes. Disability depends on the site and
severity of involvement and can
range from minor limitation of the
dexterity of the fingers to severe
disability in persons with hip or
knee involvement. The rate of progression varies, and joints may remain stable for years in an early
stage of deterioration.

❋ **LIFE SPAN** *The earliest symptoms of osteoarthritis typically
begin after age 40 and may progress
with advancing age.*

Causes

Studies indicate that osteoarthritis
is acquired and probably results
from a combination of metabolic,
genetic, chemical, and mechanical
factors. Secondary osteoarthritis
usually follows an identifiable predisposing event — most commonly
trauma, congenital deformity, or
obesity — and leads to degenerative
changes.

Clinical presentation

The most common symptom of osteoarthritis is a deep, aching joint
pain, particularly after exercise or
weight bearing, that's usually relieved by rest. Other symptoms include:
▶ stiffness in the morning and after
exercise (relieved by rest)
▶ aching during changes in weather
▶ grating of the joint during motion
▶ altered gait contractors
▶ limited movement.

These symptoms increase with
poor posture, obesity, and stress to
the affected joint.

Osteoarthritis of the interphalangeal joints produces irreversible
joint changes and node formation.
Heberden's nodes in the distal interphalangeal joints generally appear in the later stages of the disease. (See *Digital joint deformities*,
page 248.) The nodes eventually become red, swollen, and tender,
causing numbness and loss of dexterity.

Differential diagnosis

▶ Gout
▶ Malignancy
▶ Osteoporosis
▶ Rheumatoid arthritis
▶ Vasculitis

Diagnostic tests

A thorough physical examination
confirms typical symptoms, and absence of systemic symptoms rules
out an inflammatory joint disorder.
No laboratory test is specific for osteoarthritis. X-rays of the affected
joint help confirm diagnosis of osteoarthritis but may be normal in

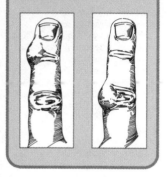

the early stages. X-rays may require many views and typically show:
▶ narrowing of joint space or margin
▶ cystlike bony deposits in joint space and margins and sclerosis of the subchondral space
▶ joint deformity due to degeneration or articular damage
▶ bony growths at weight-bearing areas
▶ fusion of joints.

Management
General
The goal of treatment is to relieve pain, maintain or improve mobility, and minimize disability. Effective treatment also reduces stress by supporting or stabilizing the joint with crutches, braces, a cane, a walker, a cervical collar, or traction. Other supportive measures include massage, moist heat, paraffin dips for hands, protective techniques for preventing undue stress on the joints, and adequate rest (particularly after activity). Occasionally, exercise may be indicated if the knees are affected.

Medication
▶ *Aspirin* or other *nonopioid analgesics* and *ibuprofen* or other *nonsteroidal anti-inflammatory drugs (NSAIDs)* may be used to treat osteoarthritis.
▶ Intra-articular injection of *corticosteroids* given every 4 to 6 months may delay the development of nodes in the hands.

Surgery
Surgical treatment is reserved for patients who have severe disability or uncontrollable pain. Surgical options include:
▶ *arthroplasty (partial or total)* — replacement of the deteriorated part of a joint with a prosthetic appliance
▶ *arthrodesis* — surgical fusion of bones, used primarily in the spine (laminectomy)
▶ *osteoplasty* — scraping and lavage of deteriorated bone from a joint
▶ *osteotomy* — change in the alignment of bone to relieve stress by excision of wedge of bone or cutting of bone.

Collaborative practice
▶ Refer the patient to an orthopedic surgeon if surgery is necessary.
▶ Refer the patient for physical therapy if indicated.

Follow-up
The patient should be monitored at regular intervals (3 to 6 months) for functional status and pain control. If the patient is frequently using NSAIDs or aspirin, periodic complete blood counts, renal function

tests, and stool for occult blood should be performed.

Complications

▶ Altered lifestyle
▶ Chronic pain
▶ Joint deformity

Patient teaching

▶ Tell the patient to get adequate rest, particularly after activity. Plan rest periods during the day, and provide for adequate sleep at night. Moderation is the key; teach the patient to pace daily activities.
▶ Encourage the patient to perform gentle, isometric range-of-motion exercises.
▶ Teach the patient to take medication exactly as prescribed, and report adverse effects immediately.
▶ Advise the patient to avoid overexertion. He should take care to stand and walk correctly, minimize weight-bearing activities, and be especially careful when stooping or picking up objects.
▶ Instruct the patient to wear proper-fitting, supportive shoes and to keep the heels from becoming worn down.
▶ Advise the patient to install safety devices at home such as guard rails in the bathroom.

Resources

▶ The Arthritis Foundation: 1-800-283-7800; *www.arthritis.org*
▶ National Institute of Arthritis and Musculoskeletal and Skin Diseases, National Institutes of Health: 1-877-22-NIAMS; *www.nih.gov/niams*

OSTEOPOROSIS

ICD-9-CM 733.0
Osteoporosis is a metabolic bone disorder in which bone absorption outpaces bone formation, causing a net loss of the bony matrix as well as the calcium that adheres to it.

Bones become porous, brittle, and abnormally vulnerable to fracture.

Causes

The cause of primary osteoporosis is unknown; however, a mild but prolonged negative calcium balance, resulting from an inadequate dietary intake of calcium, may be an important contributing factor, as may declining ovarian function and a sedentary lifestyle.

Causes of secondary osteoporosis include prolonged therapy with steroids or heparin, metabolic disorders such as hyperthyroidism, and osteogenesis imperfecta.

Risk factors include a positive family history, fair skin color, thin physique, menopause, long-term immobility (such as hemiplegia), malnutrition, lactose intolerance, Scandinavian or Asian descent, and alcohol or tobacco use.

Clinical presentation

Onset of osteoporosis is insidious; it's usually diagnosed when a fracture occurs. Weight-bearing bones are most commonly affected. Compression fracture of the thoracic spine can be asymptomatic or have pain that radiates anteriorly and is aggravated by movement.

Hip fracture generally presents as a minor fall or blow to the area followed by abrupt onset of pain, decreased range of motion of the affected hip, and external rotation of the leg. As vertebral bodies weaken, spontaneous wedge fractures, pathologic fractures of the neck and femur, Colles' fractures after a minor fall, and hip fractures are common.

Associated signs of osteoporosis are increasing deformity, kyphosis ("dowager's hump"), lordosis, and loss of height.

●●● RED FLAG *Patients with osteo-*
●●● *porosis frequently suffer minimal trauma and don't have pain*

when they sustain fracture. X-ray evaluation is needed for suspicion of fracture.

Differential diagnosis

▶ Hyperparathyroidism
▶ Hyperthyroidism
▶ Multiple myeloma
▶ Neoplasia
▶ Osteogenesis imperfecta
▶ Osteomalacia

Diagnostic tests

▶ *Height measurement* is taken annually (without shoes) in postmenopausal women.
▶ *Alkaline phosphatase* increases transiently after bone fracture.
▶ *Serum* or *urine protein electrophoresis* and *urinary-free cortisol analysis* detect metabolic disorders.
▶ High levels of *serum osteocalcin* and *urinary calcium, pyridinoline, and N-telopeptide collagen crosslinks* indicate accelerated demineralization.
▶ *Thyroid-stimulating hormone test* may detect hypothyroidism or hyperthyroidism.
▶ *Bone mineral densitometry* (BMD or DEXA scan) measures bone density; this screening test is useful in early osteoporosis.
▶ *X-rays* show typical degeneration in the lower thoracic and lumbar vertebrae. The vertebral bodies may appear flattened and denser. Loss of bone mineral becomes evident in later stages. X-rays can detect early manifestations (increased width of intervertebral spaces, accentuated cortical plates, vertical striations of vertebral bodies) as well as late manifestations (vertebral compression and multiple fractures of long bones).
▶ *Bone biopsy* isn't routinely done, but may detect metabolic bone disorders or quantify bone loss.

Management

●●● **RED FLAG** *Acute pain or suspect-*
●●● *ed fracture requires X-rays and immediate evaluation.*
Weakened vertebrae should be supported, usually with a back brace. Surgery can correct pathologic fractures of the femur by open reduction and internal fixation. Colles' fracture requires reduction with plaster immobilization for 4 to 10 weeks. Evaluate the patient's skin for redness, warmth, and new sites of pain, which may indicate new fractures.

General

Encourage weight-bearing exercise. (Build up to walking 2 miles with 1-lb weights five times per week.) The patient should avoid activities that exert stress on vertebrae and long bones. Teach the patient to avoid falls by not using scatter rugs, not rushing to answer the phone, and using handrails in the bathroom and on stairs.

Dietary recommendations include:
▶ beginning a reduction diet if overweight
▶ avoiding a high-protein diet
▶ avoiding carbonated beverages because excess phosphorus decreases serum calcium
▶ ingesting enough calcium (1,000 mg/day after age 24, 1,500 mg/day after menopause, and 2,000 mg/day for patients diagnosed with osteoporosis); all women need at least 600 IU of vitamin D daily (can be obtained by only 10 minutes a week of skin exposure to sun).

Medication

Drug therapy arrests osteoporosis but doesn't cure it.
▶ *Calcium* and *vitamin D supplements* (to reach the recommended daily allowance) to support bone formation are used in conjunction with other therapies. (See dietary recommendations above.)

Hormone replacement therapy at the lowest effective dose remains controversial; research is ongoing.

Thyroid hormone (calcitonin inhalant) prevents bone resorption, relieves pain, and may stimulate bone formation.

Biphosphonates (alendronate) form a bony matrix, which enhances calcium adherence.

Gonadotropin-releasing hormone analogue (Synarel inhalant) increases ovarian steroid production.

Selective estrogen receptor modulator (raloxifene) decreases bone demineralization.

Tamoxifen offers some protection for bone without stimulating breast changes.

Androgens, steroids, and *parathyroid hormone analogues* are being researched.

Collaborative practice

Refer the patient to a physician for back pain due to compression fractures. Refer her to a gynecologist for endometrial evaluation for abnormal vaginal bleeding. Have the patient see a physical therapist for exercises to increase strength, endurance, and proper body mechanics, and an occupational therapist to learn adaptive behaviors and correct technique for the use of braces and other devices.

Follow-up

Follow-up should be monthly during initial treatment, then quarterly. Focus on body mechanics, exercise, compliance with drug regimen, and adverse effects of drugs. The patient will need a Papanicolaou test and pelvic examination, mammography, and BMD examination annually, and vertebral X-rays every 3 years.

Complications

- Loss of independence
- Neurologic deficits due to vertebral fractures
- Severe pain

Patient teaching

- Stress the importance of physical therapy, emphasizing gentle exercise and activity.

- Promote healthy dietary options high in nutrients that support skeletal metabolism, such as calcium, vitamin D, and protein.

- Make sure the patient understands the prescribed drug regimen clearly. For example, take alendronate on an empty stomach with water and then wait at least a half-hour before ingesting food or other fluids. Otherwise, absorption drops by more than 60%.

- Advise the patient to sleep on a firm mattress and avoid excessive bed rest.

- Because an osteoporotic patient's bones fracture very easily, emphasize the importance of moving gently and carefully at all times.

- Teach good body mechanics: stoop before lifting anything and avoid twisting movements and prolonged bending.

- Instruct a woman taking estrogen in breast self-examination. Tell her to perform this examination at least once a month and to report any lumps immediately. Emphasize the need for regular gynecologic examinations. Report abnormal bleeding promptly.

●●● RED FLAG *Tell the patient to call the primary care provider to report any new or persistent signs and symptoms, including new pain, even without trauma; abnormal bleeding; and drug adverse effects (stomach pain, nausea, tarry stools).*

Resources

- National Osteoporosis Foundation: (202) 223-2226; *www.nof.org*
- Information for those who are newly diagnosed or at high risk: *www.medscape.com*
- For providers — Drug affordability: *www.needymeds.com* (contains in-

formation regarding many drug company programs that provide financial assistance for those who need their drugs)

OTITIS MEDIA

ICD-9-CM acute otitis media 382.0, acute suppurative otitis media 381.0

Inflammation of the middle ear, otitis media may be suppurative or secretory and acute or chronic. With prompt treatment, the prognosis for acute otitis media is excellent; however, prolonged accumulation of fluid within the middle ear cavity causes chronic otitis media, with possible perforation of the tympanic membrane. Chronic suppurative otitis media may lead to scarring, adhesions, and severe structural or functional ear damage.

Chronic secretory otitis media, with its persistent inflammation and pressure, may cause conductive hearing loss.

❋ **LIFE SPAN** *Acute otitis media is most common in children; it's also a problem for older adults. Incidence rises during the winter months, paralleling the seasonal rise in nonbacterial respiratory tract infections.*

Causes

Acute otitis media results from disruption of eustachian tube patency and subsequent inflammation and infection.

Acute otitis media

In the suppurative form of acute otitis media, respiratory tract infection, allergic reaction, nasotracheal intubation, or positional changes allow nasopharyngeal flora to reflux into the eustachian tube and colonize the middle ear. Suppurative otitis media usually results from bacterial infection with pneumococci, *Haemophilus influenzae* (most

common cause in children under age 6), *Moraxella catarrhalis*, beta-hemolytic streptococci, staphylococci (most common cause in children ages 6 and older), or gram-negative bacteria. Predisposing factors include the normally wider, shorter, more horizontal eustachian tubes and increased lymphoid tissue in children as well as anatomic anomalies. Chronic suppurative otitis media results from inadequate treatment of acute otitis media episodes, infection by resistant strains of bacteria or, rarely, tuberculosis.

In the secretory form of acute otitis media, eustachian tube obstruction causes buildup of negative pressure in the middle ear that promotes effusion of sterile serous fluid from blood vessels in the middle ear membrane. This may be secondary to eustachian tube dysfunction from viral infection or allergy. It may also follow barotrauma (pressure injury from inability to equalize pressures between the environment and the middle ear), which can occur during rapid aircraft descent in a person with an upper respiratory tract infection and during rapid underwater ascent in scuba diving (barotitis media). Chronic secretory otitis media follows inadequate treatment of the acute form or persistent eustachian tube dysfunction from mechanical obstruction (adenoidal tissue overgrowth, tumors) or edema (allergic rhinitis, chronic sinus infection).

Clinical presentation

Clinical features vary with the specific type of the disorder.

Acute otitis media

History may reveal tinnitus; severe, deep, throbbing pain (from pressure behind the tympanic membrane); hearing an echo; hearing popping or crackling sounds when moving the jaw; previous occurrences; and preceding illness. Elicit history of allergies, exposure to smoke, and congenital disorders.

Examination of the tympanic membrane usually shows a distorted light reflex, a bulging tympanic membrane with obscured bony landmarks (indicating suppurative acute otitis media) or a retracted tympanic membrane with prominent landmarks (indicating secretory acute otitis media), decreased motility with insufflation (air puffed into the ear), and otorrhea. This procedure is painful with an obviously bulging, erythematous tympanic membrane.

Additional symptoms include signs of upper respiratory tract infection (sneezing, coughing), hearing loss (usually mild and conductive), ear drainage, dizziness, nausea, vomiting, and constitutional symptoms (mild to high fever, irritability).

Chronic otitis media
Cumulative effects of chronic otitis media include thickening and scarring of the tympanic membrane, decreased or absent membrane mobility, cholesteatoma (a cystlike mass in the middle ear) and, in chronic suppurative otitis media, a painless, purulent discharge. The extent of conductive hearing loss varies with the size and type of tympanic membrane perforation and ossicular destruction.

●●● **RED FLAG** *If the tympanic mem-*
●●● *brane has ruptured, the patient may say the pain has suddenly stopped. Complications may include abscesses (brain, subperiosteal, epidural), sigmoid sinus or jugular vein thrombosis, septicemia, meningitis, suppurative labyrinthitis, facial paralysis, and otitis externa.*

Differential diagnosis
▶ Mastoiditis
▶ Otitis externa
▶ Parotitis
▶ Peritonsillar abscess
▶ Sinusitis

Diagnostic tests
Testing isn't routinely indicated, but when it is, examination and testing should consider the sinuses, oral cavity with emphasis on teeth, temporomandibular joint, nasopharynx for neoplasia, and cranial nerves for cranial neuralgias.

▶ *Tympanocentesis* for culture and sensitivity of middle ear effusion may help in severe cases, persistent or recurrent infections, and immunocompromised patients.

▶ *Tympanometry* may confirm suspicion of fluid behind the tympanic membrane without clinical signs.

▶ *Paranasal sinus X-rays* may reveal fracture, Wegener's granulomatosis, neoplasia, cyst, or mucocele and may differentiate acute from chronic sinusitis.

▶ *Audiometry* can quantify hearing loss and recovery.

Management
The type of otitis media dictates the treatment guidelines.

Suppurative otitis media
In suppurative acute otitis media, antibiotic therapy includes ampicillin or amoxicillin. In areas with a high incidence of beta-lactamase-producing *Haemophilus influenzae* and in patients who aren't responding to ampicillin or amoxicillin, amoxicillin/clavulanate potassium may be used.

For those who are allergic to penicillin derivatives, therapy may include cefaclor or co-trimoxazole. Broad-spectrum antibiotics can help prevent acute suppurative otitis media in high-risk patients. In patients with recurring otitis, antibiotics must be used with discretion to prevent development of resistant strains of bacteria. Severe, painful bulging of the tympanic membrane usually necessitates myringotomy.

Secretory otitis media

For acute secretory otitis media, inflation of the eustachian tube by performing Valsalva's maneuver several times per day may be the only treatment required. Otherwise, nasopharyngeal decongestant therapy may be helpful. It should continue for at least 2 weeks and sometimes indefinitely, with periodic evaluation.

Surgery

If decongestant therapy fails, myringotomy and aspiration of middle ear fluid are necessary, followed by insertion of a polyethylene tube into the tympanic membrane, for immediate and prolonged equalization of pressure. The tube falls out spontaneously after 9 to 12 months. Concomitant treatment of the underlying cause (such as elimination of allergens or an adenoidectomy for hypertrophied adenoids) may also be helpful in correcting this disorder.

Chronic otitis media

Treatment of chronic otitis media includes broad-spectrum antibiotics, such as amoxicillin/clavulanate potassium or cefuroxime, for exacerbations of acute otitis media; elimination of eustachian tube obstruction; treatment of otitis externa; myringoplasty and tympanoplasty to reconstruct middle ear structures when thickening and scarring are present; and, possibly, mastoidectomy. Cholesteatoma requires excision.

Collaborative practice

Refer the patient to an ear, nose, and throat (ENT) specialist if he has serous otitis media with a hearing loss that lasts longer than 6 weeks, extends bilaterally, or exceeds 20 decibels; vertigo or ataxia; or symptoms that worsen after 3 days of treatment. In chronic persistent infections, ENT evaluation is recommended for patients who have significant hearing loss that lasts longer than 3 weeks, infection that fails to resolve after two courses of antibiotics, cholesteatoma formation, or a ruptured tympanic membrane that fails to close.

Follow-up

For acute otitis media, see the patient 3 days after starting treatment if nonresponsive. Otherwise, see him a few days after completion of antibiotics to evaluate. For chronic otitis media see him every month, focusing on ear examination. For serous otitis media, see the patient 4 to 6 weeks after treatment for evaluation.

Complications

Acute otitis media

▶ Acute mastoiditis
▶ Ataxia
▶ Lateral sinus thrombophlebitis
▶ Meningitis

Chronic otitis media

▶ Hearing loss

Recurrent otitis media

▶ Atrophy and scarring of the eardrum
▶ Chronic mastoiditis
▶ Cholesteatoma
▶ Infection spreading to adjacent intracranial structures
▶ Otorrhea
▶ Permanent hearing loss
▶ Ruptured tympanic membrane that doesn't close

Patient teaching

▶ Explain all diagnostic tests and procedures.
▶ Teach the patient not to place cotton or plugs deep in the ear canal; however, sterile cotton may be placed loosely in the external ear to absorb drainage. To prevent infection, change the cotton whenever it gets damp, and wash hands before and after giving ear care.

▶ After tympanoplasty, observe for excessive bleeding from the ear canal. Warn the patient against blowing his nose or getting water in the ear.

▶ Explain the importance of completing a prescribed course of antibiotic treatment. If ordering nasopharyngeal decongestants, teach correct instillation.

▶ Apply heat to the ear to relieve pain. Advise the patient with acute secretory otitis media to watch for and immediately report pain and fever — signs of secondary infection.

To prevent otitis media:

▶ Teach recognition of upper respiratory tract infections and encourage early treatment.

▶ Instruct parents not to feed their infant in a supine position or put him to bed with a bottle. This prevents reflux of nasopharyngeal flora.

▶ To promote eustachian tube patency, tell the patient to perform Valsalva's maneuver several times daily.

▶ Identify and treat allergies.

●●● **RED FLAG** *Tell the patient to*
●●● *call the primary care provider to report new or persistent signs and symptoms, including headache, fever, severe pain, signs of infection (redness, swelling, drainage from ear), and disorientation.*

Resources

▶ American Academy of Pediatrics: (847) 434-4000; *www.aap.org*
▶ Patient information on otitis media: *www.medscape.com*

PARKINSON'S DISEASE

ICD-9-CM: 332.0
Parkinson's disease is a chronic, progressive, neurodegenerative central nervous system disorder characterized by tremor at rest, rigidity, and bradykinesia. Parkinson's disease strikes 1 in every 100 people over age 60.

Causes

Although the cause of Parkinson's disease is unknown, some theorize accelerated aging, a toxic or infectious cause, or an oxidative mechanism. Regardless, there's a loss of dopamine-producing neurons in the substantia nigra.

Clinical presentation

The disease is of gradual onset; history may reveal recent onset of clumsiness, falling, and a change in handwriting. The cardinal symptoms of Parkinson's disease are muscle rigidity and bradykinesia. The patient typically presents with an insidious tremor that begins in the fingers (unilateral pill-roll tremor), increases during stress or anxiety, and decreases with purposeful movement and sleep.

Muscle rigidity results in resistance to passive muscle stretching, which may be uniform (lead-pipe rigidity) or jerky (cogwheel rigidity). Bradykinesia causes the patient to walk with difficulty (gait lacks normal parallel motion and may be retropulsive or propulsive). The patient has difficulty initiating movement.

Parkinson's disease also produces a monotone voice, drooling, mask-like facies, loss of posture control (patient walks with body bent forward), and dysarthria, dysphagia, or both. Occasionally, bradykinesia may also cause oculogyric crises (eyes fixed upward, with involuntary tonic movements) or blepharospasm (eyelids completely closed). In later stages, the patient may exhibit slowed mentation progressing to dementia.

Autonomic dysfunction is evidenced by orthostatic hypotension, constipation, bladder dysfunction, and impotence.

Differential diagnosis

For diagnosis, the patient must have either rest tremor or bradykinesia, plus one of the following: rigidity, flexed posture, loss of postural reflexes, and masklike facies. Slightly hyperactive or hard-to-elicit reflexes, decreased blink reflex, and extraocular movement (EOM) (difficulty with upward gaze) are also common. If EOM elicits disturbance in ocular motility, consider progressive supranuclear palsy.

For differential diagnosis, consider:
▶ adverse drug reaction (particularly suspect neurologic agents)
▶ benign essential tumor
▶ cerebral arteriosclerosis
▶ Creutzfeldt-Jakob disease
▶ dementia
▶ depression
▶ Huntington's disease
▶ infections
▶ intracranial tumor
▶ lacunar infarctions
▶ multisystem atrophy
▶ phenothiazine or other drug toxicity
▶ progressive supranuclear palsy
▶ toxins, such as carbon monoxide, manganese, and cyanide
▶ Wilson's disease.

Diagnostic tests

No diagnostic tests exist for Parkinson's disease; however, promising research is in progress utilizing a single photon emission computed tomography and altropane or iodine[123] beta-CIT (carbomethoxy-3 [-4-iodophenyl] tropane).
▶ Conduct a *Mini–Mental Status Examination*. If the patient scores less than 20, consider a dementia disorder.
▶ In a younger person, order *liver function, serum copper,* and *ceruloplasmin tests* after a physician's

consultation to detect Wilson's disease, which causes excess copper accumulation.
▶ Consider *computed tomography scan* or *magnetic resonance imaging* to detect lacunar infarcts, brain stem atrophy, or cerebellar atrophy if you're unsure of the diagnosis or if the patient is unresponsive to drug therapy.

Management
General

Treatment is palliative; no curative treatment exists. Acute exacerbation may indicate a secondary cause, depression, or noncompliance. If the condition is drug-induced, symptoms may take months to resolve. Monitor for toxic effects of drugs.

Advise the patient to take small, frequent meals if fatigued by eating. Diet should be high in fluid and fiber intake.

Surgery

Pallidotomy may be indicated for some patients. Good to excellent mobility has been achieved in 70% of research studies of the surgery. Pallidotomy is generally restricted to one side due to the risk of performing surgery on both sides of the brain.

Medication
▶ Anticholinergics (trihexyphenidyl, benztropine)
▶ Dopamine precursors or agonists (carbidopa-levodopa, generally reserved until other drugs are tried because of decreasing effectiveness after about 5 years of treatment; pramipexole; ropinirole)
▶ Dopamine receptor agonist (bromocriptine)
▶ Synthetic cyclic primary amine (amantadine)
▶ Monoamine oxidase inhibitors (selegiline)
▶ Catechol O-methyltransferase inhibitors (tolcapone), used cautiously due to cases of liver injury

Levodopa, a dopamine replacement that's most effective during early stages, is given in increasing doses until symptoms are relieved or adverse effects appear. Because adverse effects can be serious, levodopa is commonly given in combination with carbidopa to halt peripheral dopamine synthesis. When levodopa proves ineffective or too toxic, alternative drug therapy is initiated.

Collaborative practice
Refer the patient to a neurologist for definitive diagnosis and initial drug regimen, severe disease states that are nonresponsive to drugs, and possible stereotactic neurosurgery (such as pallidotomy) to relieve symptoms. Physical therapy is complementary to increase strength and endurance and to maintain normal muscle tone and function. This includes active range of motion (ROM), passive ROM, activities of daily living, and massage to help relax muscles. Occupational therapy is important for adjustments in the home (elevated toilet seat, assistive devices for eating and dressing). Speech therapy referral should be made as soon as speech abnormalities are noticed.

Follow-up
Monitor drug treatment so dosage can be adjusted to minimize adverse effects. Evaluate the patient for depression at each visit. See the patient every 2 weeks after a change in drug therapy. During stable periods, see him monthly to quarterly. Lifelong follow-up is needed for drug therapy adjustment and physical therapy.

Complications
▶ Aspiration pneumonia
▶ Dementia
▶ Depression
▶ Dyskinesias
▶ Falls
▶ Freezing (transient paralysis)

CLINICAL PEARL *In Parkinson's disease, complications are usually the cause of death.*

Patient teaching
▶ Teach significant others that caring effectively for the patient with Parkinson's disease requires careful monitoring of drug treatment, emphasis on self-reliance, and generous psychological support.
▶ Teach the patient and his family that this is a progressive disease; the worst prognosis is for older patients with dementia.
▶ Fatigue may cause the patient to depend more on others; therefore, he should schedule rest periods; eat small, frequent meals; and use assistive devices.
▶ Teach the patient's family how to prevent pressure ulcers and contractures by proper positioning.
▶ Establish long- and short-term treatment goals, and be aware of the patient's need for intellectual stimulation and diversion.
▶ The patient with excessive tremor may achieve partial control of his body by sitting on a chair and using its arms to steady himself.
▶ Instruct the patient to minimize constipation by drinking at least 2 qt (2 L) of liquids daily and eating high-bulk foods.

RED FLAG *Tell the patient to call the primary care provider to report new or persistent signs and symptoms, including lack of improvement with management and signs of stroke, such as mental status change, facial droop, blurred vision, rapidly worsened coordination (especially if unilateral), and seizures.*

Resources
▶ American Parkinson Disease Foundation: 1-800-223-2732; *www.apdaparkinson.com*

▶ National Parkinson Foundation: 1-800-327-4545; *www.parkinson.org*
▶ Parkinson's Disease Foundation: 1-800-457-6676; *www.pdf.org*

PEPTIC ULCER

ICD-9-CM duodenal 532.9, gastric 531.9, peptic 536.8

Circumscribed lesions in the mucosal membrane, peptic ulcers can develop in the lower esophagus, stomach, pylorus, duodenum, or jejunum. About 80% of all peptic ulcers are duodenal ulcers, which affect the proximal part of the small intestine and occur most commonly in men between ages 20 and 50.

Gastric ulcers, which affect the stomach mucosa, are most common in people ages 55 to 70, especially in chronic users of nonsteroidal anti-inflammatory drugs (NSAIDs) or alcohol. *Duodenal ulcers* usually follow a chronic course, with remissions and exacerbations; 5% to 10% of patients develop complications that necessitate surgery.

Causes

Researchers recognize three major causes of peptic ulcer disease: infection with *Helicobacter pylori* (formerly known as *Campylobacter pylori*), use of NSAIDs, and pathologic hypersecretory states such as Zollinger-Ellison syndrome. Regardless of the cause, an imbalance exists between aggressive factors (such as gastric acid) and defensive factors that enhance mucosal integrity (such as mucus, prostaglandins, growth factors, blood flow, bicarbonate, and cell turnover). Gastric acid, which was once considered a primary cause, now appears mainly to contribute to the consequences of infection.

Certain drugs, including salicylates and other NSAIDs, encourage ulcer formation by inhibiting the secretion of prostaglandins (the substances that suppress ulceration). Certain illnesses, such as pancreatitis, hepatic disease, Crohn's disease, preexisting gastritis, and Zollinger-Ellison syndrome, cause hypersecretion of gastric acids.

Predisposing factors

In addition to peptic ulcer's main causes, several predisposing factors are known. They include blood type (gastric ulcers tend to strike people with type A blood; duodenal ulcers tend to afflict people with type O blood) and other genetic factors.

Exposure to irritants, such as alcohol and tobacco, may contribute by accelerating gastric acid emptying and promoting mucosal breakdown. Physical trauma, emotional stress, and normal aging are additional predisposing conditions.

Clinical presentation

Clinical features vary with the area of the GI tract that's affected.

Gastric ulcers

Heartburn and indigestion usually signal the beginning of a gastric ulcer attack. Eating food stretches the gastric wall and may cause — or, in some cases, relieve — pain and a feeling of fullness and distention. Other typical effects include weight loss and repeated episodes of massive GI bleeding.

Duodenal ulcers

Duodenal ulcers produce heartburn and well-localized midepigastric pain that's relieved by food, antacids, or antisecretory agents; weight gain because the patient eats to relieve discomfort; and a peculiar sensation of hot water bubbling in the back of the throat. Attacks usually occur about 2 hours after meals, whenever the stomach is empty, or after consumption of orange juice, coffee, aspirin, or alcohol.

Exacerbations tend to recur several times a year and then fade into remission. Vomiting and other digestive disturbances are rare.

Differential diagnosis

▶ Biliary tract disease
▶ Crohn's disease
▶ Gastritis
▶ *H. pylori* infection
▶ Malignancy
▶ Pancreatitis
▶ Variant angina

⬤⬤⬤ **RED FLAG** *A patient older than*
⬤⬤⬤ *age 50 or who presents with anorexia, weight loss, dysphagia, vomiting, or GI bleeding requires aggressive evaluation. Other red flags include a family history of cancer, positive fecal occult blood test, shortness of breath (may be due to anemia), and abnormal blood counts.*

Diagnostic tests

▶ *Serologic* H. pylori or *carbon isotope urea breath test* detects *H. pylori.* (Breath test yields up to 15% false-negative results.)
▶ *Serial fecal occult blood tests* may disclose occult blood in the stools, which requires colonoscopic evaluation. Hemoglobin and hematocrit values are decreased from GI bleeding (uncommon without hemorrhage).
▶ An elevated *fasting serum gastrin* and *secretin stimulation test* indicates Zollinger-Ellison syndrome.
▶ *Upper GI tract X-rays* show mucosal abnormalities; gastric secretory studies show hyperchlorhydria and achlorhydria. Upper GI endoscopy confirms an ulcer, and biopsy rules out *H. pylori* infection and cancer.

Management

Acute

If GI bleeding occurs, emergency treatment begins with passage of a nasogastric tube to allow for iced saline lavage, possibly containing norepinephrine. Gastroscopy allows visualization of the bleeding site and coagulation by laser or cautery to control bleeding. This type of therapy allows postponement of surgery until the patient's condition stabilizes.

Surgery is indicated for perforation, unresponsiveness to conservative treatment, and suspected cancer. Surgical procedures for peptic ulcers include:

▶ *vagotomy and pyloroplasty:* severing one or more branches of the vagus nerve to reduce hydrochloric acid secretion and refashioning the pylorus to create a larger lumen and facilitate gastric emptying
▶ *distal subtotal gastrectomy (with or without vagotomy):* excising the antrum of the stomach, thereby removing the hormonal stimulus of the parietal cells, followed by anastomosis of the rest of the stomach to the duodenum or the jejunum.

General

⬤⬤⬤ **RED FLAG** *Relief of symptoms*
⬤⬤⬤ *doesn't rule out cancer.*

Medication

Current recommendations include treating every patient at least once to eradicate *H. pylori* because the infection may occur even with other causes such as NSAID use. Although *H. pylori* infection can be eliminated, studies have demonstrated that symptomatic *H. pylori* returns in 80% of patients more than 1 year after treatment.

▶ Treatment options include acid suppression and a combination of antibiotics (three drugs twice per day for 7 to 10 days). Drug combinations include metronidazole, omeprazole, and clarithromycin; lansoprazole, amoxicillin, and clarithromycin; and ranitidine, bismuth citrate, amoxicillin, and clarithromycin.

▶ Patients taking NSAIDs may take a prostaglandin analogue (misoprostol) to minimize or prevent ulceration. A histamine-2 (H_2) receptor antagonist (cimetidine or nizatidine) or omeprazole may reduce acid secretion.

▶ If the condition is uncomplicated, the patient may try antinuclear drugs, including H_2-receptor antagonists (ranitidine, nizatidine), antacids (aluminum hydroxide), or sucralfate for 2 weeks. If the patient isn't responsive, diagnostic studies are indicated. If the patient is responsive, treat him for 8 weeks.

Collaborative practice

Refer the patient to a gastroenterologist for evaluation and GI studies for nonresponsive, recurrent symptoms or for evidence of bleeding.

Follow-up

See the patient in 2 weeks for evaluation. Perform a *Campylobacter*-like organism test biopsy, the urea breath test, or serologic tests if symptoms persist or return. If *H. pylori* returns, treat with a different drug regimen to decrease resistance.

Patients with gastric ulcer need posttreatment endoscopy at $1^1/_2$ to 3 months to detect cancer or poor healing.

Complications

▶ Gastric outlet obstruction
▶ Hemorrhage
▶ Perforation
▶ Severe back pain

● ● ● **RED FLAG** *Dizziness, syncope,*
● ● ● *hematemesis, or melena suggests hemorrhage.*

Patient teaching

▶ Teach the patient about the adverse effects of H_2-receptor antagonists and omeprazole (dizziness, fatigue, rash, mild diarrhea).

▶ Advise the patient who uses antacids, has a history of cardiac disease, or follows a sodium-restricted diet to take only antacids that contain low amounts of sodium.

▶ Tell the patient to avoid hot, spicy, and high-fat foods.

▶ Warn the patient to avoid steroids, aspirin, and NSAIDs because they decrease protective factors. For the same reason, warn the patient to avoid stressful situations, smoking, excessive intake of coffee, and ingestion of alcoholic beverages during exacerbations of peptic ulcer disease.

▶ Inform the patient of the potential adverse effects of antibiotic therapy (superinfection, diarrhea).

▶ Emphasize need for follow-up testing to confirm eradication of *H. pylori* infection.

▶ Tell the patient taking bismuth subsalicylate that this drug may cause constipation and very dark stools.

● ● ● **RED FLAG** *Tell the patient to call*
● ● ● *the primary care provider to report any new or persistent signs and symptoms, including abdominal pain that worsens or fails to respond to treatment; fever above 101° F (38.3° C); bloody or coffee-ground vomitus; and bright-red, black, tarry, or maroon-colored stools.*

Resources

▶ National Institute of Diabetes and Digestive and Kidney Diseases: *www.niddk.nih.gov*

ⓅPNEUMONIA

ICD-9-CM 486, aspiration 507.0, atypical 486, with influenza 487.0, bacterial 482.9, pneumococcal/streptococcal 481, interstitial 516.8, mycoplasma 483, Pneumocystis carinii 136.3, viral 480.9

An acute infection of the lung parenchyma, pneumonia typically impairs gas exchange. The prognosis is generally good for people who have normal lungs and adequate host defenses before the onset of pneumonia; however, pneumonia is the sixth leading cause of death in the United States.

❋ **LIFE SPAN** *Adults older than age 65 with bacterial pneumonia are at higher risk for death because clinical presentation is commonly atypical or obscured, and may not produce symptoms.*

Causes

The causes of pneumonia are reflected in the way the disease is classified.

▶ *By microbiological etiology* — Pneumonia can be viral, bacterial, fungal, protozoal, mycobacterial, mycoplasmal, or rickettsial in origin.

▶ *By type* — Primary pneumonia results from inhalation or aspiration of a pathogen and includes pneumococcal and viral pneumonia. Secondary pneumonia may follow initial lung damage from a noxious chemical or other insult (superinfection), or it may result from hematogenous spread of bacteria from a distant focus. (See *Types of pneumonia,* pages 262 to 264.)

▶ *By location* — Bronchopneumonia involves distal airways and alveoli; lobular pneumonia, part of a lobe; and lobar pneumonia, an entire lobe.

Predisposing factors

Predisposing factors to bacterial and viral pneumonia include age extremes, chronic illness and debilitation, cancer (particularly lung cancer), abdominal and thoracic surgery, atelectasis, common colds or other viral respiratory infections, chronic respiratory disease (chronic obstructive pulmonary disease [COPD], asthma, bronchiectasis, cystic fibrosis), influenza, smoking, malnutrition, alcoholism, sickle cell disease, tracheostomy, exposure to

noxious gases, aspiration, and immunosuppressant therapy.

Predisposing factors to aspiration pneumonia include old age, debilitation, nasogastric tube feedings, impaired gag reflex, poor oral hygiene, and decreased level of consciousness.

Clinical presentation

The patient history may elicit the five cardinal symptoms of early bacterial pneumonia: coughing, sputum production, pleuritic chest pain, rigors, and high fever.

Examination that yields focal dullness on percussion, increased tactile fremitus and transmission of sound, or late inspiratory crackles over the focal dullness suggests pneumonia and requires a chest X-ray or a consultation with a physician.

Differential diagnosis

▶ Atelectasis
▶ Cancer
▶ COPD
▶ Heart failure
▶ Infectious pneumonitis
▶ Pneumothorax
▶ Pulmonary contusion
▶ Pulmonary embolus
▶ Tuberculosis

Diagnostic tests

▶ *Complete blood count* may reveal leukocytosis.

▶ *Chest X-ray* showing infiltrates and sputum smear demonstrating acute inflammatory cells support the diagnosis. Chest X-ray may also reveal lobar or segmental consolidation, bronchopneumonia, pleural effusion, or air bronchogram.

▶ Positive *blood cultures* in patients with pulmonary infiltrates strongly suggest pneumonia produced by the organisms isolated from the blood cultures.

(Text continues on page 264.)

TYPES OF PNEUMONIA

Type	Causative agent	Assessment findings
Aspiration pneumonia	Aspiration of gastric or oropharyngeal contents into trachea or lungs	▶ Fever ▶ Crackles ▶ Dyspnea ▶ Hypotension ▶ Tachycardia ▶ Cyanosis ▶ Chest X-ray with infiltrates
COMMUNITY-ACQUIRED PNEUMONIAS		
Streptococcal pneumonia (pneumococcal pneumonia)	*Streptococcus pneumonia*	▶ Sudden onset of single shaking chill ▶ Fever 102° to 104° F (38.9° to 40° C) ▶ History of previous upper respiratory infection ▶ Pleuritic chest pain ▶ Severe cough ▶ Rust-colored sputum ▶ Areas of consolidation on chest X-ray (usually lobar) ▶ Elevated white blood cell (WBC) count ▶ Sputum culture possibly positive for gram-positive *S. pneumoniae*
Hemophilius influenza	*Haemophilus influenzae*	▶ Insidious onset ▶ History of upper respiratory tract infection 2 to 6 weeks earlier ▶ Fever ▶ Chills ▶ Dyspnea ▶ Productive cough ▶ Nausea and vomiting ▶ Chest X-ray with infiltrates in one or more lobes
Mycoplasma pneumonia	*Mycoplasma pneumoniae*	▶ Insidious onset ▶ Sore throat ▶ Nasal congestion ▶ Ear pain ▶ Headache ▶ Low-grade fever ▶ Pleuritic pain ▶ Erythema rash ▶ Pharyngitis

TYPES OF PNEUMONIA *(continued)*

Type	Causative agent	Assessment findings

COMMUNITY-ACQUIRED PNEUMONIAS (continued)

Type	Causative agent	Assessment findings
Viral pneumonia	Influenza virus, type A	▶ Initially beginning as upper respiratory infection ▶ Cough (initially nonproductive; later purulent sputum) ▶ High fever ▶ Chills ▶ Malaise ▶ Dyspnea ▶ Substernal pain ▶ Moist crackles ▶ Cyanosis ▶ Frontal headache ▶ Chest X-ray with diffuse bilateral broncho-pneumonia radiating from hilus ▶ Normal to slightly elevated WBC
Legionnaires' disease	*Legionella pneumophila*	▶ Flulike symptoms ▶ Malaise ▶ Headache within 24 hours ▶ Fever ▶ Shaking chills ▶ Progressive dyspnea ▶ Mental confusion ▶ Anorexia ▶ Nausea, vomiting ▶ Myalgia ▶ Chest X-ray with patchy infiltrates, consolidation, and possible effusion

HOSPITAL-ACQUIRED PNEUMONIAS

Type	Causative agent	Assessment findings
Klebsiella pneumonia	*Klebsiella pneumoniae*	▶ Fever ▶ Recurrent chills ▶ Rusty, bloody viscous sputum ▶ Cyanosis of lips and nail beds ▶ Shallow grunting respirations ▶ Severe pleuritic chest pain ▶ Chest X-ray typically with consolidation in upper lobe ▶ Elevated WBC ▶ Sputum culture and Gram stain possibly positive for gram-negative cocci, *Klebsiella*
Pseudomonas pneumonia	*Pseudomonas aeruginosa*	▶ Fever ▶ Chills ▶ Confusion ▶ Delirium ▶ Green foul-smelling sputum ▶ Chest X-ray with diffuse consolidation

(continued)

TYPES OF PNEUMONIA *(continued)*

Type	Causative agent	Assessment findings
HOSPITAL-ACQUIRED PNEUMONIAS *(continued)*		
Staphylococ-cal pneumonia (may also be community-acquired)	*Staphylococcus aureus*	▶ Cough ▶ Chills ▶ High fever 102° to 104° F (38.9° to 40° C) ▶ Pleuritic pain ▶ Progressive dyspnea ▶ Bloody sputum ▶ Tachypnea ▶ Hypoxemia ▶ Chest X-ray with multiple abscesses and infiltrate, emphysema ▶ Elevated WBC ▶ Sputum culture and Gram stain possibly positive for gram-positive staphylococci

▶ *Pleural effusions,* if present, should be tapped and the fluid analyzed for evidence of infection in the pleural space. Occasionally, a transtracheal aspirate of tracheobronchial secretions or bronchoscopy with brushings or washings may be done to obtain material for smear and culture.

▶ The patient's response to antimicrobial therapy also provides important evidence of the presence of pneumonia.

Management
Acute
Hospitalization is indicated for children younger than 4 months, for elderly patients, and for those with significant comorbidity or a severe infection.

General
Outpatient treatment involves supportive measures and follow-up to ensure effectiveness of management plan.

Medication
Antimicrobial therapy varies with the causative agent. Besides the clinical picture, it's important to know what types of respiratory infections (influenza or bacterial strains) are currently affecting your local area (community biography profile). Therapy should be reevaluated early in the course of treatment for effectiveness.

▶ *Antivirals* (amantadine) are most effective if started within 48 hours of symptom onset. For cytomegalovirus or herpes simplex virus, ganciclovir is beneficial; for *Hantavirus* and influenza B virus, ribavirin is beneficial.

▶ *Antibiotics* are ordered empirically and then adjusted as culture and sensitivity results indicate. For instance, co-trimoxazole treats *Pneumocystis carinii pneumonia* or *Haemophilus influenzae,* erythromycin treats mycoplasma, and penicillin G treats streptococcal and most aspiration pneumonias.

▶ *Cough suppressants* should be used sparingly, at bedtime, as needed for sleep.

▶ *Bronchodilator puffs* (albuterol) relieve wheezing.

Collaborative practice

Refer the patient to a physician for distressed appearance, hemoptysis, history of lung disease or immuno-compromise, unresponsiveness, or hospitalization. Refer him to an infectious disease specialist as indicated.

Follow-up

Contact the patient by phone within 48 hours; if his condition has improved, see him in 1 week. See him again in 4 to 6 weeks, and order a chest X-ray if he smokes, is over age 40, or still has symptoms.

Complications

▶ Arthralgia
▶ Bacteremia
▶ Empyema
▶ Erythema multiforme
▶ Hemolytic anemia
▶ Hypoxemia
▶ Myocarditis
▶ Pericarditis
▶ Pleural effusion
▶ Reactive airway disease
▶ Respiratory distress syndrome

Patient teaching

▶ Teach the patient that self-care measures can increase comfort, prevent complications, and speed recovery.
▶ Advise the patient of the importance of increasing fluid intake to at least 2 qt (2 L) per day and of getting adequate rest.
▶ Teach the patient how to cough and perform deep-breathing exercises to clear secretions, and advise him to do so frequently.
▶ Instruct the patient about precautionary measures — washing hands frequently, not sharing tissues or utensils, and disposing of soiled tissues properly.
▶ Teach the patient about the drugs ordered and associated adverse effects.

▶ Instruct the patient how to use a vaporizer or humidifier to thin secretions. If these devices aren't available, encourage a long steamy shower with deep breathing before bedtime.

To prevent pneumonia:
▶ Advise the patient to avoid using antibiotics indiscriminately during minor viral infections; this may result in upper airway colonization with antibiotic-resistant bacteria. If the patient then develops pneumonia, the organisms producing the pneumonia may require treatment with more toxic antibiotics.
▶ Encourage annual influenza vaccination, plus *Haemophilus pneumoniae* immunization for patients over age 65 and those with COPD, chronic heart disease, or sickle cell disease. Repeat *H. pneumoniae* immunization as indicated.

●●● RED FLAG *Tell the patient to call the primary care provider to report new or persistent signs and symptoms, including fever higher than 101° F (38.3° C) and cough producing a change in sputum color (to green, brown, or dark yellow); difficulty eating due to shortness of breath; severe throat pain and difficulty swallowing; earache or sinus pain; increasing shortness of breath and increasing orthopnea (number of pillows elevating head in order to sleep); breathing that becomes rapid or increasingly difficult, or unusual drowsiness.*

●●● RED FLAG *If the patient fails to respond, his lips become dusky or blue, or his respirations become very irregular (as occurs in Cheyne-Stokes respirations), activate emergency medical services.*

Resources

▶ American Lung Association: 1-800-LUNG-USA; *www.lungusa.org*
▶ Patient information on viral pneumonia: *www.medscape.com*

PROSTATE CANCER

ICD-9-CM primary 185, secondary 198.82, in situ 233.4 benign 222.2, uncertain 236.5

Prostate cancer accounts for 18% of all cancers; it's the second most common neoplasm found in men over age 50. Adenocarcinoma is its most common form; sarcoma occurs only rarely. Most prostatic carcinomas originate in the posterior prostate gland; the rest originate near the urethra. Malignant prostatic tumors seldom result from the benign hyperplastic enlargement that commonly develops around the prostatic urethra in elderly men. Prostate cancer seldom produces symptoms until it's advanced.

Causes

Although androgens regulate prostate growth and function and may also speed tumor growth, no definite link between increased androgen levels and prostate cancer has been found. When primary prostatic lesions metastasize, they typically invade the prostatic capsule and spread along the ejaculatory ducts in the space between the seminal vesicles or perivesicular fascia.

CULTURAL KEY *Incidence of prostate cancer is highest in Blacks and lowest in Asians.*

LIFE SPAN *Incidence of prostate cancer increases with age far more than other cancers.*

Clinical presentation

Manifestations of prostate cancer appear only in the advanced stages and include difficulty initiating a urinary stream, dribbling, urine retention, unexplained cystitis and, rarely, hematuria. Lymph node metastases can lead to lower extremity lymphedema. Skeletal metastases can present as back pain or pathologic fractures. Neurologic involvement may result in epidural compression and cord compression.

Differential diagnosis

▶ Benign prostatic hyperplasia
▶ Bladder cancer
▶ Prostatic calculi
▶ Prostatitis

Diagnostic tests

▶ A *digital rectal examination* that reveals a small, hard nodule may help diagnose prostate cancer.
▶ *Biopsy* confirms the diagnosis.
▶ *Prostate-specific antigen (PSA) levels* will be elevated in most men with prostate cancer, and serum acid phosphatase levels will be elevated in two-thirds of men with metastatic prostate cancer. Therapy aims to return the serum acid phosphatase level to normal; a subsequent rise points to recurrence.
▶ *Magnetic resonance imaging (MRI), computed tomography scan,* and *excretory urography* may also aid the diagnosis. Complete blood count that detects anemia as well as elevated acid phosphatase and alkaline phosphatase and may indicate metastasis. At that point, MRI, bone scan, and transrectal ultrasound are used to detect metastasis.

Management

RED FLAG *The urge to void and inability to void for more than 8 hours despite fluid intake is a medical emergency. If left untreated, renal damage can occur.*

General

Management of prostate cancer depends on clinical assessment, tolerance of therapy, expected life span, and the stage of the disease. Treatment must be chosen carefully because prostate cancer usually affects older men, who commonly have coexisting disorders, such as hypertension, diabetes, and cardiac disease. It's important to discuss with the patient the disease process, prognosis, and advantages and disadvantages of treatment options. It's even more important to support the patient's decisions about the extent of treatment he'll receive.

Therapy varies with each stage of the disease and generally includes radiation, prostatectomy, orchiectomy to reduce androgen production, and hormone therapy with synthetic estrogen (diethylstilbestrol) and antiandrogens, such as cyproterone, megestrol, and flutamide. Radical prostatectomy is usually effective for localized lesions.

Radiation therapy is used to cure some locally invasive lesions and to relieve pain from metastatic bone involvement. A single injection of the radionuclide strontium 89 is also used to treat pain caused by bone metastasis.

If hormone therapy, surgery, and radiation therapy aren't feasible or successful, chemotherapy (using combinations of cyclophosphamide, doxorubicin, fluorouracil, cisplatin, etoposide, and vindesine) may be tried; however, current drug therapy offers little benefit. Combining several treatment methods may be most effective.

Collaborative practice

If PSA levels are elevated or a prostatic mass is found, refer the patient to a urologist and anticipate a transurethral ultrasonogram. After being diagnosed, the patient will be referred to an oncologist for evaluation and treatment.

Follow-up

See the patient quarterly to annually, depending on the clinical picture. Incorporate specialists' recommendations into routine visits. Focus on the patient's response to treatment and changes in urination. Ask about pain in the pubic area or lower abdomen or unusual bone pain.

❀ **LIFE SPAN** *The American Cancer Society advises a yearly digital examination for men older than age 40. For black men starting at age 40 and for all others starting at age 50, a yearly blood test is recommended to detect PSA.*

Complications

▶ Cardiac failure
▶ Metastasis (particularly to bone)
▶ Urinary outflow obstruction

Patient teaching

▶ Explain the expected effects of surgery, such as impotence and incontinence, and of radiation treatments, such as diarrhea, bladder spasms, and urinary frequency.
▶ Teach the patient to do perineal exercises 1 to 10 times per hour, starting 24 hours after surgery. Have him squeeze his buttocks together, hold this position for a few seconds, and then relax.

After transurethral prostatic resection:
▶ Check for signs of urethral stricture: dysuria, decreased force and caliber of urinary stream, straining to urinate, and abdominal distention.

After radiation therapy:
▶ Check for common adverse effects, such as proctitis, diarrhea, bladder spasms, and urinary frequency. Internal radiation usually results in cystitis in the first 2 to 3 weeks.
▶ Advise the patient to drink at least 2 qt (2 L) of fluids per day but to avoid alcohol, caffeinated beverages, and decongestants because they can cause spasms and discomfort.
▶ Order analgesics (such as acetaminophen plus codeine) as needed to relieve pain.

●●● **RED FLAG** *Tell the patient to call the primary care provider to report new or persistent signs and* *symptoms, including signs and symptoms of urinary tract infection (pain or burning on urination, urinary frequency, urinary urgency, blood in the urine, cloudy or odorous urine, fever higher than 101° F [38.3° C], drainage from the penis), the urge to void and the inability to void for more than 8 hours despite good fluid intake, increased pain in the pubic or lower abdominal area, and difficulty starting a stream of urine, decreased force of the urine stream, or a feeling of incomplete emptying.*

Resources

▶ Us Too! International: 1-800-808-7866; *www.ustoo.com*
▶ American Cancer Society: 1-800-ACS-2345; *www.cancer.org*
▶ Cancer Information Service: 1-800-4-CANCER; *http://cis.nci.nih.gov*
▶ Cancer Care: 1-800-813-HOPE; *www.cancercare.org*
▶ Patient information on prostate cancer: *www.medscape.com*
▶ For patients, caregivers, and professional providers — Association of Cancer Online: *www.acor.org*

SEXUALLY TRANSMITTED DISEASES

ICD-9-CM (See *Identifying sexually transmitted diseases,* pages 270 to 275, for specific ICD-9-CM codes.) Sexually transmitted diseases (STDs) are a group of infections with similar manifestations that aren't linked to a single organism. They cause urethritis in males, and vaginitis and cervicitis in females. These primarily sexually transmitted infections have become more prevalent since the mid-1960s.

Gonorrhea and chlamydia are the most common STDs in the United States at this time. Treatment, duration of contagion, and prognosis depend on which organism is involved. The biggest risk is that a patient with one STD is at higher risk for developing another STD, the most serious being human immunodeficiency virus (HIV) infection.

Causes

STDs are spread primarily through sexual intercourse. The causative organisms are bacterial, viral, and fungal.

Clinical presentation

Signs and symptoms vary depending on the causative organism but typically include mucopurulent urethral discharge, variable dysuria, pruritus, lesions, and occasional hematuria. Subclinical STDs may be found on physical examination, especially if the patient's sexual partner has a positive diagnosis.

Both males and females may be asymptomatic or show signs of urethral, vaginal, or cervical infection on physical examination.

Differential diagnosis

See *Identifying sexually transmitted diseases,* pages 270 to 275.

Management

Recommend screening tests for anyone suspected of having an STD. All patients whose symptoms suggest infection require education about STDs and HIV, regardless of test results. Patients are usually more receptive at this time because of the perceived risk.

Complications

See *Identifying sexually transmitted diseases,* pages 270 to 275.

Patient teaching

▶ Tell women to clean the pubic area before applying vaginal medications and to avoid using tampons during treatment.

▸ Make sure the patient understands the dosage schedule for all prescribed medications clearly and follows it strictly.

▸ Teach him about the incubation, duration, transmission, recurrence, and complications of his specific STD.

▸ Teach the patient how to prevent genitourinary infections.

To prevent genitourinary infections:

▸ Tell patients to abstain from sexual contact with infected partners, to use condoms during every sexual encounter and follow appropriate hygienic measures afterward, and to void before and after intercourse. As appropriate, instruct on use of condoms and vaginal dams.

▸ Encourage patients to maintain adequate fluid intake.

▸ Advise women to avoid routinely using douches and feminine hygiene sprays, wearing tight-fitting pants and panty hose, and inserting foreign objects into the vagina.

▸ Suggest that women wear cotton underpants and remove them before going to bed.

Resources

▸ National STD Hotline: 1-800-227-8922.

▸ Planned Parenthood Foundation of America: (212) 541-7800; *www.plannedparenthood.org* (includes section for teen issues); for Spanish-speaking patients: *www.plannedparenthood.org/ESPANOL/INDEX.html*

SINUSITIS

ICD-9-CM 473.9, with influenza 487.1, acute 461.9, allergic 477.9

Sinusitis is an inflammation of the paranasal sinuses, which may be acute, chronic, allergic, or hyperplastic. Acute sinusitis usually re-

sults from the common cold and lingers in only about 10% of patients. Chronic sinusitis follows persistent bacterial infection. Allergic sinusitis accompanies allergic rhinitis. Hyperplastic sinusitis is a combination of purulent acute sinusitis and allergic sinusitis or rhinitis. The prognosis is good for all types.

Causes

Sinusitis usually results from viral or bacterial infection. The bacteria responsible for acute sinusitis are usually pneumococci, other streptococci, *Haemophilus influenzae,* and *Moraxella catarrhalis.* Staphylococci and gram-negative bacteria are more likely to occur in chronic cases or in patients in intensive care.

On rare occasions, fungi can also be an etiologic factor. *Aspergillus fumigatus* is the fungus most frequently associated with sinus disease.

Predisposing factors include a condition that interferes with drainage and ventilation of the sinuses, such as chronic nasal edema, deviated septum, viscous mucus, nasal polyps, allergic rhinitis, nasal intubation, nasogastric tubes, and debilitation related to chemotherapy, malnutrition, diabetes, blood dyscrasias, chronic use of steroids, or immunodeficiency.

Bacterial invasion commonly occurs from the conditions listed above or after a viral infection. It may also result from swimming in contaminated water.

Clinical presentation

Signs and symptoms vary with sinusitis type. In acute sinusitis, the primary symptom is nasal congestion, followed by a gradual buildup of pressure in the affected sinus. For 24 to 48 hours after onset, nasal

(Text continues on page 274.)

IDENTIFYING SEXUALLY TRANSMITTED DISEASES

Although these diseases are usually transmitted sexually, other forms of transmission are possible. For example, the etiology of bacterial vaginosis isn't completely understood, but sexual transmission is now considered unlikely. This chart provides a quick overview of diagnosis and treatment of common genital infections.

Disease and ICD-9-CM code	Clinical presentation and time from contact to symptom	Diagnosis
Bacterial vaginosis (616.10)	▶ White, malodorous, "fishy" discharge; itching; burning on urination; genital redness ▶ Time frame not applicable	Examination, culture, wet mount preparation: Clue cells, "fishy" odor produced by a drop of potassium hydroxide
Chlamydia (vaginitis 099.53; urethritis 099.41); also known as *nongonococcal urethritis*	▶ Thin, clear, malodorous discharge; postcoital bleeding; dyspareunia; or patient possibly asymptomatic ▶ Varies (1 to 3 weeks)	Examination; deoxyribonucleic acid (DNA) assay probe to check for gonorrhea and chlamydia
Gonorrhea (098.0; in eye 098.40)	▶ Yellowish-green genital discharge; burning on urination; occasionally asymptomatic in men; frequently asymptomatic in women; partner possibly diagnosed first ▶ 2 to 10 (up to 30) days	Examination; DNA probe assay to check for gonorrhea and chlamydia; possibly endocervical, conjunctival, rectal, or oral culture
Herpes simplex (054.10)	▶ Swollen, tender, painful blisters on genitals or lips ▶ Up to 2 weeks	Papanicolaou (Pap) test, examination, herpes culture
Human immunodeficiency virus (HIV) infection or acquired immunodeficiency syndrome (042)	▶ Purplish discolorations on skin, unexplained weight loss, persistent cough, anorexia, fever, fatigue ▶ 2 years or more	Tests for cancer and superinfection, as indicated by examination

Cause and treatment	Complications	Follow-up and referral
▸ Bacteria or chemical irritation; curable ▸ *Orally:* metronidazole daily for 7 days *Intravaginally:* metronidazole gel or clindamycin 2% (may use during pregnancy)	Not known	▸ If condition recurs, consider need to treat sexual partners.
▸ Mycoplasma; curable ▸ *Orally:* azithromycin in a single dose (best treatment for pregnant women) or doxycycline	Pelvic inflammatory disease (PID), sterility, tubal pregnancy, scar tissue, possible eye infections or pneumonia in neonates	▸ Follow up in 2 to 4 weeks for test of cure to determine antibody resistance or reinfection. ▸ Ensure that partners are treated.
▸ Bacterium; curable ▸ Same treatment as for Chlamydia ▸ *Disseminated infection:* ceftriaxone I.M. or I.V. q 24 hr until second day after improvement begins, then P.O. ciprofloxacin	PID, ectopic pregnancy, sterility, arthritis, blindness, eye infection in neonates	▸ Follow up in 2 to 4 weeks for test of cure to check for reinfection. ▸ Ensure that partners are treated. ▸ Report to local health authority; if a child, report to child abuse authorities.
▸ Virus; no cure ▸ *Supportive:* intermittent, cool, moist dressings with Burow's solution	Strong association with cervical cancer; severe central nervous system damage or death in infants infected during birth	▸ Follow up for recurrences and annual Pap test.
▸ Virus; no cure ▸ Supportive and antiviral	Severe medical and psychiatric problems; death	▸ Refer to a psychotherapist for counseling and to an HIV specialist.

(continued)

IDENTIFYING SEXUALLY TRANSMITTED DISEASES *(continued)*

Disease and ICD-9-CM code	Clinical presentation and time from contact to symptom	Diagnosis
Pediculosis pubis (132.2; infestation 132.9)	▶ Intense itching, pinhead blood spots on underwear; small eggs or nits (white, light gray, or honey-colored ovals on hair shaft) ▶ 3 to 14 days	Examination
Scabies (133.0)	▶ Severe nocturnal itching; raised lines in skin where mite burrows; may infest elbows, hands, web spaces, breasts, buttocks, and genitalia ▶ 4 to 6 weeks	Examination, fountain-pen ink applied to infested skin concentrates in grooves under the skin, easing identification of burrows
Syphilis (090.0-097.9)	▶ First stage: painless lesions of long duration on genitalia, fingers, lips, and breasts that resolve without treatment; second stage: rash, fever, flulike symptoms; latent stage: asymptomatic ▶ 10 to 90 days; average 21 days	Examination, rapid plasma reagin positive, fluorescent treponemal antibody positive
Trichomoniasis (131.9)	▶ Green, frothy, malodorous discharge; intense itching, burning, and redness of genitalia and thighs; dyspareunia; men usually asymptomatic ▶ Varies (1 to 4 weeks)	Pap test, examination, urinalysis, wet mount preparation: trichomonads present (motile with flagella)

Cause and treatment	Complications	Follow-up and referral
▸ Louse; curable ▸ *Topical:* permethrin, pyrethrins, lindane (follow directions on bottle); wash and dry all cloth on hot settings; if unable to wash items, dry-clean or seal in plastic bag for 2 weeks; 1:1 vinegar to water solution in hair every 15 minutes to ease nit removal	Secondary infection from scratching	▸ Follow up if unresponsive or symptoms recur. ▸ Ensure that partners are treated.
▸ Itch mite; curable ▸ *Topical:* lindane, permethrin (follow directions on bottle); itching may continue up to 14 days after successful treatment due to allergic reaction to mite and excrement; same clothing and bedding measures as for lice except no need to dry-clean and only 1 week sealed in bag	Secondary infection from scratching	▸ Follow up in 2 weeks to verify resolution. ▸ Ensure that partners are treated.
▸ Spirochete; curable until stage 3 (latent) ▸ Benzathine penicillin I.M. for primary, secondary, or latent less than 1 year; if latent more than 1 year or if unknown, benzathine penicillin I.M. weekly for 3 weeks; see Centers for Disease Control and Prevention guidelines for options	Brain damage; insanity; paralysis; heart disease; death; damage to skin, bones, eyes, liver, and teeth of fetus and neonates	▸ Venereal Disease Research Laboratory test at 3, 6, 12, and 24 months to detect relapse; if latent, test every 6 months for 2 years. ▸ Report to local health authority.
▸ Protozoa; curable ▸ Same treatment as for bacterial vaginosis ▸ *Alternative:* P.O. metronidazole in a single dose (for compliance)	Gland infections in females; prostatitis	▸ Follow up in 2 weeks. ▸ Ensure that partners are treated.

(continued)

IDENTIFYING SEXUALLY TRANSMITTED DISEASES (continued)

Disease and ICD-9-CM code	Clinical presentation and time from contact to symptom	Diagnosis
Venereal warts (*Condylomata acuminata*) (078.19)	▶ Local irritation, itching, pink or red cauliflower-like lesions; can look like ordinary warts ▶ Varies (1 to 8 months, average 2 months)	Pap test, examination, application of acetic acid (5% vinegar) to area, which will turn bluish-white (Scrapings of area turn white with acetic acid application.)
Vulvovaginal candidiasis (112.1)	▶ Severe vaginal itching, vulvar inflammation, cheesy discharge, yeastlike odor (like raw bread dough) ▶ Varies	Examination, culture, wet mount preparation

discharge may be present and later may become purulent. Associated symptoms include malaise, sore throat, headache, low-grade fever (temperature of 99° to 99.5° F [37.2° to 37.5° C]), malodorous breath, painless morning periorbital swelling, and a sense of facial fullness.

Characteristic pain depends on the affected sinus: maxillary sinusitis causes pain over the cheeks and upper teeth; ethmoid sinusitis, pain over the eyes; frontal sinusitis, pain over the eyebrows; and sphenoid sinusitis (rare), pain behind the eyes.

Purulent nasal drainage that continues for longer than 3 weeks after an acute infection subsides suggests lingering acute sinusitis. Other clinical features include a stuffy nose, vague facial discomfort, fatigue, and a nonproductive cough.

Other forms of sinusitis tend to be chronic, with symptoms similar to those of acute sinusitis, but with a continuous mucopurulent discharge. The effects of *allergic* sinusitis are predominantly those of allergic rhinitis — sneezing, frontal headache, watery nasal discharge, and a stuffy, burning, itchy nose; however, in *hyperplastic* sinusitis, bacterial growth on the diseased tissue causes pronounced tissue edema. This thickening of the mucosal lining and the development of mucosal polyps combine to produce

Cause and treatment	Complications	Follow-up and referral
▸ Virus; no cure ▸ 85% trichloracetic acid applied to lesions by primary care provider, repeated weekly until resolved ▸ Podofilox 0.5% cream (Condylox) applied to warts b.i.d. for 3 days, rest 4 days, then repeated for 4 cycles (may be used in pregnancy) ▸ If warts > 1″, referral for laser treatment, cryosurgery, or electrocautery	Highly contagious; if large enough, possible blockage of vaginal opening (Ninety percent of women with cervical cancer have evidence of venereal warts.)	▸ Follow up every 2 weeks until no visible warts; annual Pap test.
▸ Fungus; curable ▸ *Intravaginally:* 2% miconazole cream one full applicator daily h.s. for 7 days, terconazole 0.4% cream one full applicator daily for 7 days, 0.8% cream one full applicator daily for 3 days ▸ *Orally:* fluconazole in a single dose	None known	▸ For recurrent infections, consider HIV and diabetes mellitus testing.

chronic stuffiness of the nose as well as headaches.

Differential diagnosis

▸ Allergic rhinitis
▸ Chronic sinusitis
▸ Dental infection
▸ Headache — migraine, cluster, tension
▸ Nasal foreign body
▸ Otitis media
▸ Polyps
▸ Tumor or cyst
▸ Upper respiratory infection

Diagnostic tests

▸ *Nasal examination* reveals inflammation and pus, which indicate sinusitis.

▸ *Sinus X-rays* reveal cloudiness in the affected sinus, air and fluid, and thickening of the mucosal lining.
▸ *Antral puncture* promotes drainage of purulent material but is rarely done. It may also be used to provide a specimen for culture and sensitivity testing of the infecting organism.
▸ *Ultrasonography* and *computed tomography (CT) scan* aid in diagnosing suspected complications. CT scans are more sensitive than routine X-rays in detecting sinusitis.

Management

Treatment of allergic sinusitis may include identification of allergens by skin testing and desensitization by immunotherapy. If irrigation fails to relieve symptoms, one or more sinuses may require surgery.

Acute sinusitis

For acute sinusitis, local decongestants usually are tried before systemic decongestants; steam inhalation may also be helpful. Local application of heat may help to relieve pain and congestion.

Medication

Antibiotics are necessary to combat purulent or persistent infection resulting from acute sinusitis. Amoxicillin, ampicillin, and amoxicillinclavulanate potassium are the drugs of choice. Because sinusitis is a deep infection, antibiotics should be given for 2 to 3 weeks. Analgesics (ibuprofen, acetaminophen) and antihistamines (diphenhydramine) are given as needed.

In chronic and hyperplastic sinusitis, antihistamines (loratadine), antibiotics (guided by culture and sensitivity tests), and a steroid nasal spray (triamcinolone) may relieve pain and congestion. Severe allergic symptoms may require treatment with corticosteroids (cortisone) and bronchodilators (epinephrine).

Collaborative practice

Refer the patient to an otolaryngologist or another physician for a condition that's chronic, complex, or unresponsive after 3 weeks; refer him to a surgeon if necessary.

Follow-up

See the patient in 2 to 3 days to evaluate the effectiveness of treatment and again in 2 weeks.

Complications

▶ Cellulitis (orbital or facial)
▶ Central nervous system complications
▶ Osteomyelitis

Patient teaching

▶ Encourage the patient to rest and to drink plenty of fluids to promote drainage. The patient should place an extra pillow under the head and shoulders or place bricks or books under the head of the bed to promote drainage.
▶ Teach the patient to relieve pain and promote drainage by applying warm compresses.
▶ Urge the patient to finish the prescribed antibiotics, even if his symptoms disappear.
▶ Warn that vasoconstrictive nose drops and spray are associated with rebound edema if used for more than 5 to 7 days.

●●● **RED FLAG** *Tell the patient to*
●●● *call the primary care provider to report new or persistent signs and symptoms, including vomiting, chills, fever, edema of the forehead or eyelids, blurred or double vision, and personality changes.*

Resources

▶ American Academy of Otolaryngology — Head and Neck Surgery: (703) 836-4444; *www.entnet.org*
▶ American Rhinologic Society: *www.american-rhinologic.org*

● STROKE

ICD-9-CM subarachnoid hemorrhage 430, intracranial hemorrhage 431, occlusion of cerebral arteries 434, transient cerebral ischemia 435, acute but ill-defined cerebrovascular disease 436, late effects of cerebrovascular disease 438

A stroke, also known as a *brain attack* or *cerebrovascular accident*, is a sudden impairment of cerebral circulation in one or more of the blood vessels supplying the brain. A stroke interrupts or diminishes oxygen supply and commonly causes serious damage or necrosis in brain tissues. Eighty percent of strokes are caused by cerebral ischemia, and 20% result from hemorrhage. The sooner circulation returns to normal after a stroke, the better chances are for complete recovery; however, about 50% of those who survive a stroke remain permanently disabled and experience a recurrence within weeks, months, or years.

Stroke is the third most common cause of death in the United States today and the most common cause of neurologic disability. It strikes 500,000 people each year, half of whom die.

Causes

Factors that increase the risk of stroke include history of transient ischemic attacks (TIAs), atherosclerosis, hypertension, kidney disease, arrhythmias (specifically atrial fibrillation), electrocardiogram changes, rheumatic heart disease, diabetes mellitus, postural hypotension, cardiac or myocardial enlargement, high serum triglyceride levels, lack of exercise, use of hormonal contraceptives, cigarette smoking, and family history of stroke.

The major causes of stroke are thrombosis, embolism, and hemorrhage. Thrombosis is the most common cause of ischemic stroke in middle-aged and elderly people who have a higher incidence of atherosclerosis, diabetes, and hypertension. Thrombosis causes ischemia in brain tissue supplied by the affected vessel as well as congestion and edema; the latter may produce more clinical effects than thrombosis itself, but these symptoms subside with the edema. Thrombosis may develop while the patient sleeps or shortly after he awakens; it can also occur during surgery or after a myocardial infarction. The risk increases with obesity, smoking, or the use of hormonal contraceptives. Cocaine-induced ischemic

stroke is now being seen in younger patients.

Embolism, the second most common cause of ischemic stroke, is an occlusion of a blood vessel caused by a fragmented clot, a tumor, fat, bacteria, or air. It can occur at any age, especially among patients with a history of rheumatic heart disease, endocarditis, posttraumatic valvular disease, myocardial fibrillation, and other cardiac arrhythmias, or after open-heart surgery. It usually develops rapidly — in 10 to 20 seconds — and without warning. When an embolus reaches the cerebral vasculature, it cuts off circulation by lodging in a narrow portion of an artery, most commonly the middle cerebral artery, causing necrosis and edema. If the embolus is septic and infection extends beyond the vessel wall, encephalitis or an abscess may develop.

Hemorrhage — the third most common cause of stroke — may, like embolism, occur suddenly, at any age, and affects more women than men. Hemorrhage results from chronic hypertension or aneurysm, which cause sudden rupture of a cerebral artery, thereby diminishing blood supply to the area served by the artery. In addition, blood accumulates deep within the brain, further compressing neural tissue and causing even greater damage.

Strokes are classified according to their course of progression. The least severe is the TIA, or "mini stroke," which results from a temporary interruption of blood flow, most commonly in the carotid and vertebrobasilar arteries. (See *Understanding transient ischemic attacks,* page 278.) A progressive stroke, or stroke-in-evolution (thrombus-in-evolution), begins with slight neurologic deficit and worsens in a day or two. In a completed stroke,

UNDERSTANDING TRANSIENT ISCHEMIC ATTACKS

A transient ischemic attack (TIA) is an episode of neurologic deficit resulting from cerebral ischemia. The recurrent attacks may last from seconds to hours and clear in 12 to 24 hours. TIAs are commonly considered a warning sign for stroke and have been reported in more than one-half of the patients who later developed a stroke, usually in 2 to 5 years.

In a TIA, microemboli released from a thrombus may temporarily interrupt blood flow, especially in the small, distal branches of the brain's arterial tree. Small spasms in those arterioles may impair blood flow and also precede a TIA.

The most distinctive features of TIAs are transient focal deficits with complete return of function. The deficits usually involve some degree of motor or sensory dysfunction. They may progress to loss of consciousness and loss of motor or sensory function for a brief period. The patient typically experiences weakness in the lower part of the face and arms, hands, fingers, and legs on the side opposite the affected region. Other manifestations may include transient dysphagia, numbness or tingling of the face and lips, double vision, slurred speech, and vertigo.

neurologic deficits are maximal at onset.

Clinical presentation

Clinical features of stroke vary with the artery affected (and, consequently, the portion of the brain it supplies), the severity of damage, and the extent of collateral circula-

tion that develops to help the brain compensate for decreased blood supply. If the stroke occurs in the left hemisphere, it produces symptoms on the right side; if it develops in the right hemisphere, symptoms are on the left side; however, a stroke that causes cranial nerve damage produces signs of cranial nerve dysfunction on the same side as the hemorrhage.

Symptoms are usually classified according to the artery affected.
▶ *Middle cerebral artery* — aphasia, dysphasia, visual field cuts, and hemiparesis on affected side (more severe in the face and arm than in the leg) (See *Cincinnati prehospital stroke scale.*)
▶ *Carotid artery* — weakness, paralysis, numbness, sensory changes, and visual disturbances on affected side; altered level of consciousness; bruits; headaches; aphasia; and ptosis
▶ *Vertebrobasilar artery* — weakness on affected side, numbness around lips and mouth, visual field cuts, diplopia, poor coordination, dysphagia, slurred speech, dizziness, amnesia, and ataxia
▶ *Anterior cerebral artery* — confusion, weakness, and numbness (especially in the leg) on affected side; incontinence; loss of coordination; impaired motor and sensory functions; and personality changes
▶ *Posterior cerebral arteries* — visual field cuts, sensory impairment, dyslexia, coma, and cortical blindness; typically, paralysis is absent.

Symptoms can also be classified as premonitory, generalized, and focal. Premonitory symptoms, such as drowsiness, dizziness, headache, and mental confusion, are rare. Generalized symptoms, such as headache, vomiting, mental impairment, seizures, coma, nuchal rigidity, fever, and disorientation, are typical. Focal symptoms, such as

CINCINNATI PREHOSPITAL STROKE SCALE

If one of the three signs described here is abnormal, the probability of a stroke is 72%.

Facial droop
Tell the patient to show his teeth or smile. If he hasn't had a stroke, both sides of his face will move equally. If he has had a stroke, one side of his face won't move as well as the other side.

NORMAL RESPONSE

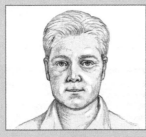

STROKE PATIENT WITH FACIAL DROOP ON RIGHT SIDE OF FACE

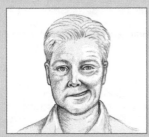

Arm drift
Tell the patient to close her eyes and hold both arms straight out in front of her for 20 seconds. If she hasn't had a stroke, her arms won't move or, if they do move, they'll move the same amount. Other findings, such as pronator grip, may be helpful.

If the patient has had a stroke, one arm won't move or one arm will drift down compared with the other arm.

NORMAL RESPONSE

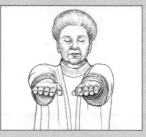

ONE-SIDED MOTOR WEAKNESS (RIGHT ARM)

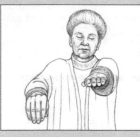

Abnormal speech
Have the patient say, "You can't teach an old dog new tricks." If he hasn't had a stroke, he'll use correct words and his speech won't be slurred. If he has had a stroke, his words will be slurred, he may use the wrong words, or he may be unable to speak at all.

Adapted with permission from Kothari, R., et al. "Early Stroke Recognition: Developing an Out-of-Hospital NIH Stroke Scale," *Academy of Emergency Medicine* 4(10):986-90, October 1997.

sensory and reflex changes, reflect the site of hemorrhage or infarct and may worsen.

Differential diagnosis

▶ Aneurysm
▶ Brain tumor
▶ Hyperglycemia, hypoglycemia
▶ Seizure
▶ Subdural hematoma
▶ Trauma

Diagnostic tests

Diagnosis of stroke is based on observation of clinical features, a history of risk factors, and the results of diagnostic tests.

▶ *Computed tomography scan* shows evidence of hemorrhagic stroke immediately but may not show evidence of thrombotic infarction for 48 to 72 hours.

▶ *Magnetic resonance imaging* may help identify ischemic or infracted areas and cerebral swelling.

▶ *Brain scan* shows ischemic areas but may not be positive for up to 2 weeks after the stroke.

▶ *Lumbar puncture* reveals bloody cerebrospinal fluid in hemorrhagic stroke.

▶ *Ophthalmoscopy* may show signs of hypertension and atherosclerotic changes in retinal arteries.

▶ *Angiography* outlines blood vessels and pinpoints occlusion or the rupture site.

▶ *EEG* helps to localize the damaged area.

▶ *Carotid Doppler study* should be done if a carotid bruit is present.

Other baseline laboratory studies include urinalysis, coagulation studies, complete blood count, serum osmolality, and electrolyte, glucose, triglyceride, creatinine, and blood urea nitrogen levels.

Management

General

Treatment options vary depending on the type of stroke the patient experiences. Early medical diagnosis of the stroke coupled with new drug treatments can greatly reduce the long-term disability secondary to ischemia.

Medication

▶ *Alteplase* (recombinant tissue plasminogen activator) is effective in emergency treatment of embolic stroke. Patients with embolic or thrombotic stroke who aren't candidates for alteplase (3 to 6 hours poststroke) should receive aspirin or heparin.

▶ *Aspirin* or *ticlopidine* can be used long-term as antiplatelet agents to prevent recurrent stroke.

▶ *Anticoagulants* (heparin, warfarin) may be required to treat crescendo TIAs not responsive to antiplatelet drugs.

▶ *Antihypertensives, antiarrhythmics,* and *antidiabetics* may be used to treat risk factors associated with recurrent stroke.

Surgery

Surgery performed to improve cerebral circulation for patients with thrombotic or embolic stroke includes endarterectomy (removal of atherosclerotic plaques from the inner arterial wall) and microvascular bypass (surgical anastomosis of an extracranial vessel to an intracranial vessel).

Collaborative practice

▶ Refer the patient immediately to a hospital if he's having symptoms of stroke.

▶ Refer the patient to a neurosurgeon or neurologist as indicated.

▶ Refer the patient to physical, occupational, or speech therapy as indicated.

▶ Consult a social worker regarding the patient's care.

▶ Refer the patient and his family to a psychologist as indicated.

▶ Refer the patient to local support groups such as the American Heart Association.

Follow-up

The patient should be seen frequently after discharge from the hospital. The frequency of visits will be related to the severity of the stroke. The patient may be seen 1 week after discharge, then every 2 to 3 weeks, then monthly, then every 3 months.

Complications

▶ Death
▶ Depression
▶ Disability
▶ Muscle atrophy

Patient teaching

▶ Explore the patient's and his family's abilities to cope with the life-altering illness. Focus on what they want and can participate in, and support all their efforts. Enlist aid when appropriate.
▶ The patient may fail to recognize that he has a paralyzed side (called unilateral neglect) and must be taught to inspect that side of his body for injury and protect it from harm.
▶ If speech therapy is indicated, encourage the patient to begin as soon as possible and follow through with the speech pathologist's suggestions. Teach his family about aspiration pneumonia and how to prevent it.
▶ Teach the patient or his family about premonitory signs of a stroke, such as severe headache, drowsiness, confusion, and dizziness. Emphasize the importance of regular follow-up visits.
▶ If aspirin has been prescribed to minimize the risk of embolic stroke, tell the patient to watch for possible GI bleeding. Make sure the patient and his family realize that acetaminophen isn't a substitute for aspirin.

▶ Stress the need to control diseases, such as diabetes and hypertension.
▶ Teach all patients (especially those at high risk) the importance of following a low-cholesterol, low-salt diet; watching their weight; increasing activity; avoiding smoking and prolonged bed rest; and minimizing stress.

Resources

▶ American Heart Association: 1-800-AHA-USA-1; *www.americanheart.org*
▶ National Institute of Neurological Disorders and Stroke: 1-800-352-9424; *www.ninds.nih.gov*
▶ National Stroke Association: 1-800-787-6537; *www.stroke.org*

TUBERCULOSIS

ICD-9-CM 011.9

An acute or chronic infection caused by *Mycobacterium tuberculosis*, tuberculosis (TB) is characterized by pulmonary infiltrates, formation of granulomas with caseation, fibrosis, and cavitation. People who live in crowded, poorly ventilated conditions are most likely to become infected with TB.

In patients with strains that are sensitive to the usual antitubercular agents, the prognosis is excellent with correct treatment; however, in patients infected with drug-resistant strains, mortality is 50%.

CULTURAL KEY *In the United States, more than 66% of reported TB cases are among nonwhite persons.*

Causes

After exposure to *M. tuberculosis*, roughly 5% of infected people develop active TB within 1 year; in the remainder, bacilli cause a latent infection. The host's immune system usually controls the tubercle bacillus by killing it or walling it up in a tiny nodule (tubercle); however, the bacillus may lie dormant within the tubercle for years and later reactivate and spread.

TB is transmitted by droplet nuclei produced when infected persons cough or sneeze. After inhalation, if a tubercle bacillus settles in an alveolus, infection occurs. Cell-mediated immunity to the mycobacteria, which develops about 3 to 6 weeks later, usually contains the infection and arrests the disease.

Although mycobacteria primarily infect the lungs, they commonly exist in other parts of the body. A number of factors increase the risk of infection reactivation, including gastrectomy, uncontrolled diabetes mellitus, Hodgkin's disease, leukemia, silicosis, acquired immunodeficiency syndrome, and treatment with corticosteroids or immunosuppressants.

If the infection becomes reactivated, the body's response characteristically leads to caseation — the conversion of necrotic tissue to a cheeselike material. The caseum may localize, undergo fibrosis, or excavate and form cavities, the walls of which are studded with multiplying tubercle bacilli. If this happens, infected caseous debris may spread throughout the lungs by the tracheobronchial tree.

Sites of extrapulmonary TB include the pleura, meninges, joints, lymph nodes, peritoneum, genitourinary tract, and bowel.

Clinical presentation

In primary infection, after an incubation period of 4 to 8 weeks, TB usually produces no symptoms but may produce nonspecific symptoms, such as fatigue, weakness, anorexia, weight loss, night sweats, and low-grade fever. The patient history should also elicit TB exposure, previous TB, other chronic diseases, and immunocompromised status. In TB reactivation, symptoms may include a cough that produces mucopurulent sputum, occasional hemoptysis, and pleuritic chest pains.

On examination, auscultation detects crepitant crackles, bronchial breath sounds, wheezes, and whispered pectoriloquy (sound transmission through the chest wall). Chest percussion detects a dullness over the affected area, indicating consolidation or pleural fluid.

Differential diagnosis

▶ Bronchiectasis
▶ Fungal infection
▶ Lymphoma
▶ Malignancy
▶ Pleural effusion
▶ Pneumonia

Diagnostic tests

▶ *Chest X-ray* shows nodular lesions, patchy infiltrates (mainly in upper lobes), cavity formation, scar tissue, and calcium deposits; however, it may not be able to distinguish active TB from inactive TB.
▶ *Tuberculin skin test* detects TB infection. Intermediate-strength purified protein derivative or 5 tuberculin units (0.1 ml) are injected intracutaneously on the forearm. The test results are read in 48 to 72 hours; a positive reaction (induration of 5 to 15 mm or more, depending on risk factors) develops 2 to 10 weeks after infection in both active and inactive TB; however, severely immunosuppressed patients may never develop a positive reaction.
▶ *Stains* and *cultures* (of sputum, cerebrospinal fluid, urine, drainage from abscess, or pleural fluid) show heat-sensitive, nonmotile, aerobic, acid-fast bacilli.

Management
General
All cases of newly diagnosed TB must be reported to the local health authority. Before initiating drug treatment, obtain baseline laboratory values — liver function studies, bilirubin, serum creatinine, complete blood count, platelet count, serum uric acid (if the patient is to receive pyrazinamide), and visual acuity plus red-green color perception (if the patient is to receive ethambutol).
Medication
▶ Daily oral doses of isoniazid, rifampin, and pyrazinamide (and sometimes ethambutol or streptomycin) for at least 6 months usually cure TB. After 2 to 4 weeks, the disease generally is no longer infectious. The patient can resume his normal lifestyle while taking the drugs.
▶ Because isoniazid sometimes leads to hepatitis or peripheral neuritis, monitor closely. To prevent or treat peripheral neuritis, give pyridoxine (vitamin B_6).
▶ Patients with atypical mycobacterial disease or drug-resistant TB may require treatment with second-line drugs, such as capreomycin, streptomycin, para-aminosalicylic acid, cycloserine, amikacin, and quinolones.
Collaborative practice
Refer the patient to a physician specializing in TB if treatment has failed after 3 months.
Follow-up
For patients who need direct observation therapy, follow-up is two to three times weekly by office staff or home visit, every 2 weeks for the next two visits, then monthly for two visits, and finally monthly for the remainder of treatment. Focus on compliance, toxicity and adverse effects of drugs. Perform a monthly chest X-ray.

For patients taking ethambutol, watch for optic neuritis; if it develops, discontinue the drug. If the patient takes rifampin, watch for hepatitis and purpura. Because isoniazid sometimes leads to hepatitis or peripheral neuritis, monitor aspartate aminotransferase and alanine aminotransferase levels monthly; if levels exceed three times normal, consider changing the drug.

After 3 months of treatment and at the conclusion of therapy, repeat the chest X-ray, acid-fast smear, and culture.

Complications
▶ Drug resistance
▶ Metastasis
▶ Secondary bacterial infection of cavitary lesions

Patient teaching
▶ Teach the patient to cough and sneeze into tissues and to dispose of all secretions properly.
▶ Remind the patient to get plenty of rest and to eat balanced meals. If the patient is anorectic, urge him to eat small meals throughout the day. Record weight weekly.
▶ Advise the patient of drug adverse effects.
▶ Emphasize the importance of regular follow-up examinations, and instruct the patient and his family about the signs and symptoms of recurring TB.
▶ Advise persons who have been exposed to infected patients to receive tuberculin tests and, if necessary, chest X-rays and prophylactic isoniazid.

RED FLAG *Tell the patient to call the primary care provider to report persistent, changing, worsening, anxiety-producing, or specific signs and symptoms, including signs of secondary infection or drug intolerance (fever, malaise, anorex-*

*ia, nausea, yellowed skin) or start-
ing to cough up blood.*

Resources

▶ American Lung Association: 1-
800-LUNG-USA; *www.lungusa.org*

▶ For providers — Drug affordability:
www.needymeds.com (contains information regarding many drug
company programs that provide financial assistance to those who
need their drugs)

URINARY TRACT INFECTION

*ICD-9-CM urinary infection 599.0
(may request organism specific
code), cystitis 595*

Cystitis and urethritis, the two
forms of lower urinary tract infection (UTI), are nearly 10 times more
common in women than in men
and affect approximately 10% to
20% of all women at least once.
Lower UTI is also a prevalent bacterial disease in children, with girls
more commonly affected.

In men and children, lower UTIs
are frequently related to anatomic
or physiologic abnormalities and
therefore require extremely close
evaluation. UTIs usually respond
readily to treatment, but recurrence
and resistant bacterial flare-up during therapy are possible. (See *Treating and preventing urinary tract infections.*)

Causes

Most UTIs result from ascending infection by a single gram-negative
enteric bacteria, such as *Escherichia
coli, Klebsiella, Proteus, Enterobac-
ter, Pseudomonas,* or *Serratia.* In a
patient with neurogenic bladder, an
indwelling urinary catheter, or a
fistula between the intestine and
bladder, UTI may result from simultaneous infection with multiple
pathogens. An anatomic or func-

tional abnormality may predispose
the patient to infection.

Recent studies suggest that infection results from a breakdown in local defense mechanisms in the
bladder that allow bacteria to invade the bladder mucosa and multiply. These bacteria can't be readily
eliminated by normal micturition.

Bacterial flare-up

During treatment, bacterial flare-up
is generally caused by the patho-
genic organism's resistance to the
prescribed antimicrobial therapy.
The presence of even a small number (less than 10,000/ml) of bacteria in a midstream urine sample obtained during treatment casts doubt
on the effectiveness of treatment.

Recurrent UTI

In 99% of patients, recurrent UTI
results from reinfection by the same
organism or from some new pathogen; in the remaining 1%, recurrence reflects persistent infection,
usually from renal calculi, chronic
bacterial prostatitis, or a structural
anomaly that may become a source
of infection.

● **CLINICAL PEARL** *The high incidence of UTI among women
may result from the shortness of the
female urethra ($1^1/_2"$ to 2" [3 to
5 cm]), which predisposes women to
infection caused by bacteria from
the vagina, perineum, rectum, or a
sexual partner.*

Men are less vulnerable to UTIs
because their urethras are longer
($7^3/_4"$ [19.7 cm]) and their prostatic
fluid serves as an antibacterial
shield.

Clinical presentation

UTIs usually produce urgency, frequency, dysuria, spasms of the
bladder, itching, burning on urination, hematuria, sensation of incomplete bladder emptying, and
fever. The urine may be dark,
cloudy, and malodorous. Other

TREATING AND PREVENTING URINARY TRACT INFECTIONS

Teach the female patient how to clean the perineum properly and keep the labia separated during voiding to collect a clean, midstream urine specimen. Explain that a noncontaminated midstream specimen is essential for accurate diagnosis.

Treatment

▶ Explain the nature and purpose of antimicrobial therapy. Emphasize the importance of completing the prescribed course of therapy or, with long-term prophylaxis, of adhering strictly to ordered dosage.

▶ Recommend taking nitrofurantoin macrocrystals with milk or a meal to prevent GI distress. If therapy includes phenazopyridine, warn the patient that this drug may turn urine red-orange.

▶ Urge the patient to drink at least eight glasses of water per day. Stress the need to maintain a consistent daily fluid intake of about 2 qt (2 L). More or less than this amount may alter the effect of the prescribed antimicrobial.

▶ Tell the patient that fruit juices, especially cranberry juice, and oral doses of vitamin C may help acidify the urine and enhance the action of the medication.

▶ Suggest warm sitz baths for relief of perineal discomfort.

Prevention

To prevent recurrent infections in men, urge prompt treatment of predisposing conditions such as chronic prostatitis.

To prevent recurrent infections in women, teach the patient to:

▶ wipe the perineum carefully from front to back and to clean it thoroughly with soap and water after defecation

▶ void immediately after sexual intercourse, drink plenty of fluids routinely, and avoid postponing urination

▶ take frequent comfort stops during long car trips, stressing the need to empty the bladder completely.

---

symptoms include lower back pain, malaise, nausea, vomiting, abdominal pain or tenderness over the bladder area, costovertebral angle tenderness, rigors, and flank pain.

The history may elicit chronic predisposing diseases (such as diabetes mellitus, multiple sclerosis, frequent UTIs, and immunocompromise), structural anomalies, methods of birth control and last menstrual period, constitutional symptoms (fever, rigor), and (in mature men) symptoms of prostatic hypertrophy.

Differential diagnosis

▶ Hematuria from noninfectious causes

▶ Pyuria secondary to a sexually transmitted disease (STD)

▶ Urethritis

▶ Vaginitis

CLINICAL PEARL *A history of gradual onset, intermittent symptoms, dysuria as urine passes over the labia (suggests candida or herpes simplex), penile discharge, vaginal discharge with bleeding, or lower abdominal pain requires aggressive evaluation to rule out STD. A finding of pyuria without significant bacteriuria also suggests STD.*

Diagnostic tests

▶ A clean midstream *urine specimen* revealing a bacterial count of more than 100,000/ml (pyuria) confirms the diagnosis. Lower counts don't necessarily rule out infection, especially if the patient is voiding frequently, because bacteria require 30 to 45 minutes to reproduce in urine.

▶ *Culture* and *sensitivity testing* determine the appropriate therapeutic antimicrobial agent. Suspect specimen contamination when multiple types of bacteria are detected. Consider urethral catheterization.

▶ *Voiding cystoureterography* or *excretory urography* may detect congenital anomalies that predispose the patient to recurrent UTIs.

▶ If the patient history and physical examination warrant, a *blood test* and *stained smear* of the discharge rules out STD (such as gonorrhea, chlamydia, syphilis, and human immunodeficiency virus).

Management
General
Encourage the patient to drink plenty of fluids (2 qt [2 L] per day).
Medication
▶ *Antimicrobials* (co-trimoxazole, fluoroquinolone) are the treatment of choice for most initial UTIs. For uncomplicated, infrequent UTIs, a 3-day antibiotic regimen is prescribed. All others receive a 10- to 14-day regimen and follow-up urine cultures for test of cure.

▶ If the urine isn't sterile, bacterial resistance has probably occurred, requiring change to a different antimicrobial. Recurrent infections due to infected renal calculi, chronic prostatitis, or structural abnormality may necessitate surgery; prostatitis also requires long-term antibiotic therapy. In patients without these predisposing conditions, long-term, low-dosage antibiotic therapy is the treatment of choice.
Collaborative practice
Refer the patient to a physician or urologist for conditions that are nonresponsive within 3 days of treatment with a bacteria-sensitive antibiotic, for frequent recurrences, for suspected anatomic abnormality, for diabetes, for a history of nephrolithiasis, or if follow-up culture detects the same pathogen.
Follow-up
See the patient in 1 to 2 weeks. Perform a urine culture at this time to verify that the infection has been eradicated.

Complications
▶ Cystitis
▶ Pyelonephritis
▶ Renal abscess

Patient teaching
▶ Tell the patient to watch for GI disturbances from antimicrobial therapy and to take drugs on an empty stomach with 8 oz (236 ml) water if possible.

▶ Explain that forcing fluids flushes bacteria out, and cranberry juice changes the pH of urine so bacteria can't survive.

▶ Instruct the patient to avoid alcohol, caffeine, and cold medications with decongestants because they can cause bladder spasms.

▶ Teach women to decrease the risk of infection by wiping from front to back after urination and by choosing a form of contraception other than a diaphragm.

▶ Tell the patient not to go long periods without voiding.

▶ Explain that voiding immediately postcoitally flushes out bacteria. If an STD is suspected, instruct the female patient to avoid intercourse.

▶ Teach comfort measures, such as taking a sitz bath, pouring warm water over the meatus during urination, washing with mild soap and water, not rubbing or scrubbing the area, and patting it dry.

●●● RED FLAG *Tell the patient to*
●●● *call the primary care provider*
to report new or persistent signs and
symptoms, including symptoms that
aren't mostly resolved within 48
hours, or high fever, chills, flank
pain, inability to urinate for more
than 8 hours despite the urge to
void, increased pain in the pubic
area or lower abdomen, and abnor-
mal vaginal discharge.

Resources

▶ Patient information on urinary
tract infections: *www.medscape.com*

7

Emergency care
Responding swiftly and accurately

Common types of emergencies 289

Common types of emergencies

The best way to deal with emergencies is to prevent them. To accomplish this, you must have full knowledge of your patient's health history, be mindful of physical and behavioral changes that foretell an emergency, and know the appropriate steps to take at any turn. This chapter details history questions to identify patient risk, precautions to avoid an emergency, signs and symptoms to guide diagnosis, and appropriate responses for situations requiring quick action. Finally, it provides patient teaching regarding when to contact a primary care provider or activate the emergency medical services (EMS).

ANAPHYLAXIS

ICD-9-CM due to: food 995.60, immunization 999.4, overdose or wrong substance given/taken 977.9
Anaphylaxis is an acute, potentially life-threatening type I (immediate) hypersensitivity reaction resulting from immunoglobulin (Ig) E–mediated mast cell or basophil degranulation. When severe, it may trigger vascular collapse, leading to systemic shock and, possibly, death.

Severe anaphylaxis causes physical distress, such as hives and respiratory distress, within seconds or minutes after exposure to the sensitizing substance. The sooner the reaction starts, the more severe it will be; death from vascular collapse and shock may occur within minutes or hours. A delayed or persistent reaction can occur for up to 24 hours after exposure to an allergen. (See *How anaphylaxis occurs,* page 290.)

Sometimes anaphylaxis takes a milder form, causing only hives or

a rash, or an intermediate form marked by a fever and swollen glands.

Causes

Anaphylaxis results from ingestion or other systemic exposure to a substance that activates a hypersensitive IgE or IgM response. Drugs that can trigger anaphylaxis include:
▶ antibiotics (most notably penicillin)
▶ sulfonamides
▶ local anesthetics (lidocaine, procaine)
▶ serums
▶ blood and blood products
▶ vaccines
▶ hormones
▶ opioid analgesics (morphine, codeine)
▶ salicylates and other nonsteroidal anti-inflammatory drugs, such as naproxen and indomethacin.

Other sensitizing substances may include diagnostic chemicals, such as sulfobromophthalein and radiographic contrast media; foods, such as nuts, legumes, berries, seafood, and egg albumin; sulfite-containing food additives, as in wines; pollens; venoms from insects (bees, wasps, hornets, and yellow jackets), spiders, snakes, and jellyfish; and products containing natural rubber latex. (See *Latex allergy screening questionnaire,* page 291.)

Clinical presentation

The patient's history may reveal frequent sneezing; feelings of weakness, fright, or impending doom, and an itchy, runny, or stuffy nose. The patient may also complain of dizziness or light-headedness, severe stomach cramps, nausea, diarrhea, and urgent urination or loss of bladder control.

Examination findings include hives, wheezing, diaphoresis, pruritic skin rash, and swelling (espe-

HOW ANAPHYLAXIS OCCURS

An anaphylactic reaction occurs only in a person who has been previously exposed, or sensitized, to a drug or other substance, called an antigen. The initial exposure leads to the production of specific immunoglobulin (Ig) E antibodies by plasma cells. IgE antibodies then bind to membrane receptors on mast cells.

The next time the person is exposed to the antigen, an antigen-antibody immune reaction may occur. The antigen binds to adjacent IgE antibodies or cross-linked IgE receptors, activating a series of cellular reactions that trigger degranulation (release of powerful chemical mediators from mast cell stores). Two other types of chemical mediators, bradykinin and leukotrienes, impair the circulatory system and drastically lower the blood pressure. Death may follow quickly.

cially of the face, neck, lips, throat, hands, and feet). Some patients develop arrhythmias, hypotension, and shock.

●●● **RED FLAG** *Signs and symptoms* ●●● *of bronchospasm and impending respiratory failure include hoarseness, dyspnea, chest tightness, difficulty speaking, anxiety, and high-pitched breath sounds (wheezing).*

Management
The first priority is to remove the underlying cause, if possible; subsequent priorities are to ensure adequate oxygenation, correct metabolic abnormalities, and support hemodynamic functions.

Immediate actions
Get emergency assistance immediately if a patient experiences signs or symptoms of anaphylaxis moments after taking a drug, eating, being bitten or stung by an insect, or exposure to a natural rubber latex product. Maintain airway patency. Observe for early signs of laryngeal edema (hoarseness, stridor, and dyspnea), which usually necessitates endotracheal tube insertion and oxygen therapy or a tracheostomy and oxygen therapy. Administer epinephrine (Adrenalin) as needed.

In cases of cardiac arrest, start cardiopulmonary resuscitation (CPR).

Keep the patient quiet. If possible, help him to an upright position to ease breathing. If he becomes dizzy, faints, or experiences nausea, have him lie down with his feet slightly elevated.

●●● **RED FLAG** *Watch for signs and* ●●● *symptoms of lip, tongue, and throat swelling and respiratory distress. If these occur, an artificial airway and supplemental oxygen should be considered.*

Pharmacologic treatment options include epinephrine subcutaneously, I.V., or I.V. drip; diphenhydramine I.V.; albuterol aerosol in saline solution; methylprednisolone I.V.; and a histamine-2 receptor antagonist (such as famotidine) I.V.

Later actions
If the patient is conscious and has normal blood pressure, give epinephrine I.M. or subcutaneously immediately to reduce airway edema; repeat every 5 to 20 minutes, as needed. Additional therapy depends on how the patient responds to initial treatment. When the acute phase of the emergency passes, consider using longer-acting steroids (prednisolone by mouth) and antihistamines (diphenhy-

LATEX ALLERGY SCREENING QUESTIONNAIRE

To determine whether your patient has a latex sensitivity or allergy, ask the following screening questions.

Allergies
▸ Do you have a history of hay fever, asthma, eczema, allergies, or rashes? If so, what type of reaction do you have?
▸ Have you experienced an allergic reaction, local sensitivity, or itching following exposure to latex products, such as balloons or condoms?
▸ Do you have shortness of breath or wheezing after blowing up balloons or after a dental visit? Do you have itching in or around your mouth after eating a banana?
▸ If you experience shortness of breath or wheezing when blowing up latex balloons, describe your reaction.
▸ Are you allergic to certain foods, especially bananas, avocados, kiwi, or chestnuts? If so, describe your reaction.

Occupation
▸ What's your occupation?
▸ Are you exposed to latex in your occupation?
▸ Do you experience a reaction to latex products at work? If so, describe your reaction.

▸ If you've had a rash develop on your hands after wearing latex gloves, how long after putting on the gloves did it take for the rash to develop?
▸ What did the rash look like?

Personal history
▸ Do you have congenital abnormalities? If yes, explain.
▸ Have you ever had itching, swelling, hives, cough, shortness of breath, or other allergic symptoms during or after using condoms, diaphragms, or following a vaginal or rectal examination?

Surgical history
▸ Have you had previous surgical procedures? Did you experience associated complications? If so, describe them.
▸ Have you had previous dental procedures? Did complications result? If so, describe them.
▸ Do you have spina bifida or a urinary tract problem that requires surgery or catheterization?

dramine) to ease breathing, or aminophylline (Aminophyllin) to treat bronchospasm.

If anaphylaxis is related to medication, consider stopping the drug and substituting another drug. Follow up within two days. Consider providing an emergency anaphylaxis kit such as EpiPen as well as medical identification jewelry.

Collaborative practice
RED FLAG *A patient in shock requires emergency medical transport to an emergency department.*

Patient teaching
RED FLAG *Tell the patient to call his primary care provider to report appearance of a rash after beginning a new medication (before taking another dose).*

RED FLAG *Tell the patient to call EMS for severe difficulty breathing (including rapid onset of progressive wheezing or stridor), facial swelling, severe mental status change, or a loss of consciousness.*

BURMS

BURNS

ICD-9-CM (for first, second, and third degree, add .1, .2, .3 suffix to site code): arm 943, back 942.04, cornea 940.4, digits 944.03, face 941, leg 945, external genitalia 942.05, tongue 947

A burn is an injury to tissues caused by a chemical, gas, electricity, abrasion, or heat. Most burns occur in the home and the workplace. Usually these are minor and can be treated on an outpatient basis.

Causes

Chemical burns result from contact, ingestion, inhalation, or injection of acids, alkalis, or vesicants (blistering agents). Alkali burns, such as from lye, are more serious than acid burns because alkalis (producing liquefaction necrosis) penetrate deeper into the skin and burn longer than acids (which produce coagulation necrosis).

Inhalation burns come from inhaling smoke (gases) or certain chemicals — especially in an enclosed space. Electrical burns arise from contact with electric current, such as from touching faulty electrical wiring or a high-voltage power line or being struck by lightning. Even contact with a relatively low current can be fatal.

Thermal burns, the most common type of burn, commonly result from residential fires, motor vehicle accidents, children playing with matches, improperly stored gasoline, space heater mishaps, handling explosives or firecrackers, and scalding accidents.

Clinical presentation

Signs and symptoms vary with the type of burn. History reveals when the burn happened, the location of contact (arms, or lungs by inhala-

tion), characteristics of the agent (name, concentration, quantity, and mechanism of action [acid or alkali]), what therapeutic action was taken, and whether the burn was an intentional act.

External chemical burns

External chemical burns may turn the skin red or discolored, raw, white, and soft. The patient may report severe pain and general weakness, although he'll feel no pain at all if the burn has completely destroyed nerve endings. Dyspnea or loss of consciousness may also occur.

Inhalation burns

A patient with inhalation burns may present with cough, dyspnea, hoarseness, light-headedness, nausea, chest pain, loss of consciousness, and a burning sensation of the eyes or mouth. Examination may reveal facial burns, soot in the nares and mouth, and laryngeal edema.

Electrical burns

In electrical burns, history may reveal severe pain or no pain at either the entrance or exit burn. An electrical burn can damage the nervous system, the cardiovascular system, and the kidneys. It may lead to arrhythmias and possible cardiac arrest, renal failure, and massive bleeding. If the spinal cord is damaged, electrical burns can lead to seizures, coma, respiratory arrest, and even paralysis

A *lightning burn* may cause swollen, charred, or reddened skin around the entrance wound and a burn pattern resembling a tree branch. Permanent neurologic changes, including neuralgia and paresis, may also result.

CLINICAL PEARL *In cases of an electrical burn, check for burns in areas of the skin where metal, such as jewelry, watches, and zip-*

pers, may have been in contact with the skin.

Thermal burns

Signs and symptoms of thermal burns will vary according to the depth of tissue injury. In general, all burns (except inhalation) are classified by depth. *First-degree (superficial) burns* injure only the epidermis — the top layer of the skin. Examples include minor sunburn and burns from brief contact with a hot iron. The burned area is usually tender, reddened, painful, and has little or no swelling and no blistering. Erythema resolves in 1 to 2 days without scarring.

Second-degree (partial-thickness) burns damage both the epidermis and the dermis (the skin layer below the epidermis). Examples include deep sunburns, short exposure to flame, and burns caused by hot liquids. These burns usually cause pronounced pain, and the blisters or the epidermis may be broken in the burned area. The skin will be edematous, and the burn may weep. The skin may appear red, streaked, or splotchy; although it may heal in 10 days to 4 weeks, it remains discolored.

Third-degree (full-thickness) burns extend through the epidermis and dermis and into the subcutaneous tissue layer. These burns may also involve muscle, bone, and interstitial tissue. The skin appears leathery and charred with no blisters present. Full-thickness burns are painless because the nerve endings in the dermis have been destroyed. Extensive full-thickness burns generally require skin grafting.

Diagnosis

Diagnosis involves determining the *size* and *classification* of the burn. A burn's *size* is determined by measuring the percentage of body surface area (BSA) covered by the burn using the Rule of Nines chart. In infants and children, the Lund-Browder chart is used to estimate burn size. (See *Using the Rule of Nines and the Lund-Browder chart,* pages 294 and 295.)

Burns may be *classified* into three categories according to the size of the burn and its depth. *Major* burns meet the following criteria:
) third-degree burns on more than 10% of BSA
) second-degree burns on more than 25% of BSA in adults (more than 20% in children)
) burns of hands, face, feet, or genitalia
) burns complicated by fractures or respiratory damage
) electrical burns
) all burns in poor-risk patients.

Moderate burns are classified as:
) third-degree burns on 2% to 10% of BSA
) second-degree burns on 15% to 25% of BSA in adults (10% to 20% in children).

Minor burns are classified as:
) third-degree burns on less than 2% of BSA
) second-degree burns on less than 15% of BSA in adults (10% in children).

Management

Burn management depends on the type and severity of the burn. The first priority in an emergency, including burns, is to assess the patient's airway, breathing, and circulation. Institute emergency resuscitative measures and activate the emergency medical services system and transport the patient to the hospital as necessary. He may require endotracheal intubation and mechanical ventilation if his respiratory status deteriorates, especially with facial and neck burns. Monitor for cardiac arrhythmias, especially in the patient who received an elec-

(Text continues on page 296.)

USING THE RULE OF NINES AND THE LUND-BROWDER CHART

You can quickly estimate the extent of an adult patient's burn by using the Rule of Nines. This method divides an adult's body surface area into percentages. To use this method, mentally transfer your patient's burns to the body chart shown below, then add up the corresponding percentages for each burned body section. The total, an estimate of the extent of your patient's burn, enters into the formula to deter-mine his initial fluid replacement needs.

You can't use the Rule of Nines for infants and children because their body section percentages differ from those of adults. For example, an infant's head accounts for about 17% of the total body surface area compared with 9% for an adult. Instead, use the Lund-Browder chart.

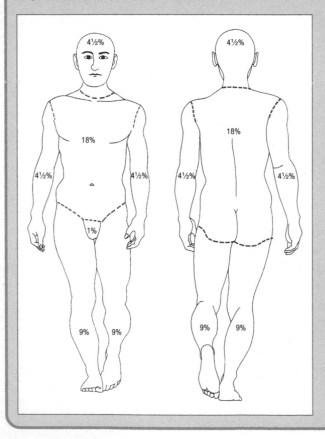

Lund-Browder chart

To determine the extent of an infant's or child's burns, use the Lund-Browder chart shown here.

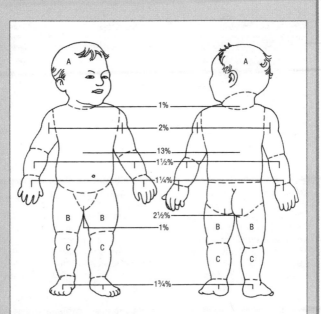

Relative percentages of areas affected by growth

	At birth	0 to 1 year	1 to 4 years	5 to 9 years	10 to 15 years	Adult
A: HALF OF HEAD						
	9½%	8½%	6½%	5½%	4½%	3½%
B: HALF OF THIGH						
	2¾%	3¼%	4%	4¼%	4½%	4¾%
C: HALF OF LEG						
	2½%	2½%	2¾%	3%	3¼%	3½%

> ### CLINICAL PEARL
> ## ELECTRICAL BURN CARE
>
> Keep these tips in mind when caring for a patient with an electrical burn:
>
> ▸ Be alert for ventricular fibrillation as well as cardiac and respiratory arrest caused by the electrical shock; begin cardiopulmonary resuscitation immediately.
> ▸ Get an estimate of the voltage that caused the injury.
> ▸ Tissue damage from an electrical burn is difficult to assess because in-
>
> ternal destruction along the conduction pathway usually is greater than the surface burn would indicate. Locate the entrance and exit wounds caused by the electrical burn.
> ▸ An electrical burn that ignites the patient's clothes may also cause thermal burns.

trical burn. (See *Electrical burn care.*) Remove the source of the burn and items that retain heat, such as clothing or jewelry.

Chemical burns

Usually, a chemical burn is immediately rinsed with copious amounts of water; rinsing should continue for at least 15 minutes. If the agent that caused the burn was a dry chemical, the substance should be brushed off prior to rinsing. Some chemicals react when mixed with water and shouldn't be rinsed. Refer to the Material Safety Data Sheet (MSDS) for treatment of the specific chemical involved in the burn.

●●● **RED FLAG** *When cleaning a* ●●● *patient with chemical burns, it's important to pay particular attention to skin folds where chemical agents can become trapped.*

Thermal burns

First-degree burns. Immediately apply a cool compress or immerse the burned area in cool water; allow compress to remain in place or continue immersion until pain is relieved. *Don't* put ice or ice water on the burn because this will cause rapid chilling and further tissue injury. *Don't* put ointments, creams, butter, or sprays on the burn be-

cause they trap heat within the burned tissue, thereby increasing tissue damage.

Aloe vera gel, applied topically, may help reduce the discomfort of sunburn. The patient may take aspirin, acetaminophen, or ibuprofen for symptomatic relief of superficial burns. He should be instructed to return to the facility if the skin blisters.

Second-degree burns. Cover moderate and major partial-thickness burns with a clean, dry, sterile bed sheet (because of drastic reduction in body temperature, don't cover large burns with saline-soaked dressings) and prepare the patient for transport to the hospital for further treatment. For minor partial-thickness burns, apply a cool compress or immerse the burned area in cool water.

●●● **RED FLAG** *To prevent hypother-* ●●● *mia, don't cool more than 20% of an adult's body surface area or 10% of a child's body. Cover the burn with a dry, nonstick, sterile dressing.*

Treatment of blisters is commonly left to the discretion of the caregiver; if the blister is small and has a thick wall, it's usually left intact; if it's thin-walled and appears liable to rupture, it should be lanced and covered with a nonadherent dressing.

Pharmacologic treatment options include oral opioid analgesics as needed for pain relief and tetanus prophylaxis as indicated. Silver sulfadiazine (Silvadene) cream may be applied to allow better wound healing and reduce the risk of infection. Silver sulfadiazine cream shouldn't be used on the face and is contraindicated in patients who are pregnant, breast-feeding, or allergic to sulfonamides.

CLINICAL PEARL *Systemic antibiotics are unnecessary for second-degree burns unless secondary cellulitis develops.*

Third-degree burns. Cover the burn with a clean, dry, sterile bed sheet, treat the patient for shock and prepare him for immediate transport to the hospital.

Collaborative practice

Surgical consultation is indicated if burns are greater than 10% of body surface or third-degree burns are greater than 3% of body surface. Hospital admission and surgical consultation are needed for patients with circumferential burns and burns involving the perineum, hand, or organs of sensation. Hospital admission is required if smoke inhalation injury is suspected, for electrical and chemical burns, chemical burns of the eye, major second-degree burns, and third-degree burns.

Patient teaching

▶ Instruct the patient to check for signs and symptoms of infection and impaired circulation.
▶ If the burn involves an extremity, instruct the patient to keep the limb elevated.
▶ Instruct the patient to change the dressing on second-degree burns

daily for 5 to 7 days; before replacing the dressing, the wound should be gently cleaned with soap and water and silver sulfadiazine cream should be reapplied in a layer thick enough to cover the burn. When the wound has healed, he should apply moisturizing cream to prevent skin cracking.
▶ Instruct the patient regarding burn prevention — appliances properly installed with grounding, rubber gloves and dry shoes used when working with electric circuits, unused wall sockets capped, and extension cords unplugged when not in use.

RED FLAG *Tell the patient to call his primary care provider to report pain persisting beyond 48 hours or signs or symptoms of infection (redness, increasing pain, swelling, purulent drainage, and fever above 101° F [38.3° C]).*

CARDIOPULMO-NARY ARREST

ICD-9-CM 427.5 cardiac arrest, 799-1 respiratory arrest

Cardiopulmonary arrest — occurring when the patient stops breathing and his heart contractions cease — suppresses cardiac output. As a result, the brain and all other organs are deprived of a circulating blood supply and the oxygen needed to function.

Cardiopulmonary arrest leads to irreversible brain damage within 4 to 6 minutes and death within 10 minutes, depending on the patient's condition, the nature of the arrest, and the elapsed time between onset of symptoms and initiation of cardiopulmonary resuscitation (CPR).

Regardless of whether it's performed properly, CPR can cause rib or sternum fracture, separation of the ribs from the sternum, pneumothorax, hemothorax, lung contusion, and liver or spleen laceration. Multiple organ dysfunction syndrome after cardiac arrest may lead to acute respiratory distress syndrome, disseminated intravascular coagulation, shock, and neurologic deficits.

Causes

Cardiopulmonary arrest may occur from conditions affecting the airways, the brain, or the heart. Immediate causes of cardiopulmonary arrest include ventricular fibrillation, ventricular asystole (cardiac standstill), and electromechanical dissociation. These problems usually result from coronary artery disease or its complications.

Ventricular fibrillation and ventricular asystole may result from heart damage caused by a previous myocardial infarction or from toxic doses of sympathomimetic drugs (such as dobutamine and dopamine), antiarrhythmic drugs (such as quinidine and disopyramide), or parasympathomimetic drugs (such as neostigmine). Cocaine abuse has also been linked to cardiac arrest.

Other causes of cardiopulmonary arrest include:
▶ vagal stimulation associated with diagnostic procedures such as colonoscopy
▶ hypothermia, acidosis, and hypokalemia, which can induce ventricular fibrillation and, in turn, cardiopulmonary arrest
▶ foreign body airway obstruction
▶ depression of the respiratory center resulting from such conditions as stroke, head injury, neuromuscular disorders, drug overdose, and electrical shock.

Clinical presentation

Cardiopulmonary arrest is the absence of breathing and an absent pulse. Some patients have no heart rhythm or have a heart rhythm but no pulse (electromechanical dissociation), as shown on an electrocardiogram (ECG). Lack of a pulse always indicates cardiac arrest regardless of which heart rhythm appears on the ECG monitor.

Management

If the patient shows signs or symptoms of cardiopulmonary arrest, check his airway, breathing, and circulation. Perform CPR as needed. Activate the emergency medical services (EMS) system and prepare the patient for transport to the hospital. Depending on the type of cardiac arrhythmia, the patient may require defibrillation or synchronized cardioversion.

During hospitalization, if the patient continues to have dangerous arrhythmias despite antiarrhythmic drug therapy, he may be a candidate for an implantable cardioverter-defibrillator (ICD). This small pulse generator is implanted in the patient's chest, and a leadwire (or wires) is positioned transvenously in the endocardium of the right ventricle. The lead senses the heart rate and delivers shocks or antitachycardia pacing to halt the arrhythmia so that the heart resumes proper rhythm. The device can be programmed to suit the patient's specific needs.

●●● **RED FLAG** *A patient in car-*
●●● *diopulmonary arrest requires emergency medical transport to an emergency department. Follow up within 24 hours if cardiopulmonary arrest is due to a secondary cause; follow up within 1 week of hospital discharge for cardiac disease.*

Patient teaching

●●● **RED FLAG** *Tell the patient to*
●●● *call his primary care provider or to activate the EMS system to report chest pain that changes in*

character or increases in frequency and duration.

Teach the patient about preventive measures and lifestyle changes to help prevent cardiopulmonary events in the future. Provide education related to medications and medical devices (such as ICD) as appropriate.

CONCUSSION

ICD-9-CM 850.9, with loss of consciousness 850.5, due to blast/high impact 869.0

A relatively minor brain injury, a concussion may result from a direct blow to the head, such as when a person slips on ice and hits his head on the sidewalk, or it may come from an acceleration-deceleration injury, as commonly occurs in a head-on motor vehicle collision. In this injury, the head is hurled forward and then stops abruptly as it hits the windshield. The brain, however, keeps moving, hitting against one side of the skull and then rebounding against the opposite side. There's no penetrating trauma, but a transient loss of consciousness of at least a few seconds may have occurred.

Most patients recover from concussion within 48 hours and don't suffer lasting damage. Patients may complain of memory loss, persistent headaches, insomnia, and dizziness that may (uncommonly) last for months after the injury.

Some concussions may be accompanied by intracranial bleeding that can lead to permanent injury or death if not treated promptly. Repeated concussions have a cumulative effect on the brain and can result in permanent brain damage.

Causes

Usually, a concussion results from a direct blow to the head. The shock wave from an explosion can also cause concussion.

Clinical presentation

The patient history may reveal confusion or disorientation, and a brief loss of consciousness. Examination may elicit unsteady gait, slurred speech, a vacant stare, dazed appearance, incoordination, delayed motor responses, and irritability. The patient may report dizziness, nausea and vomiting, severe headache, and blurred or double vision. He may be unable to remember what happened just before or after the injury.

Diagnosis

Concussion differs from more serious head injuries by the following criteria:
▶ no loss of consciousness or brief loss of consciousness at the time of the injury
▶ no nausea or vomiting
▶ no change in mental status from the time of incident until the time seen
▶ no focal neurologic deficit
▶ possibly minimal to moderate headache.

For up to 1 year after a concussion, some patients experience delayed effects, or *postconcussion syndrome*. Signs and symptoms include lack of usual energy, double vision, memory loss, irritability, emotional lability, poor concentration, reduced libido, loss of inhibitions, difficulty relating to others, intolerance to noise, easy intoxication by alcohol, and dizziness, giddiness, or lightheadedness. Postconcussion effects usually subside over time.

Management

A finding that doesn't fit the definition of concussion should be referred to a physician. *Subacute subdural hematoma* takes 24 hours to

USING THE GLASGOW COMA SCALE

The Glasgow Coma Scale provides an easy way to describe the patient's mental status and detect changes. A score of 15 indicates that the patient is alert and oriented and can follow simple commands. A decreased score may signal an impending neurologic crisis. A score of less than 8 indicates severe neurologic damage.

Test	Score
EYES OPEN	
Spontaneously	4
To speech	3
To pain	2
No response	1
BEST MOTOR RESPONSE	
Obeys	6
Localizes pain (reaches toward pain to remove cause)	5
Flexion-withdrawal (moves away from pain)	4
Abnormal flexion (decorticate rigidity)	3
Extension (decerebrate rigidity)	2
No response	1
BEST VERBAL RESPONSE	
Oriented	5
Disoriented	4
Inappropriate words	3
Incomprehensible sounds	2
No response	1

2 weeks for symptoms to develop; patients at high risk are the elderly and those with alcohol-induced brain atrophy. *Chronic subdural hematoma* is usually detected more than 2 weeks after the injury and results from liquefaction of the hematoma.

After a head injury, determine whether the patient is alert. If he's awake and alert, assess his orientation. The Glasgow Coma Scale quickly ascertains neurologic status. (See *Using the Glasgow Coma Scale.*)

Try to determine whether loss of consciousness occurred during or after the accident. If so, the patient may require a computed tomography scan to determine the extent of injury.

Monitor vital signs every 5 minutes until the extent of the injury is known. The first sign of increasing intracranial pressure is a change in mental status. Later signs include increasing blood pressure with decreasing pulse. (See *Grading sports-related concussions.*)

A patient with a simple concussion can usually recover at home,

GRADING SPORTS-RELATED CONCUSSIONS

Concussion grades	Clinical presentation	Immediate actions	Minimum time before returning to sport
Grade 1	No loss of consciousness; mental status change < 15 minutes	▸ Examined on scene by first responder; recheck every 5 minutes for 15 minutes. ▸ Second grade 1 on same day: remove from activity.	▸ Grade 1 once within previous 24 hours: 15 minutes ▸ Grade 1 twice in same day: 1 week
Grade 2	No loss of consciousness; mental status change > 15 minutes	▸ Remove from activity; monitor frequently; additional testing as indicated.	▸ Grade 2: 1 week ▸ Grade 1, then grade 2 on same day: 2 weeks
Grade 3	Loss of consciousness or seizure	▸ Emergency medical services transport to emergency department	▸ Brief loss of consciousness: 1 week ▸ Prolonged loss of consciousness: 2 weeks ▸ Second grade 3 in lifetime: 1 month

as long as someone observes him closely for at least 24 hours; symptoms of intracranial bleeding usually occur within 24 hours. The patient must be observed closely for the initial 2 hours, every 2 hours for the following 8 hours, and every 4 to 6 hours for 16 hours thereafter. Each time, check for change in mental status, bruising below the eyes or behind the ears, severe head pain, or dizziness. The patient's condition should be followed up within 24 hours.

Collaborative practice

Patients with loss of consciousness, persistent vomiting, or changed neurologic status (such as in vision or personality) should be taken to the emergency department. Inform emergency medical services personnel of pertinent information, including the patient's condition when

you first saw him, his medical history, allergies, and the name of his primary care provider.

Patient teaching

▸ Advise the patient to eat lightly, especially if nausea or vomiting occurs. Occasional vomiting is common and nausea usually subsides in a few days. Aggressive evaluation is needed if the patient vomits more than three times within the 24-hour period immediately following the trauma.

▸ Advise the patient to avoid taking pain medications for 2 hours after the injury. If pain is severe enough to require it, the patient needs to be evaluated. After 2 hours, he may take acetaminophen for a headache. To avoid the risk of GI bleeding, don't give aspirin.

▶ Warn the patient not to drink alcohol for at least 24 hours.

●●●
●●● RED FLAG *Tell the family to call the patient's primary care provider to report marked changes in behavior, seizure activity, clear fluid leaking from ear or nose, bruising below the eyes or behind the ears, severe head pain, vomiting more than three times in 24 hours, difficulty waking, confusion, or difficulty walking or talking in the initial 48 hours after the trauma. After 48 hours, worsening symptoms of postconcussion syndrome should be reported.*

●●●
●●● RED FLAG *If a child with a concussion is inconsolable, lethargic, or extremely restless for more than 10 minutes, the parent or caregiver should notify the primary care provider immediately.*

CORNEAL ABRASION

ICD-9-CM external 930.9, eyelid 930.1, eyeball 930.8

Commonly caused by a mechanical or chemical insult, a corneal abrasion is a scratch on the surface epithelium of the cornea. Corneal abrasions are among the most common eye injuries. With treatment, the prognosis is usually good.

Causes

A corneal abrasion usually results from a foreign body, such as a cinder or a piece of dust, dirt, or grit that becomes embedded under the eyelid. Even if tears wash out the foreign body, it may still injure the cornea.

A small piece of metal may become lodged in the eye of a worker who didn't wear eye protection. The metal forms a rust ring on the cornea as well as an abrasion. Corneal abrasions may occur in persons who fall asleep wearing hard contact lenses or daily wear soft lenses. A corneal scratch produced by a fingernail, a piece of paper, or other organic substance may cause a persistent lesion. The epithelium doesn't always heal properly, and a recurrent corneal erosion may develop, with delayed effects more severe than those of the original injury.

Clinical presentation

Corneal abrasions typically present with a history of unilateral eye discomfort when blinking, a foreign body sensation and, because the cornea is richly endowed with nerve endings from the trigeminal nerve (cranial nerve V), pain disproportionate to the size of the injury. A history of eye trauma or prolonged wearing of contact lenses also suggests corneal abrasion. Examination may reveal photophobia, difficulty keeping the eye open, redness, and increased tearing. A corneal abrasion frequently affects visual acuity, depending on the size and location of the injury.

Diagnosis

When evaluating eye pain, consider a foreign body and keratitis (bacterial, viral, fungal) as well as corneal laceration or perforation. Staining the cornea with fluorescein stain confirms the diagnosis: The injured area appears yellow-green when examined with a cobalt blue light. Slit-lamp examination discloses the depth of the abrasion. Examining the eye with a flashlight may reveal a foreign body on the cornea; the eyelid must be everted to check for a foreign body embedded under the lid. Before beginning treatment, test the patient for visual acuity to provide a medical baseline and a legal safeguard.

●●●
●●● RED FLAG *Pain, significantly decreased vision, sluggish*

pupillary reaction, and a cloudy cornea indicate glaucoma. Pain, decreased vision, sluggish pupillary reaction, but with a dull and swollen iris, suggest iritis. Erythema and edema around the lacrimal duct, combined with mucopurulent discharge on palpation of the lacrimal sac, indicate lacrimal duct obstruction.

Management

CLINICAL PEARL *Penetrating or complex lid injuries, intraocular foreign body, significant loss of vision, acute ocular pain, or corneal laceration or perforation should be protected by a nonpressure eye shield before the patient is transported for emergency ophthalmologic evaluation. Don't instill antibiotic eyedrops or ointment. Check the status of tetanus immunization to determine the necessity for tetanus prophylaxis.*

Chemical splashes should be irrigated with tap water immediately; consult the Material Safety Data Sheet to determine the chemical agent that caused the abrasion. If the chemical can't be verified, the poison control center should be contacted. If a specific treatment can't be verified, irrigate the patient's eye and move him to an emergency medical facility immediately.

Foreign bodies are initially treated by simply trying to remove them. Attempt removal using a sterile gauze pad moistened with sterile normal saline. Initial application of a tight pressure patch prevents further corneal irritation when the patient blinks, excluding an abrasion caused by contact lenses. The patch should be worn for 24 to 48 hours. Most corneal abrasions heal in less than 36 hours with a pressure patch.

Pharmacologic treatment options include instilling broad-spectrum antibiotic eyedrops or ointment (gentamicin) in the affected eye four times per day for 2 days to prevent infection or instilling short-acting cycloplegic eyedrops (cyclopentolate) to relieve ciliary spasm. Oral analgesics (acetaminophen) may be used for pain relief. Follow up daily until healing is complete, focusing on signs of infection or loss of vision. If improvement isn't significant in 24 hours, refer the patient to an ophthalmologist.

Collaborative practice

Patients with one or more of the emergency conditions listed above should be referred immediately for ophthalmologic evaluation.

RED FLAG *Corneal ulcers are an emergency; patients with corneal ulcers should be referred for immediate ophthalmologic evaluation. Typically, corneal ulceration begins with pain (aggravated by blinking) and photophobia, followed by increased tearing. Eventually, central corneal ulceration produces pronounced visual blurring. The eye may appear injected (red). If a bacterial ulcer is present, purulent discharge may be present.*

Patient teaching

▸ Tell the patient with an eye patch to leave the patch in place for at least 24 hours. Warn him that wearing a patch alters depth perception and, therefore, advise caution in everyday activities, such as climbing stairs and stepping off a curb.
▸ Reassure the patient that the corneal epithelium usually heals in 24 to 48 hours.
▸ Warn the patient not to rub the affected eye.
▸ Teach the patient the proper way to instill ophthalmic drugs.
▸ Stress the importance of instilling prescribed antibiotic eyedrops as

directed because an untreated corneal infection can lead to ulceration and permanent loss of vision.
▶ Emphasize the importance of safety glasses to protect workers' eyes from flying debris.
▶ Review instructions for wearing and caring for contact lenses.

FOREIGN BODY IN EYE

ICD-9-CM external 930.9, eyelid 930.1, eyeball 930.8

A foreign body lodged in the eye is the most common type of eye injury encountered in primary care. Besides causing pain, it can lead to discomfort, inflammation, and infection. If the foreign body scratches the surface lining of the cornea, a corneal abrasion occurs. If the eye doesn't heal properly, a persistent wound or ulcer can develop, and the cornea may become permanently scarred.

Causes

Typically, the foreign body is a tiny piece of dirt or metal, a cinder, or a bit of dust. Usually, the patient blinks the object into a position along the eyelid, where it can be removed with a clean gauze pad or tissue.

Clinical presentation

A foreign body in the eye can cause mild, unilateral pain as well as redness, tearing, a burning sensation, and photophobia. The patient may report a foreign body sensation; this feeling may persist even after the particle is removed because the eye remains irritated. With a corneal abrasion, the patient is more likely to complain of impaired vision.

Diagnosis

Observation of a foreign body in the eye under light and magnification confirms the diagnosis. Fluorescein stain highlights the ocular foreign body. Consider the possibility of an intraocular foreign body, corneal abrasion, corneal laceration or perforation, or keratitis (bacterial, viral, or fungal).

Management

Immediate actions

Check the superior and inferior cul-de-sac for foreign bodies. Evert the upper eyelid to enhance visualization (roll the eyelid backward over a smooth object such as a pen).

Pharmacologic options include:
▶ local analgesia (proparacaine) for pain control during removal of the foreign body
▶ antibiotic ophthalmologic ointment twice daily for 2 to 3 days after removal of the foreign body to prevent infection.

Verify tetanus immunization status. The patient may require tetanus prophylaxis.

If the patient complains of feeling a foreign body in the eye but the particle isn't visible, help him rinse the eye under a gentle stream of clean, warm running water while moving the eye in different directions to help flush out the particle.

If the particle remains in the eye after flushing, gently pull the lower eyelid down and examine the inside of the lid. Then ask the patient to look up. If you can see the foreign object on the inside of the lid, remove it with the corner of a moistened sterile gauze pad or a clean cloth or tissue. Never use an instrument such as tweezers or a dry cotton swab to remove a foreign body in the eye. Tweezers could cause injury if they graze the eyeball; dry cotton fibers from a swab may stay in the eye, causing irritation.

Depending on the amount of abrasion, patching may be indicated for 24 hours. If eye irritation continues or the particle is still in the eye, ask the patient to close his eye. Then cover the eye with several gauze pads and tape the pads in place. Rubbing may force a sharp object deeper into the eye or scratch delicate eye tissues.

••• RED FLAG *Never try to remove*
••• *an object that's embedded or impaled in the eyeball. Doing so could force the object deeper into the eye, causing further damage. Instead, place a protective shield over the eye. Don't put pressure on the eyeball. Don't let the patient rub the eye. Keep the patient calm, and immediately transport him to an ophthalmologist or emergency department.*

Later actions

If the particle is deeply embedded, an ophthalmologist will anesthetize the eye to remove the particle with a foreign body spud (a spadelike device). After removal, antibiotic eyedrops are instilled in the eye every 3 to 4 hours. The patient is advised to wear a pressure patch to prevent further irritation of the cornea during blinking. Follow up within 24 hours.

••• RED FLAG *A tiny piece of metal*
••• *that becomes lodged in the eye may quickly form a rust ring on the cornea, causing a corneal abrasion. Typical victims of this injury are metal workers who don't wear protective eyewear. To remove a rust ring, the ophthalmologist uses an ophthalmic burr.*

Collaborative practice

Refer the patient to an ophthalmologist if he has an intraocular foreign body, significant loss of vision, progressive pain, redness or discharge, acute ocular pain, or corneal lacera-

tion or perforation. Don't instill antibiotic eyedrops or ointment; instead, patch the eye with a protective shield and avoid putting pressure on the eye.

Patient teaching

▶ Caution the patient not to rub the eye.
▶ Advise the patient to wear protective glasses.

● INSECT BITES AND STINGS

ICD-9-CM chigger 133.8, fire ant/ spider/snake/venomous insect 989.5
At the very least, bites from mosquitoes, ticks, spiders, and other insects can be annoying. At worst, they can cause anaphylaxis, respiratory failure, and death. In addition, many insects can transmit diseases.

Causes

Ticks actively seek warm-blooded hosts and feed on their blood. Spiders bite if they're disturbed. A black widow or brown recluse spider bite can cause an anaphylactic reaction that leads to shock, respiratory arrest, and death. This reaction may result from either a toxin released during the bite or an allergy to the bite. (See "Anaphylaxis," page 289.) Mosquitoes can transmit malaria and West Nile Virus; wood ticks and dog ticks can transmit Rocky Mountain spotted fever, and deer ticks can transmit Lyme disease. (See *How to recognize ticks and spiders*, page 306.)

Clinical presentation

An insect bite may cause localized pain, itching, and swelling. An insect's stinger may be left in the skin, or a bite or puncture mark may be visible. Other signs and symptoms of insect bites vary be-

HOW TO RECOGNIZE TICKS AND SPIDERS

Knowing how to spot certain ticks and spiders can protect you and those around you from potentially dangerous bites. Use this guide to help you to recognize dangerous insects.

Deer tick

Common throughout the United States, the deer tick is responsible for transmitting Lyme disease. The deer tick matures in stages. Between the larval and adult stage, it's as small as a pencil point. An adult deer tick is about ⅛" (0.3 cm) in size. After seeking and attaching itself to a host, the deer tick swells five to seven times its original size.

Wood tick

The flat, brown-speckled wood tick is found in woods and fields throughout North America. It attaches to humans and feeds on their blood. The wood tick may inject a poison that can cause acute paralysis or transmit Rocky Mountain spotted fever, a potentially fatal disease.

Brown recluse spider

The brown recluse spider is small and light brown, with three pairs of eyes. The hallmark of a brown recluse spider is a violin-shaped darker area found on the cephalothorax. This spider is about

1" (2.5 cm) long, including the legs. Found in the south-central part of the United States, it favors dark areas, such as barns and woodsheds, and most commonly bites between April and October. The brown recluse spider injects a poison that causes its victim's blood to clot within 2 to 8 hours after the bite.

Black widow spider

The female black widow spider is glossy and coal-black with a red or orange hourglass mark on its underside; it's ½" (1.3 cm) in length, with legs 1½" (3.8 cm) long. Common throughout the United States, especially in warmer climates, the black widow spider is usually found in dark areas, such as outdoor privies and woodsheds. Its venom is toxic to the nerves and muscles of a human victim, causing muscle spasms in the arms and legs, rigidity of stomach muscles, and ascending paralysis that leads to difficulty swallowing and breathing; circulatory collapse may follow. The male black widow spider doesn't bite.

cause specific poisons act on specific areas of the body.

Tick bites

Tick bites are painless at first and may cause itching at the site. If the tick isn't removed or the head is left in the body, the site will become irritated and, possibly, infected. Some people experience tick paralysis, which causes weakness, pain in the feet or legs, or respiratory failure. It's frequently unnoticed because the deer tick is only as big as the

period at the end of this sentence, and its bite produces no sensation. If the bite victim has been infected with Lyme disease, a bull's-eye rash may appear within a few days. During the next few weeks, months, or even years, severe symptoms may occur. (See "Lyme disease," page 151.)

Spider bites

Black widow spider bites cause an immediate sharp, stinging pain followed by a dull, numbing pain. The bitten area begins to swell, and tiny red bite marks appear. Within 10 to 40 minutes after the bite, stomach muscles become rigid and severe abdominal pain occurs. Both problems subside within 48 hours. Muscle spasms in the arms and legs also occur.

Some people experience a systemic reaction from a black widow spider bite. This reaction causes extreme restlessness, dizziness, sweating or chills, pallor, seizures (especially in children), nausea, vomiting, headache, eyelid swelling, hives, itching, and fever.

Bites from brown recluse spiders cause little or no pain at first. However, these bites usually become painful over time. About 2 to 8 hours after the bite, a small, red puncture wound forms a small blister. The center becomes dark and hard 3 to 4 days later. In 2 to 3 weeks, a sore develops. Some people have systemic reactions, which may include fever, chills, nausea, vomiting, fatigue, muscle pain, and pinpoint red spots on the skin.

Scorpion and tarantula bites

Bites from scorpions and tarantulas may cause severe signs and symptoms, especially pain. Expect to see puncture marks and some redness and swelling at the site. The patient may have muscle pain and cramps in the arms, legs, shoulders, and back. Although symptoms usually subside after 6 to 12 hours, some patients experience life-threatening effects, such as circulatory or respiratory failure.

Bee, wasp, and ant stings

Local reactions to bee, wasp, or ant stings include local edema and are a problem if the reaction involves the mouth or throat (due to possible respiratory compromise) or the eye (due to possible long-term in-

juries, such as cataracts, iris atrophy, and refractive changes).

Toxic reactions are defined as more than nine stings in one episode; they can cause nausea, syncope, diarrhea, edema, involuntary muscle spasms, headache, and seizures. Toxic reaction is differentiated from an anaphylactic response because multiple stings are needed to precipitate the reaction, which is notable for the absence of urticaria or bronchospasm and the increased incidence and severity of diarrhea.

A patient experiencing an anaphylactic response may demonstrate an inverse relation between the severity of the reaction and the length of time from the initial sting to the time of systemic reaction; less time to react equals a more severe reaction. Delayed reaction is uncommon; it presents with constitutional signs (fever, malaise, headache, urticaria, lymphadenopathy, and polyarthritis) up to 2 weeks after the sting.

Management

Immediate actions

If the patient is in distress, first check his airway, breathing, and circulation. Give cardiopulmonary resuscitation as needed.

●●● RED FLAG *Anyone bitten by a* **●●●** *toxic spider or scorpion should go to an emergency department (ED) immediately to receive antivenin. Clean the bite area with soap and water and apply a cold pack or ice to the bite to help relieve discomfort and delay the effects of the venom. The bitten arm or leg should be splinted and kept lower than the patient's heart.*

After an insect bite, watch for the following signs and symptoms, which may indicate a systemic reaction from a toxin or an allergic reaction:

❱ weakness

- extreme restlessness
- nausea
- vomiting
- dizziness
- difficulty breathing (which may signal respiratory failure).

Firmly grasp the tick at its head with tweezers, and then slowly and gently pull out the tick. Don't apply oil or ointment because the tick is more likely to inject into the skin as it suffocates. Don't pull out a tick with your hand because doing so could leave the tick's head embedded in the skin. Don't try to remove the tick with a lighted match or cigarette.

Clean the wound with an antiseptic or rubbing alcohol. If the patient or a caregiver is unable to remove the entire tick, including the head, it needs to be removed by a health care provider.

After a spider bite, the patient should receive tetanus immunization. For black widow bites, *Latrodectus mactans* antivenin should be given when symptomatic treatment is unsuccessful. The manufacturer recommends the use of a skeletal muscle relaxant as well. Skin testing must be performed before administration to check for possible anaphylactic response to antivenin. For brown recluse bites, give systemic steroids (methylprednisolone I.V. followed by oral prednisone for 5 days). Acute monitoring, including laboratory tests and urine output, is needed to detect renal failure that may require dialysis. For severe local or toxic hymenoptera stings, consider short-term oral steroid use and oral antihistamines (diphenhydramine) to decrease inflammatory response.

Treatment for less severe insect or spider bites depends on which species inflicted the bite. A mild reaction is no cause for alarm and can be treated conservatively with cold compresses and acetaminophen. To relieve minor discomfort from an insect bite, apply ice or ice water to the bite. This stops the swelling, decreases pain, and slows absorption of toxins. A paste of baking soda and water or a cloth dampened with aloe vera juice may also be applied.

Later actions

A patient with symptoms of Lyme disease may receive an antibiotic. Typically, adults receive oral tetracycline four times per day and children receive oral amoxicillin three times per day for 10 to 21 days. When given in the early stages of Lyme disease, these drugs can minimize later complications. In later stages, high-dose antibiotics (penicillin I.V. for 2 to 3 weeks or ceftriaxone I.V. for 2 weeks) are indicated. (See "Lyme disease," page 151.)

❋ **LIFE SPAN** *Children react more strongly to toxins from insect, scorpion, tick, and spider bites because they're smaller than adults. Such a bite in a child is considered a medical emergency.*

Follow up with an office visit within 1 week of discharge from the hospital, or within 2 days if emergency treatment only was required. Consider providing an emergency anaphylaxis kit such as EpiPen as well as medical identification jewelry.

Collaborative practice

The patient with symptoms of a systemic reaction or involvement of three or more body systems requires immediate transport to the nearest ED. Notify emergency medical services personnel of pertinent information, including the patient's condition when first bitten, duration between bite and arrival of emergency transport, his medical history, and allergies.

Patient teaching

▶ Instruct the patient to seek medical help for bites or stings if he has a history of allergic reaction or has signs and symptoms of a systemic reaction.

▶ Advise patients with a history of allergic reactions to carry an Epi-Pen.

▶ If possible, have the patient bring the insect or spider to the ED to confirm its identity.

MAMMAL BITES

ICD-9-CM by site (with tendon involvement, add suffix .2): arm 884, ear 872, buttock 877, leg 891, face 873.4, foot 892, lip 873.43
Although seldom fatal, bites from animals or humans can cause injuries ranging from bruises and superficial scratches to severe crush injuries, deep puncture wounds, tissue loss, and severe damage to blood vessels. In the United States, 60% to 90% of animal bites come from dogs, about 10% come from cats, and the third most common bites are from humans. Surprisingly, human bites are the most to be feared due to the great variety of infectious bacteria and viruses normally present in the human oral cavity.

A dog bite may cause crush injuries, dislocation of involved joints, and muscle, tendon, and nerve damage. Cat bites usually aren't as serious; their sharp teeth, however, can cause deep puncture wounds that damage muscles, tendons, and bones. Because these tissues have a limited blood supply, the risk of infection is 30% to 50% greater than that associated with dog bites.

Infection is more likely if the wound isn't tended promptly, if there's a crush injury, or if the hand is involved. Clenched-fist injuries are the most serious because damaged joint capsules increase the risk of developing osteomyelitis and septic arthritis.

Unfortunately, many animals — usually wild ones — carry the rabies virus in their saliva and can transmit it by biting or by licking an open wound. Rabies is rare in the United States, but it's always fatal unless treated. The risk of getting rabies from a dog is low but possible. Bats, skunks, and raccoons cause nearly all cases of rabies in the United States. Human bites can infect other humans with diseases, such as herpes simplex virus, cytomegalovirus, syphilis, tuberculosis and, possibly, human immunodeficiency virus.

Causes

Animal bites commonly occur when a sick or injured animal is trying to protect itself or when an animal is protecting its food, territory, or young. Human bites most commonly result from fights among school-age children and young adults.

Clinical presentation

A dog bite may cause bleeding, pain, tenderness, swelling, and decreased sensation at the injury site. A large dog usually inflicts a more severe wound than a smaller dog. A cat bite may cause small, deep puncture wounds.

A human bite may induce bleeding, which may be scant or profuse. If the bite results in a puncture wound or a tear, bleeding may occur immediately, with bruising and swelling appearing later.

Management
Immediate actions

If the bite wound isn't bleeding heavily (as with a puncture wound), wash it vigorously with soap and water for 5 to 10 minutes. Apply a clean pressure dressing and

GUIDE TO POSTEXPOSURE RABIES PROPHYLAXIS

To make decisions about rabies treatment, consider the details of the exposure, the animal's species and vaccination status, and the prevalence of rabies in the region. The wound should be thoroughly cleaned with soap and water. All bites by an animal of questionable health or vaccination status require prompt evaluation. This table provides general guidelines for the next actions to take. Note that the Food and Drug Administration (FDA) considers all three types of rabies vaccines equally safe and effective.

Animal species	Condition of animal at time of attack	Treatment of exposed human
WILD		
Bat Raccoon Skunk Other carnivores	▸ Considered rabid unless proved negative (the animal should be killed and the head tested immediately; observation isn't recommended)	▸ Rabies immune globulin, human (RIG*) and human diploid cell vaccine (HDCV) or rabies vaccine, adsorbed (RVA**)
DOMESTIC		
Cat Dog	▸ Healthy and available: 10 days of isolation and observation	▸ None
	▸ Unknown (escaped)	▸ Consult public health officials and a health care provider; if treatment is indicated, give RIG* and HDCV or RVA**
OTHER		
Gnawing animals (such as hamsters, rabbits, and beavers) Livestock	▸ Rabies suspected or known	▸ Consider individually RIG* and HDCV or RVA**

*RIG should be administered at the beginning of treatment. This product isn't FDA-approved for intradermal use.

**HDCV or RVA are equally effective. HDCV is the only rabies vaccine approved by the FDA for intradermal use.

elevate the extremity if bleeding continues.

▓▓▓ RED FLAG *Don't scrub a bite wound; you could bruise the tissue. Don't suture wounds that* are at an increased risk of becoming infected, such as deep puncture bites and hand wounds. Apply an ice pack to the wound site for 20 minutes to decrease edema and pain.

Pharmacologic treatment options include:

▶ over-the-counter analgesics (acetaminophen, ibuprofen) for local pain.

▶ tetanus prophylaxis for patients who've been immunized in the past but haven't had a booster within the past 5 years; tetanus toxoid and tetanus immune globulin for patients who haven't had an initial immunization series.

▶ rabies prophylaxis given without delay if rabies is considered possible; consult a physician before starting (See *Guide to postexposure rabies prophylaxis.*)

▶ antibiotics for infection, as indicated.

Later actions

Splint clenched-fist injuries and elevate; use X-rays to rule out fractures. Follow up within 2 to 3 days.

Animal bites

If the puncture wounds are simple and don't involve the hands, no other treatment is necessary. Moderate to severe wounds should be debrided, and the patient should be given antibiotic therapy prophylaxis. If no signs or symptoms of infection appear after 3 days, the wound may be closed with sutures or tape strips.

Human bites

Obtain wound cultures to rule out gram-negative organisms. The patient should receive penicillin and a beta-lactamase-resistant penicillin such as amoxicillin. Wound closure should be delayed for 3 days; the wound may then be closed only if no infection is evident.

Collaborative practice

Collaborate with the physician for all bites in which rabies is suspected. Refer facial and ear wounds and clenched-fist injuries to a reconstructive surgeon. Other bites that should be referred include wounds on the hands, feet, or genital area,

and large bite wounds contaminated with debris such as bits of a tooth.

Patient teaching

▶ Advise anyone who has witnessed an animal bite to tell the authorities where the incident occurred and the animal owner's name, if possible. If the animal was wild, tell them the animal's location at the time of the bite. Authorities will try to capture the animal and confine it for 10 days of observation. If it appears rabid, it will be killed and its brain tissue tested for rabies.

▶ Tell the patient that symptoms of infection usually appear after 24 hours. At least once daily, observe for signs of infection (fever higher than 101° F [38.3° C], redness, increased swelling, red streaks in the skin, or cloudy, yellow, or green drainage) or a lump in the wound that grows.

●●● RED FLAG *Tell the patient to*
●●● *call his primary care provider to report signs of infection.*

OPEN TRAUMA WOUNDS

ICD-9-CM 879.8
Open trauma wounds (abrasions, avulsions, crush wounds, lacerations, missile injuries, and punctures) are injuries that commonly result from home, work, or motor vehicle accidents, or from acts of violence.

Clinical presentation

In all open wounds, assess the extent of injury, vital signs, level of consciousness (LOC), obvious skeletal damage, local neurologic deficits, and general patient condition. Obtain an accurate history of the injury from the patient and witnesses, including such details as mechanism and time of injury, alterations in LOC, and treatment provided. If the injury involved a weapon, notify the police as mandated by law.

Assess for peripheral nerve damage — a common complication in lacerations and other open trauma wounds — as well as for fractures and dislocations. Signs of peripheral nerve damage vary with wound location as follows:

▶ *radial nerve* — weak forearm dorsiflexion, inability to extend thumb in a hitchhiker's sign

▶ *median nerve* — numbness in the tip of the index finger; inability to place the forearm in a prone position; weak forearm, thumb, and index finger flexion

▶ *ulnar nerve* — numbness in the tip of the little finger, clawing of hand

▶ *peroneal nerve* — footdrop, inability to extend the foot or big toe

▶ *sciatic and tibial nerves* — paralysis of ankles and toes, footdrop, weakness in leg, and numbness in sole.

Management

Most open wounds require emergency treatment. Stop bleeding by applying direct pressure on the wound. If the wound is on an extremity, elevate it if possible and apply pressure to pulse points proximal to the wound. Don't apply a tourniquet unless it's necessary to save the patient's life because doing so may cause tissue damage that requires amputation.

Increased respirations, decreasing LOC, thirst, and cool, clammy skin all indicate blood loss and shock, and emergency medical services (EMS) should be activated. For all types of open wounds, follow up in 2 to 3 days.

Abrasions

Abrasions are open surface wounds of the epidermis and, possibly, the dermis that result from friction; nerve endings are exposed. Abrasions present as scratches, reddish welts, or bruises, accompanied by pain and a history of friction injury. Obtain a history to distinguish the injury from a second-degree burn.

Clean the wound gently with a topical germicide, and irrigate it. Avoid vigorous scrubbing of abrasions, which increases tissue damage. Remove all imbedded foreign objects. Apply a local anesthetic (lidocaine) if cleaning is painful. Apply a light, water-soluble antibiotic ointment (bacitracin) to prevent infection. If the wound is severe, apply a loose protective dressing that allows air to circulate.

If appropriate, give tetanus prophylaxis for patients who've been immunized in the past but haven't had a booster within the past 5 years, or tetanus toxoid and tetanus immune globulin for patients who haven't had an initial immunization series.

Puncture wounds

Simple puncture wounds of extremities are small-entry wounds that aren't likely to involve damage to underlying structures or have retained foreign objects. They commonly have ragged edges, occur on the face or fingers, and may be caused by a human or animal bite. If you suspect damage to underlying structures or the presence of a foreign object, immediately refer the patient to an emergency department (ED).

●●● **RED FLAG** *Don't remove impal-*
●●● *ing objects before transporting the patient to the ED. If an eye is involved, call an ophthalmologist immediately.*

Check the patient history for bleeding tendencies and use of anticoagulants, and check the description of the injury, including force and depth of entry. Thoroughly clean the injured area with soap and water. Irrigate all minor wounds with saline solution after removing foreign objects. Apply a dry, sterile dressing.

Provide tetanus prophylaxis of tetanus toxoid in patients who have been immunized in the past but haven't had a booster within the past 5 years, or tetanus toxoid and tetanus immune globulin in patients who haven't had an initial immunization series.

Lacerations

Lacerations are open wounds resulting from penetration by a sharp object or from a severe blow with a blunt object. Apply pressure and elevate the injured extremity to control bleeding. Irrigate with saline solution. Debride necrotic margins and close the wound using strips of tape or sutures unless contamination is likely.

Grossly contaminated lacerations or lacerations more than 8 hours old. Order a course of a broad-spectrum antibiotic. Don't close the wound, but do apply a sterile dressing and splint. After 5 to 7 days, close the wound with sutures or tape strips if it appears uninfected and shows healthy granulated tissue.

All other lacerations. Check the patient history for bleeding tendencies and anticoagulant use. Determine the approximate time of the injury and estimate the amount of blood lost. Assess for neuromuscular, tendon, and circulatory damage.

Give tetanus toxoid in patients who have been immunized in the past but haven't had a booster within the past 5 years, or tetanus toxoid and tetanus immune globulin in patients who haven't had an initial immunization series. Stress the need for follow-up and suture removal.

●●● RED FLAG *If sutures become*
●●● *infected, culture the wound and scrub with surgical soap preparation. Remove some or all sutures, and give a broad-spectrum antibiotic. Instruct the patient to soak the wound in warm, soapy water for 15 minutes three times per day and to return for a follow-up visit every 2 to 3 days until the wound heals. If the injury is the result of foul play, report it to the authorities as required by law.*

Collaborative practice

Many open wounds require emergency medical transport to the ED, including:

▶ an avulsion injury
▶ crush injury
▶ deep puncture wound
▶ wound that may contain a retained object
▶ wound in which underlying structures may be damaged
▶ wound with ragged edges
▶ missile injury such as a gunshot wound.

Inform EMS personnel of pertinent information, including the patient's condition when you first saw him, his medical history, allergies, and the name of the primary care provider. All lacerations that are gaping or are more than $1/4''$ (0.6 cm) long involving the face or areas of possible functional disability, such as the elbow or hand, need to be seen by a physician or a reconstructive surgeon in the ED.

Patient teaching

▶ For puncture wounds, instruct the patient to apply warm soaks daily and to report signs or symptoms of infection.
▶ For lacerations, instruct the patient to elevate the injured extremity for 24 hours after injury to reduce edema. Tell him to keep the dressing clean and dry and to report signs or symptoms of infection.

POISONING

ICD-9-CM due to acids 983.1, caustic alkalis 983.2, toxic petroleum products 981

Poisoning may involve a variety of substances. In most cases, the poisonous substance is ingested. With an ingested poison, the main concern is the possibility of systemic effects. Poisoning can result in organ failure or death, depending on the substance and the extent of exposure. Most poisoning episodes can be managed in primary care settings.

Ingested poisons fall into three general categories:
● corrosive (caustic) substances, such as household bleaches, metal polishes, antirust solutions, paint and varnish removers, drain cleaners, refrigerants, fertilizers, and photographic chemicals
● petroleum-based substances, such as floor polish and wax, furniture polish and wax, gasoline, kerosene, and lighter fluid
● substances that are neither corrosive nor petroleum-based.

Most accidental poisons are of the third type. For example, medications left unattended and in a child's reach may result in accidental poisoning.

Causes

Poisonings can be accidental or purposeful (as in a suicide attempt). Most accidental poisonings involve children younger than age 6 and, because most toxic substances taste unpleasant, the child usually spits them out, thereby limiting the child's exposure to the toxic substance. One exception, however, is antifreeze, which tastes sweet. The patient history must be focused and specific but nonjudgmental because purposeful poisonings are cries for

help and caregivers of accident victims usually feel guilty or distraught.

●●● **RED FLAG** *The patient suspect-*
●●● *ed of having tried purposeful poisoning should be closely watched and requires emergency psychiatric evaluation.*

Clinical presentation

Signs and symptoms of poisoning vary with the type and amount of poison swallowed. Typically, the ingestion is suspected soon after it happens, and signs and symptoms will be absent. Many substances will never produce signs and symptoms because they're of low toxicity. History may reveal nausea and vomiting, stomach cramps, headache, weakness, and burning sensations in the mouth, throat, or stomach.

Examination may reveal:
● abdominal gas
● abnormally fast or slow pulse
● a dull, masklike facial expression
● an altered state of consciousness, delirium, or mental disturbances
● burned or damaged skin
● changes in skin color, particularly around the lips or fingernails
● change in urine or stool color
● clumsiness
● complete or partial paralysis
● coughing
● diaphoresis
● diarrhea, possibly with stomach cramps
● drooling or excessive salivation
● excessively dilated or constricted pupils
● facial twitching
● loss of voluntary muscle control
● muscle spasms
● respiratory changes or difficulty breathing
● seizures
● unusual breath odor
● vision or hearing problems.

CLINICAL PEARL
WHAT THE PATIENT'S BREATH MAY REVEAL

Some swallowed poisons affect the patient's breath, as described in this table. If you suspect your patient has been poisoned, smell his breath and report peculiar breath odor to the primary care provider or emergency medical services personnel.

Odor	Possible poison
Alcohol-like	Alcohol
Bitter almonds	Cyanide
Garliclike	Phosphorus, arsenic
Gasoline-like	Petroleum-like products
Pearlike	Chloral hydrate
Shoe polish-like	Nitrobenzene
Stale tobacco	Nicotine
Sweet	Acetone
Violets	Turpentine

If such signs or symptoms are present but no one witnessed the poisoning, instruct someone at the site to check for telltale signs that a poisoning has occurred, such as:
▶ an open medicine or household chemical container
▶ spilled liquid, powder, or pills
▶ liquid, powder, or pills in the patient's mouth or on the teeth
▶ stains on the patient's clothing
▶ burns or swelling on the hands or mouth
▶ a peculiar odor on the patient's breath, body, or clothes. (See *What the patient's breath may reveal.*)

Management
Immediate actions
If the patient shows signs or symptoms of poisoning, check his airway, breathing, and circulation (ABCs). Administer cardiopulmonary resuscitation as needed. Check vital signs every 5 minutes, apply pulse oximetry, and provide oxygen via facemask until the nature of the poison is known.

CLINICAL PEARL *Call the poison control center immediately. Have the following information ready when you call:*
▶ the patient's age and weight
▶ the name of the poison and its ingredients (or if it's a plant, the type of plant) and the amount of poison the patient has swallowed, if you know
▶ the time the poisoning occurred
▶ the patient's signs and symptoms
▶ a medical condition the patient suffers from — for instance, diabetes mellitus, high blood pressure, heart disease, or epilepsy — and what medications the patient takes regu-

larly. Follow the instructions of the poison control center exactly.

Aiding a conscious patient

After establishing the status of the patient's ABCs, maintain the airway by suctioning secretions, performing aspiration precautions, and placing an oral airway if needed. If the patient is experiencing a seizure, take appropriate steps. (See "Seizure disorder.")

Contact the poison control center immediately for suspected ingestion of a nonfood. The poison control center has information available on drugs, household products, plants, and foods that can be dangerous.

Giving ipecac syrup

Since November 2003, the American Academy of Pediatrics (AAP) no longer recommends the routine use of syrup of ipecac. The first action should be to call the poison control center. If the patient must be taken to a hospital emergency department (ED) immediately, send the following materials with him:
▶ a container of the patient's vomitus. It can be tested to determine the nature of the poison. Also notify emergency medical services (EMS) personnel if the patient has vomited undigested tablets; if possible, estimate how many tablets the patient took by inspecting the vomitus.
▶ the poison container and its remaining contents to help identify the poison and estimate how much the patient swallowed. Send enough of a poisonous plant to allow accurate identification — for example, an entire mushroom or a branch with leaves, flowers, and berries.

Collaborative practice

Refer the patient to the ED when indicated by the poison control center or for symptoms of concern. Notify emergency medical services personnel of data given to the poison control center, plus psychiatric history, pertinent social history, current and past medication usage, and prior hospitalizations. Initiate emergency psychiatric consultation for suspected purposeful poisoning.

Patient teaching

Based on the latest AAP recommendations, advise the parents to safely dispose of any syrup of ipecac they may currently have in their home.

●●● **RED FLAG** *Instruct parents to*
●●● *childproof their homes by keeping all medicines in safety-cap bottles, labeling all containers and storing only edible substances in food and drink containers, and locking away all medicines and toxins, such as cleaning supplies, drain cleaners, paints and thinners, auto products, and garden sprays.*

● SEIZURE DISORDER

ICD-9-CM 780.39, atonic 345, febrile 780.31, repetitive 780.39

Seizure disorder, or epilepsy, is a condition of the brain characterized by recurrent seizures — paroxysmal events associated with abnormal electrical discharges of neurons in the brain. Primary seizure disorder is idiopathic without apparent structural changes in the brain. Secondary seizure disorder, characterized by structural changes or metabolic alterations of the neuronal membranes, causes increased automaticity.

Seizure disorder affects 1% to 2% of the population; approximately 2 million people live with seizure disorder. The incidence is highest in childhood and old age. The prognosis is good if the patient adheres strictly to the prescribed treatment.

Causes

In about one-half of seizure disorder cases, the cause is unknown. In children, fever may bring on generalized seizures. Other possible causes include:

▶ anoxia (after respiratory or cardiac arrest)

▶ birth trauma (such as inadequate oxygen supply to the brain, blood incompatibility, or hemorrhage) or perinatal infection

▶ brain tumor

▶ cerebral aneurysm rupture

▶ electrolyte abnormalities

▶ head injury or trauma

▶ infectious diseases, such as meningitis, encephalitis, or brain abscess

▶ metabolic disorders, such as hypoparathyroidism or hypoglycemia.

In addition, alcohol and drug withdrawal can cause nonepileptic seizures.

Clinical presentation

Assessment findings depend on the type of seizure and may vary with the underlying cause. The hallmark of seizure disorders is recurring seizures, which can be classified as partial or generalized. Some patients are affected by more than one type of seizures. (See *Seizure types*, pages 318 and 319.)

Management

Immediate actions

The top priority in this medical emergency is to keep the patient from harm and to observe him during the seizure. Your observations will help determine what type of seizure the patient has had and which brain area was involved.

If you're with a patient who experiences an aura, help him into bed or onto the floor, and then place a pillow, blanket, or other soft material under his head. Loosen his clothing, and move sharp or hard objects out of the way.

During a seizure, stay with the patient and be ready to intervene in case airway obstruction or other complications occur. If possible, have another person obtain appropriate equipment (soft pillow and blanket, for example) and activate emergency medical services (EMS). Note the time of seizure onset.

Don't try to restrain the patient or restrict his movements during a seizure. The force of the patient's movements can cause a fracture. If a patient seems to be in the beginning of the tonic phase of a tonic-clonic seizure (marked by muscle contraction and stiffening of the body), insert an oral airway into his mouth, if available, so that his tongue won't block his airway.

●●● RED FLAG *If an oral airway*
●●● *isn't available, don't try to hold the patient's mouth open or place your hands inside his mouth because you may be injured. When his jaw becomes rigid, don't try to force an oral airway (or other hard object) into place because this may cause further injury, such as broken teeth.*

To allow secretions to drain, turn the patient onto his side during the seizure (or during the clonic phase of a generalized tonic-clonic seizure, when respirations resume). If respirations don't return, check the patient's airway for an obstruction. Then check breathing and circulation, and begin cardiopulmonary resuscitation as needed.

Postseizure care

Protect the patient by providing a safe area where he can rest. When he awakens, reassure and reorient him. Assess his vital signs and neurologic status. Then record the following information:

▶ time the seizure started and stopped

▶ what happened just before the seizure (such as an aura or a strange mood)

SEIZURE TYPES

The various types of seizures — partial, generalized, status epilepticus, and unclassi-fied — have distinct signs and symptoms.

Partial seizures

Arising from a localized area of the brain, partial seizures cause focal symp-toms. These seizures are classified by their effect on consciousness and whether they spread throughout the mo-tor pathway, causing a generalized seizure.

▶ A *simple partial seizure* begins locally and generally doesn't cause an alteration in consciousness. It may present with sensory symptoms (lights flashing, smells, and auditory hallucinations), au-tonomic symptoms (sweating, flushing, and pupil dilation), and psychic symp-toms (dream states, anger, and fear). The seizure lasts for a few seconds and oc-curs without preceding or provoking events. This type can be motor or sen-sory.

▶ A *complex partial seizure* alters con-sciousness. Amnesia for events that oc-cur during and immediately after the seizure is a differentiating characteristic. During the seizure, the patient may fol-low simple commands. This type of seizure usually lasts for 1 to 3 minutes.

Generalized seizures

As the term suggests, generalized seizures cause a generalized electrical abnormality within the brain. They can be convulsive or nonconvulsive and in-clude several types:

▶ *Absence seizures* occur most common-ly in children, although they may affect adults. They usually begin with a brief change in level of consciousness, indi-cated by a blinking or rolling of the eyes, a blank stare, and slight mouth move-ments. The patient retains his posture and continues preseizure activity without difficulty. Typically, each seizure lasts from 1 to 10 seconds. If not properly treated, seizures can recur as frequently as 100 times per day. An absence seizure is a nonconvulsive seizure, but it may progress to a generalized tonic-clonic seizure.

▶ *Myoclonic seizures* are brief, involun-tary muscular jerks of the body or ex-tremities, commonly occurring in the ear-ly morning.

▶ *Clonic* seizures are characterized by bi-lateral rhythmic movements.

▶ where the seizure began (what part of the body, what side)
▶ what happened during the seizure (for example, what type of muscle movements the patient made and whether he lost consciousness or fell down, made noises, drooled, lost bowel or bladder control, stopped breathing, frothed at the mouth, or made repetitive move-ments)
▶ what happened after the seizure (for instance, whether the patient was confused or groggy, fell asleep, complained of a headache, remem-bered having had the seizure, and experienced residual weakness).

If the patient is known to have di-abetes mellitus, obtain a blood glu-cose level and administer 50 ml of dextrose 50% in water by I.V. push as indicated.

A bolus of thiamine may be given if chronic alcoholism or withdrawal is suspected. If the seizure is pro-longed and the patient shows signs of oxygen deprivation, initiate re-suscitation measures immediately.

▸ *Tonic* seizures are characterized by a sudden stiffening of muscle tone, usually of the arms, but possibly including the legs.

▸ *Generalized tonic-clonic seizures* typically begin with a loud cry, precipitated by air rushing from the lungs through the vocal cords. The patient then loses consciousness and falls to the ground. The body stiffens (tonic phase) and then alternates between episodes of muscle spasm and relaxation (clonic phase). Tongue biting, incontinence, labored breathing, apnea, and subsequent cyanosis may occur. The seizure stops in 2 to 5 minutes, when abnormal electrical conduction ceases. When the patient regains consciousness, he's confused and may have difficulty talking. If he can talk, he may complain of drowsiness, fatigue, headache, muscle soreness, and arm or leg weakness. He may fall into a deep sleep after the seizure.

▸ *Atonic seizures* are characterized by a general loss of postural tone and a temporary loss of consciousness. They occur in young children and are sometimes called "drop attacks" because they cause the child to fall.

Status epilepticus
Status epilepticus is a continuous seizure state that can occur in all seizure types. The most life-threatening example is generalized tonic-clonic status epilepticus, a continuous generalized tonic-clonic seizure. Status epilepticus is accompanied by respiratory distress leading to hypoxia or anoxia. It can result from abrupt withdrawal of anticonvulsant medications, hypoxic encephalopathy, acute head trauma, metabolic encephalopathy, or septicemia secondary to encephalitis or meningitis.

Unclassified seizures
The unclassified seizures category is reserved for seizures that don't fit the characteristics of partial or generalized seizures or status epilepticus. Events that lack the data necessary for making a definitive diagnosis are included in the category of unclassified seizures.

Follow-up and prevention
After the patient has been stabilized, determine and treat the underlying cause of the seizure. Extensive evaluation, including magnetic resonance imaging (MRI), is indicated for an adult patient following a first seizure. MRI is the preferred procedure because it's best for detecting subtle changes; if this isn't available, a computed tomography scan with and without contrast may be used.

Follow-up depends on the etiology of the seizure and is needed for recurrent seizures. If drug therapy fails, surgical removal of a demonstrated focal lesion may be performed to prevent seizures from recurring. A vagus nerve stimulation device, which acts on the brain the way a pacemaker acts on the heart, may also be used to manage seizures. The device, which is implanted in the chest and neck, sends electrical signals to the brain to inhibit seizure activity. Potential adverse effects of the vagus nerve stimulation device include voice changes, throat discomfort, and shortness of breath.

Collaborative practice

Status epilepticus is a medical emergency. Call for EMS and report pertinent information, including the patient's condition when you first saw him, his medical history, allergies, and the name of his primary care provider. Refer the patient to a neurologist or neurosurgeon if a condition in addition to epilepsy is considered.

Patient teaching

▶ Most patients experience a period of decreased mental functioning when a seizure ends. Reassure the patient that this is a normal post-seizure occurrence and will soon resolve.
▶ Stress the need for compliance with the prescribed drug therapy.
▶ Teach the patient about adverse effects of medication.
▶ Warn the patient against drinking alcoholic beverages.

SPRAINS AND STRAINS

ICD-9-CM 848.9

A sprain is a complete or incomplete tear in the supporting ligaments surrounding a joint that usually follows a sharp twist. A strain is an injury to a muscle or tendinous attachment. Both injuries usually heal without surgical repair.

Clinical presentation

In assessing sprains and strains, it's important to err on the side of caution; pain over a bone is considered a fracture until proven otherwise. A sprain causes local pain (especially during joint movement), swelling, loss of mobility (which may not occur until several hours after the injury), and a black-and-blue discoloration from blood extravasating

into surrounding tissues. A sprained ankle is the most common joint injury. A sprain causes maximal pain when the ligament is stretched. For example, inversion and plantar flexion of the foot commonly causes pain in a sprained ankle.

A strain may be acute, resulting from vigorous muscle overuse or overstress, or chronic, resulting from repeated overuse. An acute strain causes a sharp, transient pain (the patient may report hearing a "snapping noise") and rapid swelling. When severe pain subsides, the muscle is tender; after several days, ecchymoses appear. A chronic strain causes stiffness, soreness, and generalized tenderness several hours after the injury.

In sprain or strain, history usually reveals a recent injury or chronic overuse. The patient history and examination may reveal more serious injuries, such as inability to bear weight due to pain, joint instability, tenderness localized to a particular bone, increasing pain or edema, or signs of vascular compromise (pallor or cyanosis, paresthesia, "pins and needles" sensation, inability to move the joint).

Sprains are graded based on their severity:
▶ *Grade I* — partial or complete tear of the ligament, causing local tenderness, minimal edema; usually able to bear weight. Treatment is usually symptomatic with elastic compression support to control edema. Intermittent removal of immobilization, with active range-of-motion (ROM) exercises, progresses as tolerated. Strengthening exercises start at 2 to 3 weeks, depending on patient tolerance.
▶ *Grade II* — partial or complete tear of ligaments, causing painful weight bearing and minimal ligament function during examination. Treatment is the same as for Grade I, plus im-

mobilization and non–weight bearing with an air splint or cast; treatment may switch to hinged-joint immobilization at 2 weeks.

▶ *Grade III* — ligamentous laxity, instability, and complete interruption in alignment causing inability to bear weight and, commonly, obvious deformity. After evaluation by an orthopedic surgeon, treatment usually consists of a cast worn for 3 weeks. After 3 weeks, physical therapy, including ROM exercises, strengthening exercises, and proprioception training, begins. However, the orthopedic surgeon may cast for up to 6 weeks or perform surgical repair.

●●● **RED FLAG** *Pain within 2″ (5.1*
●●● *cm) proximal or distal to the joint plus bone tenderness within 2¹/₂″ (6.4 cm) of the bone indicates the need for X-rays to check for fracture.*

●●● **RED FLAG** *Orthopedic referral is*
●●● *needed for a patient unable to bear weight on the affected extremity from immediately after the trauma until the time of examination.*

●●● **RED FLAG** *All new bony abnor-*
●●● *malities, regardless of size, require urgent orthopedic referral. If such a referral is unavailable, refer the patient to the emergency department (ED).*

Management

Treatment of sprains focuses on controlling pain and swelling plus immobilizing the injured joint to prevent further injury and allow healing. Immediately after the injury, use rest, ice, compression, elevation (RICE) therapy. Apply an elastic bandage wrap or, if the sprain is severe, a soft cast or splint. The goal is pain-free full range of motion. Codeine or another analgesic may be necessary if the injury is severe. Chronic strains usually don't need treatment, but heat application, nonsteroidal anti-inflammatory drugs (such as ibuprofen) or an analgesic-muscle relaxant (such as cyclobenzaprine) can relieve discomfort.

Control swelling by resting as much as possible and intermittently applying ice for 12 to 48 hours. To prevent frostbite, place a towel between the ice pack and the skin, leaving it in place for no more than 20 minutes at a time. Immobilize the joint, and control swelling by using an elastic bandage as directed. For a sprained ankle, apply the bandage from the toes to midcalf. Position the limb with the affected joint elevated above the level of the heart as much as possible for 2 to 3 days; pillows can be used for elevation during sleep.

Patients with sprains or strains are usually treated on an outpatient basis, so provide gait training and verify proper technique with crutches to reduce the risk of permanent axillary nerve damage and falls. After 48 hours, a heating pad set at WARM replaces the ice packs, using the same schedule for pain relief and to enhance resorption of edema.

Call the primary care provider if pain worsens or persists; a later X-ray may reveal a fracture that wasn't originally visible. Follow up within 1 week and then as needed if the patient is greatly improved. Refer to an orthopedist in 2 weeks if little improvement is noted.

Collaborative practice

Urgent orthopedic or ED evaluation is needed for Grade III sprains or strains (obvious deformity, inability to bear weight on the joint, or joint instability). (See *Muscle-tendon ruptures,* page 322.)

Patient teaching

▶ Inform the patient that an immobilized sprain usually heals in 4 to

> **CLINICAL PEARL**
> **MUSCLE-TENDON RUPTURES**
>
> Perhaps the most serious muscle-tendon injury is a rupture of the muscle-tendon junction. This type of rupture may occur at such a junction, but it's most common at the Achilles tendon, which extends from the posterior calf muscle to the foot. An Achilles tendon rupture produces a sudden, sharp pain and, until swelling begins, a palpable defect. Such a rupture typically occurs in men between ages 35 and 40, especially during physical activities, such as jogging or tennis.
>
> To distinguish an Achilles tendon rupture from other ankle injuries, the primary care provider performs this simple test: With the patient prone and his feet hanging off the foot of the table, the primary care provider squeezes the calf muscle. If this causes plantar flexion, the tendon is intact; if it causes ankle dorsiflexion, it's partially intact; if there's no flexion at all, the tendon is ruptured.
>
> An Achilles tendon rupture usually requires surgical repair, followed first by a long leg cast for 4 weeks and then by a short cast for an additional 4 weeks.

6 weeks, after which the patient can gradually resume normal activities. Occasionally, however, torn ligaments don't heal properly and cause recurrent dislocation, requiring surgical repair.

▶ Teach the patient to reapply the elastic bandage by wrapping from below to above the injury, forming a figure eight. For a sprained ankle, he should apply the bandage from the toes to midcalf. Tell the patient to remove the bandage before going to sleep and to loosen it if it causes the limb to become pale, numb, or painful.

▶ Inform the patient who's an athlete that he may tape his wrists and ankles before sports activities to prevent injury; make sure he knows the proper procedure for doing so.

▶ Advise the patient to avoid excessive physical stress and to wear appropriate gear for activity. Inform him of the risks associated with specific activities (for example, sports).

▶ Emphasize rationale for appropriate conditioning, warm-up, and cool-down exercises.

SUBCONJUNCTIVAL HEMORRHAGE

ICD-9-CM 372.72

Subconjunctival hemorrhage is a local blood vessel rupture that causes a flat, bright-red hemorrhage under the conjunctiva of the eye. It's a self-limited, benign condition that clears within 3 weeks.

Causes

Subconjunctival hemorrhage may result from minor trauma or from a Valsalva's maneuver, such as coughing, sneezing, vomiting, or attempting to defecate.

Clinical presentation

The condition is asymptomatic although it does present a startling appearance. Consider conjunctivitis if symptoms are present.

Management

Subconjunctival hemorrhage condition resolves spontaneously within 3 weeks. Aggressive evaluation is needed to locate other sites of bleeding. Hematologic studies — prothrombin time, partial thromboplastin time, and International Normalizing Ratio — are required if the patient is taking anticoagulants. Follow up for new or worsening symptoms.

Collaborative practice

Refer the patient to an ophthalmologist if blood appeared after trauma to the area or if there are persistent recurrences, pain, blurring or vision loss, discharge, blood in the pupil or iris, or if the hemorrhage covers more than 25% of the sclera.

Patient teaching

▶ Reassure the patient that the redness should resolve within 3 weeks.
▶ Instruct the patient not to touch the affected eye.
▶ Instruct the patient to call his primary care provider if extreme pain or vision changes develop.

8
Precautions

Preventing the spread of contagious disease

324 •

Centers for Disease Control and Prevention isolation precautions

The Centers for Disease Control and Prevention (CDC) and the Hospital Infection Control Practices Advisory Committee developed the CDC *Guideline for Isolation Precautions in Hospitals* to help hospitals maintain up-to-date isolation practices. The 1997 guidelines contain two tiers of precautions, standard precautions and transmission-based precautions.

STANDARD PRECAUTIONS

The first tier of the CDC isolation precautions, called *standard precautions,* is used when caring for all hospital patients, regardless of their diagnoses or presumed infections. Standard precautions are the primary strategy for preventing nosocomial infection; these precautions replace the earlier, universal precautions. They should be followed at all times and with every patient.

Standard precautions, if followed correctly, provide protection from:
▶ blood
▶ all body fluids, secretions, and excretions — except sweat — regardless of whether they contain visible blood
▶ skin that isn't intact
▶ mucous membranes.

TRANSMISSION-BASED PRECAUTIONS

The second tier of the CDC isolation precautions is *transmission-based precautions.* These precautions are instituted when caring for patients with known or suspected highly transmissible infections that necessitate more stringent precautions than those described in the standard precautions.

Transmission-based precautions are categorized as airborne precautions, droplet precautions, or contact precautions.

Airborne precautions
Airborne precautions, if followed correctly, reduce the risk of airborne transmission of infectious agents. Microorganisms carried through the air can be dispersed widely by air currents, making them available for inhalation or deposit on a susceptible host in the same room as, or some distance away from, the infected patient.

Airborne precautions include special air-handling and ventilation procedures to prevent the spread of infection. These precautions require the use of respiratory protection, such as a mask — in addition to standard precautions — when entering an infected patient's room. (See *Indications for airborne precautions,* page 326.)

Droplet precautions
Droplet precautions, if followed correctly, reduce the risk of transmitting infectious agents in large-particle (exceeding 5 micrometers) droplets. Such transmission involves the contact of infectious agents to the conjunctivae or nasal

INDICATIONS FOR AIRBORNE PRECAUTIONS

Disease	Precautionary period
Chickenpox (varicella)	Until lesions are crusted and no new lesions appear
Herpes zoster (disseminated)	Duration of illness
Herpes zoster (localized in immuno-compromised patient)	Duration of illness
Measles (rubeola)	Duration of illness
Smallpox (variola major)	Duration of illness, until all scabs fall off
Tuberculosis (TB) — pulmonary or laryngeal, confirmed or suspected	Depends on clinical response; patient must be on effective therapy, be improving clinically (decreased cough and fever and improved findings on chest radiograph), and have three consecutive negative sputum smears collected on different days, or TB must be ruled out

or oral mucous membranes of a susceptible person. Large particle droplets don't remain in the air and generally travel short distances of 3′ (0.9 m) or less.

Droplet precautions require the use of a mask—in addition to standard precautions—to protect the mucous membranes. (See *Indications for droplet precautions*.)

Contact precautions

Contact precautions, if followed correctly, reduce the risk of transmitting infectious agents by direct or indirect contact. Direct-contact transmission can occur through patient care activities that require physical contact. Indirect-contact transmission involves a susceptible host coming in contact with a contaminated object, usually inanimate, in the patient's environment.

Contact precautions include the use of gloves, a mask, and a gown—in addition to standard precautions—to avoid contact with the infectious agent. Stringent hand washing is also necessary after removing the protective items. (See *Indications for contact precautions*, pages 328 and 329.)

INDICATIONS FOR DROPLET PRECAUTIONS

Disease	Precautionary period
Adenovirus infection in infants and young children	Duration of illness
Diphtheria (pharyngeal)	Until off antibiotics and two cultures taken at least 24 hours apart are negative
Influenza	Duration of illness
Invasive *Haemophilus influenzae* type B disease, including meningitis, pneumonia, and sepsis	Until 24 hours after initiation of effective therapy
Invasive *Neisseria meningitidis* disease, including meningitis, pneumonia, epiglottiditis, and sepsis	Until 24 hours after initiation of effective therapy
Mumps	For 9 days after onset of swelling
Mycoplasma pneumoniae infection	Duration of illness
Parvovirus B19	Maintain precautions for duration of hospitalization when chronic disease occurs in an immunodeficient patient. For patients with transient aplastic crisis or red-cell crisis, maintain precautions for 7 days.
Pertussis	Until 5 days after initiation of effective therapy
Pneumonic plague	Until 72 hours after initiation of effective therapy
Rubella (German measles)	Until 7 days after onset of rash
Streptococcal pharyngitis, pneumonia, or scarlet fever in infants and young children	Until 24 hours after initiation of effective therapy

INDICATIONS FOR CONTACT PRECAUTIONS

Disease	Precautionary period
Acute viral (acute hemorrhagic) conjunctivitis	Duration of illness
Clostridium difficile enteric infection	Duration of illness
Diphtheria (cutaneous)	Duration of illness
Enteroviral infection, in diapered or incontinent patient	Duration of illness
Escherichia coli disease, in diapered or incontinent patient	Duration of illness
Hepatitis A, in diapered or incontinent patient	Duration of illness
Herpes simplex virus infection (neonatal or mucocutaneous)	Duration of illness
Impetigo	Until 24 hours after initiation of effective therapy
Infection or colonization with multidrug-resistant bacteria	Until off antibiotics and culture is negative
Major abscesses, cellulitis, or pressure ulcer	Until 24 hours after initiation of effective therapy
Parainfluenza virus infection, in diapered or incontinent patients	Duration of illness
Pediculosis (lice)	Until 24 hours after initiation of effective therapy
Respiratory syncytial virus infection, in infants and young children	Duration of illness
Rotavirus infection, in diapered or incontinent patient	Duration of illness
Rubella, congenital syndrome	Precautions during any admission until infant is 1 year old, unless nasopharyngeal and urine cultures negative for virus after age 3 months
Scabies	Until 24 hours after initiation of effective therapy

INDICATIONS FOR CONTACT PRECAUTIONS *(continued)*

Disease	Precautionary period
Shigellosis, in diapered or incontinent patient	Duration of illness
Smallpox	Duration of illness; requires airborne precautions
Staphylococcal furunculosis, in infants and young children	Duration of illness
Viral hemorrhagic infections (Ebola, Lassa, Marburg)	Duration of illness
Zoster (chickenpox, disseminated zoster, or localized zoster in immunodeficient patient)	Until all lesions are crusted; requires airborne precautions

Reportable diseases and infections

Certain contagious diseases must be reported to local and state public health officials and, ultimately, to the CDC. Typically, these diseases fit one of two categories — those reported individually on definitive or suspected diagnosis and those reported by the number of cases per week.

The most commonly reported diseases include:
▶ gonorrhea
▶ hepatitis
▶ measles
▶ salmonellosis
▶ shigellosis
▶ syphilis
▶ viral meningitis.

In most states, the patient's primary care provider must report communicable diseases to health officials. In hospitals, the infection control practitioner or epidemiologist reports them. Therefore, you should know the reporting requirements and procedure so that you can report these diseases to the appropriate person within your facility. Fast, accurate reporting helps to identify and control infection sources, prevent epidemics, and guide public health policy. (See *CDC's list of reportable diseases and infections,* page 330 and 331.)

CDC's LIST OF REPORTABLE DISEASES AND INFECTIONS

The Centers for Disease Control and Prevention (CDC), the Occupational Safety and Health Administration, the Joint Commission on Accreditation of Healthcare Organizations, and the American Hospital Association all require health care facilities to document and report certain diseases acquired in the community or in hospitals and other health care facilities.

Generally, the health care facility reports diseases to the appropriate local authorities. These authorities notify the state health department, which in turn reports the diseases to the appropriate federal agency or national organization.

The list of diseases that appears below is the CDC's list of nationally reportable infectious diseases for 2003. Each state also keeps a list of reportable diseases appropriate to its region.

- Acquired immunodeficiency syndrome
- Anthrax
- Botulism (food-borne, infant, other [wound and unspecified])
- Brucellosis
- Chancroid
- *Chlamydia trachomatis,* genital infections
- Cholera
- Coccidioidomycosis
- Cryptosporidiosis
- Cyclosporiasis
- Diphtheria
- Ehrlichiosis (human granulocytic, human monocytic, human [other or unspecified agent])
- Encephalitis/meningitis: arboviral California serogroup viral, eastern equine, Powassan, St. Louis, western equine, West Nile)
- Enterohemorrhagic *Escherichia coli* (O157:H7, Shiga toxin positive [serogroup non-O157], Shiga toxin positive [not serogrouped])
- Giardiasis
- Gonorrhea
- *Haemophilus influenzae,* invasive disease
- Hansen's disease (leprosy)
- *Hantavirus* pulmonary syndrome
- Hemolytic uremic syndrome, postdiarrheal
- Hepatitis, viral, acute (hepatitis A acute, hepatitis B acute, hepatitis B virus perinatal infection, hepatitis C acute)
- Hepatitis, viral, chronic (chronic hepatitis B, hepatitis C virus infection [past or present])
- Human immunodeficiency virus (adult ≥ 13 years, pediatric < 13 years)
- *Legionella* infections (legionnaires' disease)
- Listeriosis
- Lyme disease
- Malaria
- Measles
- Meningococcal disease
- Mumps
- Pertussis
- Plague
- Poliomyelitis (paralytic)
- Psittacosis (ornithosis)
- Q fever
- Rabies (animal, human)
- Rocky Mountain spotted fever
- Rubella (German measles) and congenital syndrome
- Salmonellosis
- Severe acute respiratory syndrome
- Shigellosis
- Streptococcal disease, invasive, Group A
- Streptococcal toxic shock syndrome
- *Streptococcus pneumoniae,* drug-resistant, invasive disease
- *Streptococcus pneumoniae,* invasive, in children ages < 5 years
- Syphilis (primary; secondary; latent; early latent; late latent; latent unknown duration; neurosyphilis; late nonneurologic)

REPORTABLE DISEASES AND INFECTIONS *(continued)*

- Syphilis, congenital (syphilitic still-birth)
- Tetanus
- Toxic shock syndrome
- Trichinosis
- Tuberculosis
- Tularemia
- Typhoid fever
- Varicella (morbidity)
- Varicella (deaths only)
- Yellow fever

9
Primary care procedures
Performing them with confidence

Key procedures   333

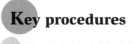

Key procedures

ABSCESS INCISION AND DRAINAGE

CPT code: 10060 I&D of abscess; 10080 I&D of pilonidal cyst, simple; 10081 I&D of pilonidal cyst, complicated; 10140 I&D of hematoma or seroma, or fluid collection

An abscess is a local collection of pus in a cavity formed by the breakdown of tissue and surrounded by inflamed tissue. Abscesses typically result from *Staphylococcus aureus* or a streptococcal infection. Males and children have a higher incidence of abscess formation.

Specific types of abscesses include furuncles, paronychia, pilonidal cysts, and perianal cysts. Furuncles, or boils, occur in hair follicles or sweat glands. Paronychia progress from cellulitis to abscesses over time and involve one or more fingernails or toenails. Pilonidal cysts result from ingrown hairs close to the anus and may have sinus openings. Perianal cysts typically result from a rectal fistula.

Equipment

Antiseptic skin cleaner (such as povidone-iodine) • topical anesthetic (such as ethyl chloride or a tissue freezing kit) • 1% to 2% lidocaine with or without epinephrine • 3- to 10-ml syringe • 25G to 30G ½" needle • 16G to 18G needle • 4" × 4" sterile gauze pads • 1 scalpel • sterile drape • sterile gloves • sterile curved hemostats • iodoform gauze • culture swab • sterile scissors • tape • protective eyewear if abscess contents appear under pressure

Essential steps

▶ Explain the procedure to the patient and address questions or concerns he may have.
▶ Obtain informed consent.
▶ Wash your hands.
▶ Position the patient comfortably with the abscess exposed.
▶ Clean the site and surrounding area with antiseptic skin cleaner.
▶ Apply the sterile drape, and put on sterile gloves.
▶ Anesthetize the area by freezing the surface with topical anesthetic or injecting the perimeter with lidocaine solution.
▶ With the scalpel, make an incision deep and wide enough to allow purulent material to drain easily and to prevent premature closure.
▶ Insert the culture swab deep into the wound to collect material for culturing. Alternatively, use a 16G or an 18G needle and syringe to withdraw fluid for culturing before incising.
▶ Use curved hemostats to explore the cavity and break down membranes leading to other fluid-filled compartments.
▶ After expressing all purulent material, pack the cavity with iodoform gauze, leaving at least ¼" (0.6 cm) of gauze extending outside the wound.
▶ Dress the wound with sterile gauze.
▶ Administer broad-spectrum antibiotic prophylaxis.
▶ Give an opioid analgesic the first day.
▶ After day 1, administer a non-steroidal anti-inflammatory drug such as ibuprofen.

Complications

▶ Cellulitis
▶ Gangrene
▶ Pain
▶ Recurrence
▶ Scarring

Special considerations

▶ Don't inject lidocaine into the abscess because lidocaine loses its effectiveness in an acidic environment.
▶ Biopsy breast abscesses, excluding subareolar abscesses.
▶ For paronychia under the nail, use a hot sterile needle to bore through the nail and facilitate drainage. Partial removal of the nail may be necessary.
▶ For a pilonidal cyst, position the patient in the left lateral or lithotomy position. Probe the sinus tracts with a cotton-tipped applicator. If the abscess is more than 5 mm deep, refer the patient to a surgeon. If it's less than 5 mm deep, perform elliptical excision for pilonidal sinus. (See "Elliptical excision," page 348.)

Patient teaching

▶ Advise the patient to return for follow-up in 2 days.
▶ Tell the patient with a pilonidal cyst to take a sitz bath four times per day. Tell him to clean and irrigate the area with a flexible shower hose or water from a squeeze bottle and to leave the wound open to air to promote drainage and healing. Explain that the wound must heal from the inside outward, which can take up to 3 months.

●●●**RED FLAG** *Instruct the patient to*
●●● *call his primary care provider for signs of infection, such as increasing redness, swelling, pain, and warmth; cloudy yellow, green, or brown drainage; opening of wound; foul odor; red streak from wound area; and fever.*

ANESTHESIA: TOPICAL AND LOCAL

No specific code assigned (usually included in the CPT code of the procedure being performed)
Anesthesia causes loss of sensation, thereby permitting surgical repair (such as incision and drainage), laceration repair, biopsy, foreign-body removal, and dislocation reduction. It's indicated for a procedure that causes pain that an anesthetic could eliminate and is contraindicated in patients who are allergic to a specific anesthetic. Factors that affect the type, amount, and duration of anesthetic needed include local blood supply, presence of infection, effects of certain chronic diseases, size of the affected area, and diameter and conduction of nerve fibers as well as psychological factors, such as anxiety and pain threshold.

Equipment
Topical
A eutectic mixture of local anesthetic (EMLA) is used for topical treatment of intact skin where no additional treatment is necessary. Ice or ethyl chloride are used for topical anesthesia in patients with intact skin who will be undergoing a procedure lasting less than 3 seconds.

●●●**RED FLAG** *Penetration occurs*
●●● *more quickly in diseased tissue, and effect penetrates less than 5 mm. EMLA is contraindicated for mucous membranes and genitalia.*

Local
Medication appropriate for location and size of the area requiring numbing ● antiseptic skin cleaner such as povidone-iodine solution (Betadine) ● gloves ● appropriate-sized syringe for site ● 25G to 30G ½" to 1" needle ● anesthetic without a vasoconstrictor for poorly vascularized or infected areas or im-

munocompromised patients • anesthetic with a vasoconstrictor such as epinephrine for a clean wound in a highly vascular area (to reduce bleeding and systemic absorption)
• 4″ × 4″ sterile gauze pads

CLINICAL PEARL *A vasoconstrictor (epinephrine) is contraindicated for use:*
▶ *in extremities (digits, nose, ear, or penis)*
▶ *in patients with vascular disorders, diabetes, or thyrotoxicosis*
▶ *in areas with compromised blood flow (such as a skin flap).*

Essential steps

▶ Explain the procedure to the patient and address questions or concerns he may have.
▶ Obtain informed consent.
▶ Verify that the patient isn't allergic to iodine, topical medications, or local anesthetics.
▶ Wash your hands.
Topical
▶ Remove oils from skin with soap, acetone, or alcohol.
▶ Apply EMLA and an occlusive dressing for 1 to 2 hours.
   For a procedure lasting less than 3 seconds:
▶ Rub the skin firmly with ice for 10 seconds, or spray with ethyl chloride for no longer than 2 seconds (to reduce risk of blistering).
Local
▶ Position the patient with the affected area exposed.
▶ Put on gloves.
▶ Clean the site and surrounding area with povidone-iodine solution.
▶ Draw up anesthetic into the appropriate sized syringe, using an 18G needle. Then replace the needle with a 25G to 30G needle.
▶ Identify the appropriate injection site. For digital anesthesia, use anterior and posterior web spaces of digit, close to the bone.

▶ Insert the needle at a 45-degree angle.
▶ Ask the patient if he notices a change in sensation. If he reports pain, indicating direct contact with the nerve, withdraw the needle 1 mm.
▶ Aspirate to make sure there's no blood return. If there is, the needle is in a blood vessel. Withdraw the needle slightly and reinsert in another area.
▶ Inject 1 to 2 ml of lidocaine while partially withdrawing the needle. Then redirect the needle across the surface, advance it, and inject another 0.5 ml while withdrawing the needle. This method distributes the anesthetic uniformly, providing the optimal effect.
▶ Massage the area gently. Maximum effect should occur in 5 to 15 minutes.

Complications
Ice or ethyl chloride
▶ Blistering from excessive freezing
Local
▶ Allergic reaction
▶ Anaphylaxis
▶ Arrhythmia (from systemic absorption)
▶ Ischemia
▶ Mental status changes

Special considerations
▶ The duration of EMLA is 2 hours after removal of the dressing.
▶ Ice or ethyl chloride is useful for such procedures as skin tag clipping and before injecting a local anesthetic.
▶ Topical anesthesia is indicated for nosebleeds and eye injuries and before painful procedures on mucous membranes.
▶ Topical lidocaine and cocaine (a vasoconstrictor) start working in less than 5 minutes. A dose of 1 to 2 drops of tetracaine (0.5%) is indicated before examination of an eye

injury and has an onset of action of 5 to 8 minutes. These drugs readily penetrate mucous membranes. Topical phenylephrine (0.005%) can also cause vasoconstriction. Most topical anesthetics have a duration of action of 30 to 45 minutes.

● Duration of anesthetic for nerve block is 30 minutes to 1 hour; duration increases if a vasoconstrictor (such as epinephrine) is also used.

Patient teaching

● Assure the patient that full sensation usually returns within 2 hours.

●●● RED FLAG *Instruct the patient to call his primary care provider for changes in sensation for more than 2 hours or signs of infection, such as increasing redness, swelling, pain, and warmth; cloudy yellow, green, or brown drainage; opening of wound; foul odor; red streak from wound area; and fever.*

CORNEAL ABRASION TREATMENT

CPT code: 65205 removal of foreign body, external eye, conjunctival, superficial; 65210 removal of foreign body, external eye, conjunctival, embedded; 65220 removal of foreign body, external eye, conjunctival, corneal without slit lamp; 99070 eye tray: supplies and material provided by doctor over and above what's usually included in office visit; ICD-9: 918.1

Injury to the covering of the cornea results in a corneal abrasion. The cornea has five layers: the epithelium (outer), Bowman's layer, stroma (middle), Descemet's layer, and endothelium (inner). The abrasion can result from chemical or mechanical injury (trauma), typically a contact lens or other foreign body in the eye. Injury limited to the epithelium heals without scarring; if

the injury extends to Bowman's layer, scar tissue may form. Signs and symptoms include pain, the feeling that there's something in the eye, photophobia, tearing, blurred vision, and blepharospasm; the conjunctiva may also appear red from vascular response to the injury.

Equipment

Snellen chart ● topical ophthalmic anesthetic (such as 0.5% proparacaine or 0.4% benoxinate, unless the patient is allergic to ester anesthetics) ● sterile fluorescein sodium strips ● sterile cotton-tipped applicators ● bright white light source (penlight) ● Wood's light or other source of cobalt-blue light ● 8- to 10-power magnification (magnifying glass, ophthalmoscope on the +20 to +40 diopter setting) ● isotonic irrigant (sterile saline or other eye irrigation solution such as Dacriose) ● sterile eye patches and 1″ paper tape ● cycloplegic drops for severe pain such as 1 drop of 1% cyclopentolate HCl (2% for heavily pigmented eyes)

●●● RED FLAG *Don't use fluorescein solution in place of fluorescein sodium strips because its use increases the risk of infection.*

Essential steps

● Explain the procedure to the patient and address questions or concerns he may have.

● Obtain informed consent.

● Obtain a history of allergies, injury, and contact lens and protective eyewear use.

● Perform vision screening.

● Examine the patient's pupillary reflex, extraocular movements, anterior and posterior chambers, and fundi.

● Have the patient remove contact lenses.

● Wash your hands and follow standard precautions.

▶ Inspect the eye and eyelid for erythema, drainage, and foreign objects.

▶ Place the patient in the supine position, with his head turned laterally to the affected side.

▶ Irrigate the eye copiously with ophthalmic irrigant.

▶ Tell the patient that the anesthetic causes a burning sensation at first. Then open the affected eye and instill 1 to 2 drops of ophthalmic anesthetic solution.

▶ Inspect the eye using the penlight and compare it with the unaffected eye. The sclera should appear intact, the anterior chamber free of mucus or blood, the iris normal in size and shape, the pupil normal in size and shape, and the pupils equally reactive to light. If the eye deviates from those findings, refer the patient to an ophthalmologist.

▶ Evert the upper lid by placing a cotton-tipped applicator on the upper lid, grasping the lashes, and turning the lid inside out over the applicator to expose the posterior surface of the upper lid. If available, use eyelid retractors to expose the conjunctiva.

▶ Examine for signs of trauma, foreign bodies, infection, sty, or inverted eyelash. (For foreign bodies, see "Removal of foreign body from the eye," page 359.)

▶ Moisten a fluorescein strip with 1 to 2 drops of sterile normal saline solution; you may use the patient's own tears instead. Don't use too much solution or too much staining will occur, making it difficult to identify a defect.

▶ Retract the lower lid and touch the fluorescein strip to the conjunctiva.

▶ Instruct the patient to blink to distribute the stain.

▶ Use Wood's light to examine the entire cornea and to identify areas of bright green concentrated fluorescence on the conjunctiva. The fluorescence indicates the location of the abrasion.

▶ If you don't find a defect or if you note vertical streaking on the cornea, suspect a foreign body embedded on the conjunctiva of the eyelid, and examine the entire conjunctiva.

●●● RED FLAG *If you still can't find the cause of the patient's signs and symptoms, refer him to an ophthalmologist.*

▶ Gently rinse the eye with sterile saline solution to flush stain from the conjunctiva.

▶ Consider administering cycloplegic drops for severe pain. Instill antibiotic ointment for prophylaxis against infection. Don't administer more anesthetic because it could decrease the rate of healing, resulting in scarring.

▶ Encourage the patient to keep the eye closed (to reduce discomfort) and to avoid rubbing it.

▶ Consider covering the affected eye with an eye patch to promote patient comfort. Have the patient close both eyes and firmly tape two eye patches (the first patch folded in half) over the affected eye.

● CLINICAL PEARL *Don't patch the eye in a patient with only a small peripheral defect (less than 1/4" [0.6 cm]), in children younger than age 5, or in cases of suspected infection.*

▶ Administer ophthalmic antibiotics for prophylaxis, such as tobramycin or sulfacetamide ointment, for 3 days.

▶ Administer tetanus toxoid if the patient hasn't received immunization within the past 5 years.

▶ Schedule a return office visit in 24 hours for reevaluation and for removal of the eye patch, if applicable.

▶ Document the size and location of all abrasions. Illustrations can help, but be careful that the illustration doesn't seem to magnify the size of the lesion. During subsequent examinations, document the degree of healing.

Complications

▶ Conjunctivitis
▶ Infection
▶ Permanent visual impairment
▶ Scarring
▶ Uveitis

Special considerations

▶ Look carefully for a foreign body in the cul-de-sac if you note a pattern of multiple vertical lines during conjunctival staining.
▶ Perform Seidel's test if you suspect leakage of intraocular fluid. To do so, place a fluorescein strip directly over the site and look for a flow of green liquid.
▶ Don't use topical corticosteroids; they may interfere with healing.
▶ If appropriate, encourage the patient to use protective eyewear at work and during recreational activities.
▶ Use a slit lamp for eye examination only if you're skilled in the technique.

Collaborative practice

Refer the patient to an ophthalmologist immediately for:
▶ acute vision loss
▶ a herpes lesion
▶ an intraocular foreign body
▶ blunt or sharp trauma to the eye
▶ corneal infection
▶ deterioration of vision or acute vision loss
▶ signs of infection
▶ a metallic foreign body
▶ a foreign body that can't be irrigated out
▶ noncompliance (for instance, a child who may need sedation)
▶ chemical burns (after immediate copious irrigation for 15 minutes

with tap water from a shower or hose)
▶ possible globe penetration (signs include hyphema, lens opacity, and pupil irregularity)
▶ dendritic, large, or centrally located defects found on fluorescein examination
▶ an abrasion that isn't healing well within 24 hours or completely healed within 48 hours.

Patient teaching

▶ Advise the patient that he can take pain medicine, such as acetaminophen, to alleviate pain.
▶ Tell the patient that he must monitor his progress every day until his eye is completely healed to catch such complications as infection at an early, treatable stage.
▶ Tell him not to rub his eyes; doing so could disrupt new layers of epithelial granulation and delay healing.
▶ Tell the patient who isn't wearing an eye patch to rest his eye, especially if he has a history of amblyopia.

🌼 **LIFE SPAN** *Advise the caregiver of a pediatric patient who isn't wearing an eye patch that the child should rest his eye.*
▶ Advise the patient to avoid contact lens use for 3 weeks.

▓▓▓ **RED FLAG** *Instruct the patient to call his primary care provider for symptoms that persist or recur, acute changes in vision, and signs of infection (rapidly increasing redness, swelling, pain, and warmth; cloudy appearance of the eye; yellow, green, or brown drainage; and fever).*

⬤ CYST INJECTION, GANGLION

CPT code: 20550 injection, tendon sheath, ligament trigger point or ganglion cyst; 20600 arthrocentesis, aspiration, or injection of a small joint, bursa, or ganglion cyst (leg, fingers, toes); 20605 intermediate joint, bursa, or ganglion cyst (temporomandibular, acromioclavicular, wrist, elbow, ankle, olecranon bursa)

A ganglion cyst is a tumor that develops on or in a tendon sheath. Most commonly, the cause is chronic or recurrent inflammation from frequent strains or contusions at the site. Joints contain a thick, gel-like material. When this gel leaks from the joint into the weakened tendon sheath, it forms a cyst. Indications for removing the cyst are relieving discomfort and increasing joint mobility.

Injection of an anesthetic, with or without a steroid, into the ganglion cyst provides pain relief and usually increases range-of-motion. However, benefits may not be permanent.

Equipment

For injection: Antiseptic skin cleaner such as povidone-iodine • sterile drape • sterile gloves • 3- and 10-ml syringes • 18G 1½″ needle • 22G or 25G 1½″ needle • 1% lidocaine (single-dose vials preferred because they contain no preservatives, decreasing the risk of allergic reaction) • culture tube • corticosteroid, short-acting (such as hydrocortisone 20 mg), intermediate (such as methylprednisolone 4 mg), or long-acting (such as dexamethasone 0.6 mg) • sterile 4″ × 4″ gauze pads • tape

Essential steps

▶ Explain the procedure to the patient and address questions or concerns he may have.
▶ Check the patient's history for allergies, especially to iodine and latex.
▶ Obtain informed consent.
▶ Wash your hands.

▶ Position the patient comfortably with the cyst clearly exposed.
▶ Clean the site and surrounding area with povidone-iodine solution.
▶ Apply the sterile drape, and put on sterile gloves.
▶ Use a small-gauge needle with the 3-ml syringe to draw up 2.5 ml of 1% lidocaine and 0.5 ml of corticosteroid. Agitate gently.
▶ Using the 10-ml syringe with the 18G needle, insert the needle into the cyst and aspirate. If the aspirate appears cloudy, send the specimen for culture and sensitivity and continue the procedure; if the return is bloody, remove the needle, apply a dressing, and end the procedure.
▶ Unscrew the syringe and replace it with the second syringe that contains lidocaine and corticosteroid, and aspirate for blood. If no blood appears, inject the medications.
▶ Remove the needle and apply a pressure dressing.

Complications

▶ Atrophy of subcutaneous tissue
▶ Corticosteroid flare
▶ Infection
▶ Recurrence
▶ Sepsis

Special considerations

▶ If the cyst recurs, consider excising it instead of administering a second injection.

Patient teaching

▶ Instruct the patient to leave the dressing on for 12 hours. Explain that redness, swelling, and warmth are normal. Tell him to rest and elevate the joint for 24 hours.
▶ If the cyst recurs, suggest cyst removal.
▶ Recommend a nonopioid analgesic, such as acetaminophen or ibuprofen, for pain.
▶ Tell the patient to follow up in 1 week.

●●● **RED FLAG** *Tell the patient to call*
●●● *his primary care provider for*
signs of infection, such as increasing
redness, swelling, pain, and warmth;
cloudy yellow, green, or brown drain-
age; opening of wound; foul odor;
red streak from wound area; and
fever.

DEFIBRILLATION

CPT code: 92950 cardiopulmonary
resuscitation (CPR)
Always an emergency procedure,
defibrillation delivers a controlled,
untimed transcutaneous electric
charge to the myocardium, depolarizing the heart muscle and commonly allowing the sinoatrial node
to resume its inherent rhythm. Its
effectiveness depends on the
amount of elapsed time from cardiac arrest to defibrillation; the patient's chances of survival decrease
with a delay in defibrillation. Indications for defibrillation include
ventricular fibrillation and pulseless
ventricular tachycardia. Conditions
that may contribute to lethal arrhythmias include hypoxia, severe
acidosis, and electrolyte imbalance.
If possible, treat the underlying
cause while resuscitation effort continues.

Equipment

Defibrillator or universal automated
external defibrillator (AED) with an-
terior-posterior or transverse paddles (manual or external automatic
defibrillator) ● conductive medium
pads or gel ● electrocardiogram
(ECG) monitor with recorder ● I.V.
line and solution ● oxygen administration and suction equipment ●
oral or nasal airway or endotracheal
intubation equipment ● handheld
resuscitation bag with 100% oxygen
adapter and face mask ● transvenous or transthoracic pacemaker
system ● emergency drugs, such as

epinephrine, atropine, lidocaine, vasopressors

Essential steps

▶ Establish that the patient is unresponsive.
▶ Call for help, and activate the
emergency response system
▶ Open the airway, and assess for
absence of spontaneous breathing.
▶ Provide two full ventilations.
▶ Assess for absence of carotid
pulse (adult and child) or brachial
pulse (infant).
▶ Initiate CPR until a monitor and
defibrillator are available.
▶ Expose the chest wall.
▶ Apply the ECG monitor leads to
the chest wall (avoiding paddle
placement sites) or use "quick-
look" paddles to determine cardiac
rhythm. Quick-look paddles allow
for single-lead interpretation of cardiac rhythm.
▶ For ventricular fibrillation or
pulseless ventricular tachycardia,
prepare to defibrillate.
▶ Apply conductive pads to chest
wall, using transverse or anterior-
posterior placement. If conductive
pads aren't available, apply conductive gel to the paddles and place in
the transverse position.
▶ Turn on the defibrillator.
▶ Select the appropriate energy level
for defibrillation according to
whether a monophasic or biphasic
defibrillator will be used. (See
Biphasic defibrillators.)
▶ Make sure the paddles or pads are
correctly placed.
▶ Warn those present in the room to
step back from the patient. Quickly
scan the area to make sure that
everyone and all unnecessary
equipment are clear of the patient.
▶ Charge the defibrillator for manual defibrillation or allow the AED to
determine its charge (follow the
AED instructions and stand clear of
the patient when the AED is analyz-

BIPHASIC DEFIBRILLATORS

Most facility defibrillators are mono-phasic; that is, they deliver a single current of electricity that travels in one direction between the two pads or paddles on the patient's chest. To be effective, they require a high amount of electric current.

Biphasic defibrillators differ from monophasic units because the electric current discharged from the pads or paddles travels in a positive direction for a specified duration and then reverses and flows in a negative direction for the remaining time of the electrical discharge. These units deliver two currents of electricity and lower the defibrillation threshold of the heart muscle, making it possible to successfully defibrillate ventricular fibrillation

(VF) with smaller amounts of energy. Instead of 200 joules, an initial shock of 150 joules is usually effective. The biphasic defibrillator is adjustable for differences in impedance or the resistance of the current through the chest, which helps reduce the number of shocks needed to terminate VF. Biphasic technology utilizes lower energy levels and fewer shocks, and thus reduces the damage to the myocardial muscle. Biphasic defibrillators, when used at the clinically appropriate energy level, may be used for defibrillation and — when placed in the synchronized mode — for synchronized cardioversion. Pad or paddle placement is the same as with the monophasic defibrillator.

ing the rhythm and when discharging the shock).
▶ Make sure the rhythm is still ventricular fibrillation or pulseless ventricular tachycardia.
▶ Activate the discharge buttons on the paddles of the manual defibrillator and keep the paddles on the chest wall until the paddles discharge.
▶ Assess the rhythm on the monitor and check the patient for a pulse.
▶ If defibrillation doesn't succeed, repeat three countershocks at increasing energy levels in rapid succession, after making sure everyone and all nonessential equipment are clear of the patient.
▶ If the three rapid countershocks don't succeed, reinitiate CPR, provide manual ventilation, administer emergency drugs, and continue to defibrillate according to advanced cardiac life support (ACLS) protocol while transporting the patient to an acute care facility.

▶ If defibrillation succeeds, assess the patient's vital signs, peripheral pulses, level of consciousness, and respiratory effort; administer emergency cardiac medications, oxygen or ventilation, and I.V. fluids; and continue cardiac monitoring while transporting the patient to an acute care facility.
▶ Obtain a postdefibrillation ECG rhythm strip or 12-lead ECG.
▶ Document the patient's rhythm before defibrillation, time of each defibrillation, energy levels used, results of each defibrillation, and all other resuscitation measures used.

Complications
▶ Burns
▶ Chest wall injury
▶ Death

Special considerations
▶ Make sure you're familiar with the defibrillator before using it.

● As needed, treat hypoxia, hypothermia, and acidosis — potential problems associated with ineffective defibrillation.

● Select correct energy levels sequentially from 200 to 360 joules per ACLS protocol for external defibrillation, or the biphasic energy equivalent, in adults.

LIFE SPAN *Use 2 joules/kg when using a defibrillator in a pediatric patient.*

● Announce "Charging defibrillator; stand clear" when charging the defibrillator.

● Maintain about 25 lb of pressure on each paddle during defibrillation.

● Don't defibrillate over a pacemaker or implanted cardioverter-defibrillator generator because doing so may interfere with the device's functioning.

RED FLAG *If the patient is wearing a transdermal nitroglycerine patch, make sure you remove it prior to defibrillation.*

DIAPHRAGM FITTING

CPT code: 57170 diaphragm or cervical cap fitting with instructions
The diaphragm is a barrier method of contraception that mechanically blocks sperm from entering the cervix. It consists of a soft latex rubber dome supported by a round metal spring on the outside. Its effectiveness ranges from 80% to 93% for new users and increases to 97% for long-term users. Diaphragm use is indicated for patients who prefer or require reversible contraception without medication. Contraindications include a history of toxic shock syndrome, vaginal stenosis, pelvic abnormalities, uterine prolapse, large cystocele or rectocele, allergy to spermicidal jellies or natural rubber latex, or being less than 6 weeks postpartum.

Equipment

Diaphragm fitting rings ● diaphragm ● water-soluble lubricant (such as K-Y gel) ● diaphragm introducer (optional) ● gloves ● goggles

Essential steps

● Explain the procedure to the patient and address questions or concerns she may have.

● Check the patient for a history of allergies, especially to natural rubber latex.

● Instruct the patient to undress below the waist, and assist her into the dorsal lithotomy position.

● Wash your hands, and put on gloves.

● Insert your index and middle fingers as if performing a pelvic examination.

● Measure from the symphysis bone to the posterior of the cervix by touching the posterior fornix with your middle finger and raising your hand until the index finger touches the pubic arch.

● Use your thumb to hold your hand in place directly under the pubic bone.

● While maintaining your thumb position, withdraw your hand from the patient.

● Place one end of the diaphragm rim or fitting ring on the tip of the middle finger with the opposite side lying just in front of the thumb. This will give you the approximate diameter of the diaphragm. Diaphragms are manufactured in sizes of 60 to 90 mm, with the average being 75 to 80 mm. (See *Proper diaphragm measurement.*)

● Lubricate the rim or dome of the fitting ring or diaphragm to lessen the discomfort of insertion. (See *Inserting the diaphragm*, page 344.)

◗ Check the diaphragm to ensure that it fits snugly against the vaginal walls. Follow the edges of the diaphragm ring, feeling for gaps. Several insertions and removal of diaphragms in varying sizes may be required until the proper size is found.

◗ To remove the diaphragm, insert your index finger under the symphysis pubis and hook the diaphragm under the proximal rim. Gently pull the diaphragm down and out.

◗ Teach the patient how to insert and remove the diaphragm. Then leave the patient with the diaphragm in place so that she can practice inserting and removing it in private, leaving it in when she's done.

◗ Examine the patient to see whether she inserted the diaphragm correctly and if so, allow her to walk around for a few minutes to make sure she can't feel it.

Complications

◗ Pregnancy from not using spermicidal jelly or from improperly placing the diaphragm (the result of poor technique or such body changes as a weight gain or loss of more than 15 lb [6.8 kg] or surgery)

◗ Teratogenic effects from the spermicide nonoxynol-9 if the patient becomes pregnant

●●● RED FLAG *Indications for ceasing to use a diaphragm include recurrent urinary tract infections, discomfort, or ulceration from an improper fit. If the patient reports one or more of these symptoms, however, make sure you inform her about alternate methods of contraception in addition to advising her to cease using the diaphragm.*

Special considerations

◗ Although you shouldn't use spermicidal jelly for the demonstration, explain to the patient that she'll

PROPER DIAPHRAGM MEASUREMENT

To determine the correct size of the diaphragm, extend and hold together your index and middle fingers and insert them into the patient's vagina. With the middle finger touching the posterior fornix, raise your hand until your index finger touches the pubic arch. Press your thumb against your hand directly under the pubic bone.

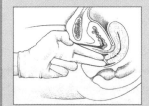

Keep your hand in that position and smoothly withdraw it. The correctly sized diaphragm is the one that fits with one end of the diaphragm rim on the tip of the middle finger and the opposite side of the rim lying just in front of the thumb tip.

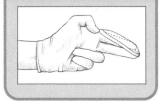

need to use it whenever she uses the diaphragm.

◗ You can obtain diaphragm fitting rings free from such companies as Ortho Pharmaceutical in sizes that increase in 5-mm increments.

◗ Several types of diaphragms are available. The arching spring (the most common diaphragm in the United States) has a firm rim, needs

INSERTING THE DIAPHRAGM

Instruct the patient as you insert the diaphragm, identifying structures and associated feelings to prepare her for self-insertion. Lubricate the rim or dome of the fitting ring or diaphragm to lessen the discomfort of insertion.

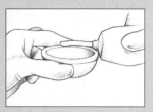

Hold the vulva open with one hand. Fold the diaphragm in half with the other hand by pressing the opposite sides together.

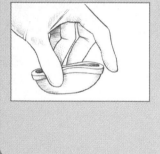

Slide the folded diaphragm into the vagina and toward the posterior cervicovaginal fornix.

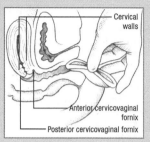

Cervical walls

Anterior cervicovaginal fornix

Posterior cervicovaginal fornix

The diaphragm should fit from below the symphysis and cover the cervix. The proximal rim should fit behind the pubic arch with minimal pressure. Note that the cervix is palpable behind the diaphragm. The cervix feels like a "nose."

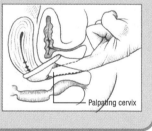

Palpating cervix

no introducer, is typically easier to insert, and is helpful to patients who have less pelvic support, cystocele, rectocele, or retroverted uterus. The coil spring has a flexible rim and needs no introducer but requires good internal support and the cervix in the midplane or anterior position. The flat spring has flat-plane flexibility and may need an introducer; this type is recommended for smaller women, those with a

narrow pelvic shelf, and women who have never been pregnant.

Patient teaching

▶ Advise the patient to return in 1 to 2 weeks to assess for correct placement.
▶ Emphasize to the patient the importance of using the diaphragm with spermicidal jelly every time she has intercourse. Explain that she should apply about a teaspoon

of spermicidal jelly (such as nonoxynol-9) to the concave surface and a thin layer around the rim.
▶ Teach her to insert one rim behind the pubic bone and the opposite rim behind the cervix and to confirm placement by feeling the cervix behind the dome.
▶ For subsequent coitus, she should leave the diaphragm in place and insert more spermicidal jelly into the vagina; she shouldn't douche.
▶ Tell her to leave the diaphragm in place at least 6 hours after the last session of intercourse but less than 24 hours.
▶ Advise the patient to wash the diaphragm with mild soap and dry it after each use, and inspect it at least once a month for holes and wear of the latex.
▶ Emphasize that diaphragms don't prevent sexually transmitted diseases.

●●● **RED FLAG** *Emphasize that the*
●●● *patient is to call you if she experiences symptoms of toxic shock syndrome, including fever greater than 101° F (38.3° C), nausea, vomiting, diarrhea, sore throat, body aches, rash, or feeling dizzy, faint, or weak.*

DISLOCATION REDUCTION

CPT codes: 23650 closed treatment of shoulder dislocation, with manipulation; 24600 closed treatment of elbow dislocation; 26700 closed treatment of metacarpophalangeal dislocation, single, with manipulation; 26770 closed treatment of interphalangeal joint dislocation, single, with manipulation; 27550 closed treatment of knee dislocation
Dislocation is the partial or complete displacement of one bone from another. It can occur spontaneously due to a structural defect,

traumatic injury, or joint disease. A dislocated joint is reduced when the normal position is restored. Reduction decreases pain, helps prevent structural defects and lost or decreased use of the joint, and facilitates healing.

Equipment

Cleaning solution such as alcohol or povidone-iodine solution • 3 ml lidocaine without epinephrine • 5-ml syringe with 25G needle

Essential steps

▶ Explain the procedure to the patient and address questions or concerns he may have.
▶ Obtain informed consent.
▶ Obtain radiographic confirmation to rule out fractures and to determine the direction of dislocation.
▶ Wash your hands.
▶ If necessary, use an assistant to help stabilize the patient.

☀ **LIFE SPAN** *For a pediatric patient, the parents usually provide the best assistance when stabilizing the patient.*

▶ As needed, use an oral opioid or muscle relaxant or both, but have naloxone (Narcan) available and monitor the patient's vital signs and airway patency during and after the procedure.

Finger or toe reduction

▶ Use a digital nerve block. Clean the digit with povidone-iodine or alcohol. Infiltrate up to 3 ml of lidocaine (without epinephrine), using a 25G needle for field anesthesia. (See "Anesthesia: Topical and local," page 334.)
▶ Grasp and stabilize the proximal segment in one hand.
▶ With your other hand, grasp and apply firm and steady longitudinal traction to the distal segment in the direction of angulation.
▶ Slowly move the distal segment in the opposite direction of the angula-

tion while continuing to apply steady traction and pressure to the dorsal side.

▶ Continue moving the distal segment toward the neutral position until reduction occurs.

▶ Check joint stability.

▶ Apply an aluminum finger splint with tape to maintain the joint in position of function; you can tape a stable joint to the adjacent finger.

▶ As needed, obtain an X-ray to confirm positioning of the joint.

Shoulder reduction

The most commonly used method of shoulder reduction is called *manual reduction*.

▶ With the patient in a supine position, grasp and support his upper arm above the elbow with both hands and support the forearm under your own arm against your body. Make sure the arm is adducted, externally rotated, and flexed.

▶ Apply firm, steady distracting axial traction to the arm, pulling it distally. ("Distracting" means to pull away from the skeletal attachment.)

▶ While maintaining traction, slowly ease the arm into the shoulder until reduction occurs. You may also need to provide some internal or external rotation or slight pressure directed anteriorly from beneath the upper arm.

▶ As needed, ask an assistant to apply countertraction to stabilize the patient. Do this by wrapping a bed sheet around the patient's upper torso and having the assistant apply countertraction from the side opposite the affected shoulder.

▶ Obtain anteroposterior and axillary lateral X-rays to confirm reduction.

▶ Apply a sling and swath to prevent shoulder external rotation and abduction.

▶ Shoulder immobilization may be required for 2 to 4 weeks.

A secondary method for shoulder dislocation is called the *Stimson technique*.

▶ Use this method for patients with recurrent dislocations. Place the patient in a prone position on the examination table with the involved extremity hanging off the table toward the floor.

▶ Apply steady traction to the distal extremity, either manually or with a 10- to 15-lb (4.5- to 6.8-kg) weight attached to the patient's wrist. Reduction should occur within a few minutes. You may need to provide some rotation or flexion of the extremity.

Patella reduction

▶ Place the patient in a supine position. Apply steady manual pressure to the lateral aspect of the patella with one hand while slowly extending the knee with the other hand until reduction occurs.

▶ Rule out patella fracture or rupture of the patellar or quadriceps tendon.

▶ Apply a knee immobilizer to prevent knee flexion.

✳ **LIFE SPAN** *For radial head subluxation in children (nursemaid's elbow):*

▶ *rule out elbow, shoulder, and clavicle fracture or dislocation*

▶ *seat the child in the parent's lap, and explain to the parent that the child may experience brief pain with the procedure but then should experience immediate relief of symptoms once reduction occurs*

▶ *grasp the patient's wrist and distal forearm in one hand and support the elbow with the opposite hand, with the thumb over the radial head*

▶ *supinate the forearm, rotating the hand palm up*

▶ *flex the elbow until you feel a snap over the radial head, indicating that the orbicular ligament has reduced*

▶ a sling or immobilization should not be required.

Complications

▶ Malpositioning or failure to maintain reduction
▶ Neurologic compromise
▶ Opioid overdose
▶ Vascular compromise

Special considerations

⣿ RED FLAG *Don't attempt reduction of a large joint or a joint with a concurrent fracture unless acute vascular or neurologic compromise threatens the limb. Instead, refer the patient to an orthopedist or send him to the emergency department for reduction. Dislocations of the elbow, hip, knee (femorotibial), and ankle also require emergency referral unless acute neurovascular compromise exists. Most dislocations should be referred to an orthopedist after reduction.*

Patient teaching

▶ Instruct the patient to call or return at once if redislocation, loss of normal sensation of the limb (numbness and tingling), or increased pain occur.
▶ Explain that the joint will probably swell for 24 to 48 hours after the injury and that keeping the joint elevated and applying ice for 20 minutes intermittently should minimize pain and swelling.
▶ Promote the use of anti-inflammatory medication, which will help decrease pain and swelling.
▶ Tell the patient with a patella or shoulder dislocation — especially a patient younger than age 30 — that the risk of recurrence is high; explain the need for possible surgical treatment.

⣿ DOPPLER ULTRA-SONOGRAPHY

CPT code: 93922 noninvasive physiologic studies of upper- or lower-extremity arteries, single-level, bilateral (includes ankle/brachial indices, Doppler waveform analysis, volume plethysmography, and transcutaneous oxygen tension measurement)

Doppler ultrasonography consists of an audio unit, volume control, and a transducer that detects the movement of red blood cells. It's used to determine arterial blood flow when blood perfusion may be compromised (for instance, in a cool, edematous, pale, cyanotic, or apparently pulseless extremity) and to determine placement for an arterial insertion.

Equipment

Doppler • ultrasound transmission gel (not water-soluble lubricant) • marking pen • soft cloth and antiseptic solution or soapy water

Essential steps

▶ Explain the procedure to the patient and address questions or concerns he may have.
▶ Wash your hands.
▶ Position the patient comfortably with the affected area accessible.
▶ Mark the selected artery with the marking pen.
▶ Apply a small amount of coupling or transmission gel to the ultrasound probe.
▶ Position the probe on the skin directly over the selected artery.
▶ Set the volume control to the lowest setting. If your model doesn't have a speaker, plug in the earphones and slowly raise the volume.
▶ To obtain the best signal, tilt the probe at a 45-degree angle from the

artery, making sure to apply gel between the skin and the probe. Slowly move the probe in a circular motion to locate the center of the artery and the Doppler signal — a hissing noise at the heartbeat. Don't move the probe rapidly because this will distort the signal.

▶ After you've assessed the pulse, clean the probe with a soft cloth soaked in antiseptic solution or soapy water. Don't immerse the probe or bump it against a hard surface.

Complications

No complications are associated with Doppler ultrasonography.

Special considerations

▶ Don't place the Doppler probe over an open or draining lesion.
▶ Be sure to remove all conductive gel from the patient's skin.
▶ Be aware that failure to position the transducer properly can interfere with results.

Patient teaching

▶ Tell the patient that he won't feel pain but that the gel may feel cold.
▶ Explain the results and the patient's options.
▶ Provide additional teaching based on test results, diagnosis, and prognosis: for example, teach the patient appropriate measures to prevent thrombosis (smoking cessation, elevation of the affected area, exercise, or weight reduction).

ELLIPTICAL EXCISION

CPT codes: 11400-406 excision benign lesions on trunk, arms, or legs; 11420-426 on scalp, neck, hands, feet, or genitalia; 11600-606 excision malignant lesions on trunk, arms, or legs; 11620-626 on scalp, neck, hands, feet, or genitalia; (add 22 or 09922 for unusual or complex excision)

In elliptical (also called *fusiform*) excision, the clinician can remove a skin lesion too large for a cutaneous punch and then suture the area closed, leaving behind a linear scar (larger lesions require a different form of excision and require skin flaps or grafts for closure). The location of the incision usually depends on the location of natural skin tension lines, which correspond with wrinkle lines. If such lines aren't readily apparent, gently pinching the skin in several directions should bring them out (this technique may not work with children and adolescents).

The goal of such surgery is to remove the lesion and leave as small a cosmetic defect as possible by following skin tension lines and, for lesions on the face, facial expressions. When deciding where to make the excision, the clinician must consider the depth of the skin; the impact of the excision on adjacent structures; the length, width, and orientation of the resulting scar; and the scar's effect on function. Placement of a shoulder incision, for instance, depends more on creating a scar that won't pull apart than on appearance. Ideally, the procedure will transform the oval-shaped wound left by the excision into a thin-line closure. Depending on the lesion's depth, the sutures may be absorbable or nonabsorbable or both. (See *Choosing suture materials*.)

Equipment

Marker • sterile gloves • sterile drape • masks • protective eyewear • antiseptic • 2″ × 2″ or 4″ × 4″ gauze pads • anesthetic • #11 scalpel • straight or curved iris scissors • forceps or hook • specimen container with 10% formalin

CHOOSING SUTURE MATERIALS

Sutures can be absorbable or nonabsorbable. Absorbable sutures are strands of suture material that eventually dissolve. Nonabsorbable sutures must be removed because the body can't dissolve them. This chart outlines various types of suture material and their indications for use.

Type of material	Indications for use
ABSORBABLE	
Plain gut	Rarely used due to its high tissue reactivity
Chromic catgut	Oral mucosa, vermilion border
Polyglycolic acid	Superficial closure of skin and mucosa
NONABSORBABLE	
Silk	Tying off blood vessels
Nylon	Use and size of suture vary with location of wound:
	▶ 6-0 for eyelids and face
	▶ 5-0 for forehead, neck, and other delicate skin
	▶ 4-0 for neck, scalp, extremities, and back
	▶ 3-0 for running suture of scalp

• electrocautery unit • sutures • suture needles

Essential steps

▶ Explain the procedure to the patient and address questions or concerns he may have.
▶ Obtain informed consent.
▶ Note the area in a circle at its clinical margins. Imagine a concentric circle around the first circle that includes the margin for normal skin. Use the marker to draw a final ellipse that's three times as long as it is wide.
▶ Wash and dry your hands, put on sterile gloves and a mask, and use eye protection.
▶ Administer the anesthetic, injecting it in a ring to obtain field anesthesia. Make sure that you anesthetize beyond the demarcated margins in anticipation of undermining.

▶ Use a gauze pad to apply antiseptic to the area, starting at the center and spiraling outward. Then drape the area to allow a clear view of the surgical site.
▶ Hold the scalpel like a pencil at a 90-degree angle, with the anterior belly of the blade in contact with the previously marked line. Apply three-point traction with the other hand, using firm, confident, vertical pressure at the corner of the ellipse. (See *Using three-point traction*, page 350.)
▶ Press down gently with the scalpel, and draw it through the skin in one firm, constant stroke, keeping the blade perpendicular to the skin surface (to avoid beveling the wound and margins.) You don't have to cut through the skin's full thickness with a single stroke, but make sure you can see upper sub-

USING THREE-POINT TRACTION

Making an elliptical excision requires you to maintain firm traction to the skin surface in more than one direction. This illustration shows how to apply three-point traction to maintain multidirectional traction when making an elliptical excision. The arrows indicate the direction in which traction is being applied.

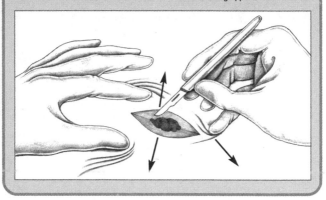

cutaneous fat before trying to remove the specimen.

▶ Rarely, you may encounter a highly active blood vessel. If this happens, remove the blade and cauterize the affected site before continuing.

▶ After making the incisions, use a straight or curved iris scissors and forceps or hook and gently elevate one end of the fusiform ellipse.

▶ Insert the scissors through the subcutis and complete the incision through the subcutis along both sides of the specimen. Undermine the base completely and elevate the specimen. (See *Undermining.*)

▶ Place the specimen in a specimen container.

▶ Cauterize as needed to stop bleeding, but don't cauterize too much or the wound won't heal as quickly.

▶ Suture the wound closed. (See "Suturing simple lacerations," page 369.)

Complications

▶ Infection
▶ Keloids
▶ Pain
▶ Scarring

Special considerations

●●● RED FLAG *Refer the patient to a*
●●● *reconstructive surgeon for facial lesions greater than 1/4" (0.6 cm); refer to a dermatologist for deep lesions.*

▶ Keep in mind that wounds closed by approximation of the skin edges heal by primary intention.

▶ To speed healing and prevent crust formation, cover the wound with an occlusive or a semiocclusive dressing (particularly important for wounds created by a procedure).

Patient teaching

▶ Instruct the patient to keep the sutures dry.

UNDERMINING

Undermining, the technique of freeing the skin from underlying tissues, can decrease tension on the wound edge and is critical for obtaining acceptable cosmetic results after wound repair. Proper undermining minimizes scarring and keloid formation.

The level of undermining that should be done depends on the anatomic location of the wound and the natural plane of the wound. In general, undermine an area about the size of the widest part of the wound.

Blunt undermining

In blunt undermining, advance the scissors with the tips closed and then force them open. This causes blunt dissection of the underlying tissues.

Sharp undermining

In sharp undermining, a less-frequently used technique, use short, cutting strokes with a scalpel to separate the skin from underlying tissues.

Undermining tips

▶ Keep in mind that undermining increases the risk of bleeding. Make sure you can see the source of bleeding and can cauterize it safely.
▶ Treat the wound edge gently. Handle it with a single-pronged skin hook instead of forceps.

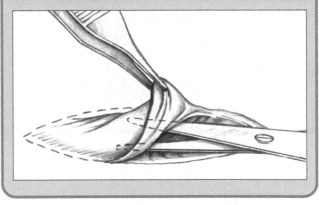

▶ Instruct him to remove the initial dressing in 24 hours and then clean it twice per day and cover it with ointment. The three-layer dressing consists of petroleum jelly or triple antibiotic ointment, a nonadherent dressing, and gauze followed by a tape covering. After the first day, tell him to replace the initial dressing with a smaller gauze bandage, being careful not to place the gauze itself directly over the wound (fibers in the gauze can get trapped in the wound edge, become matted, and delay healing).
▶ For suture removal, have the patient return in 3 to 6 days for a face wound, 7 to 10 days for an ear wound, and 10 to 12 days for a trunk or an extremity wound.

●●● RED FLAG *Tell the patient to call*
●●● *his primary care provider for signs of infection, such as increasing redness, swelling, pain, and warmth; cloudy yellow, green, or brown drainage; opening of wound;*

foul odor; red streak from wound area; and fever.

FRACTURE IMMOBILIZATION

CPT codes: 29065 application, plaster, shoulder to hand (long arm); 29075 application, plaster, elbow to finger (short arm); 29085 application, plaster, hand and lower forearm (gauntlet); 29345 application, plaster, thigh to toes (long leg); 29355 application, plaster, thigh to ankle (cylinder); 29405 application, plaster, below knee to toes (short leg); 29425 application, plaster, walking or ambulatory type; 29440 adding walker to previously applied cast.

Fractures must be properly immobilized to minimize discomfort, avoid any undue motion, ward off possible further injury, and allow time for proper healing of bones and ligaments.

Equipment

Disposable gloves ● bucket of cool water ● tubular stockinette ● rolls of cast padding ● rolls of Fiberglas or plaster of Paris (from 1' to 6' rolls) ● sheet, towel, or gown to cover patient ● cast shoe for short-leg casts ● bandage scissors

Essential steps

▸ Explain the procedure to the patient and address questions or concerns he may have.
▸ Obtain X-rays as appropriate.
▸ After the X-ray has been read, prepare the patient for immobilization.
▸ Measure a length of stockinette about 6" (15 cm) longer than the area you need to cast; this will allow for shortening of the stockinette as you pull it over the limb and for some overlap at each end to turn down after you apply the cast

material. Cut a thumbhole for an arm cast.
▸ Roll on the cast padding, overlapping by one-half the roll width with each turn. Start distally and roll proximally, leaving no gaps or wrinkles. Extend the padding about 2" (5 cm) beyond the end of the planned cast. Apply extra padding over bony prominences and wounds and where the edge of the cast will be located.
▸ Maintain the limb in a neutral position unless otherwise indicated to correct the deformity. Preferred joint angles are 45 to 75 degrees of flexion for metacarpal, 10 degrees of flexion for distal interphalangeal, abduction for the thumb, 35 degrees of extension for the wrist, 90 degrees of flexion for the elbow, 10 to 15 degrees of flexion for the knee, 90 degrees of flexion for the ankle, and neutral for the subtalar.
▸ Wearing gloves, submerge a roll of casting material in water for a few seconds until saturated, briefly squeeze out excess water, and roll the first layer immediately. Start distally and roll proximally. Don't pull while wrapping; simply roll it on, overlapping the roll width by one-half with each turn. Gently mold with both hands around bony prominences, but don't squeeze hard enough to leave an impression in the cast.
▸ After applying the first layer, turn down the ends of the stockinette.
▸ Roll on the second layer of casting material, again overlapping by one-half with each turn. Take an extra turn or two over large joints, such as the knee and ankle, to provide extra reinforcement. If you reach the end of the cast before finishing the roll, continue back down the limb distally. Two or three layers are usually enough for upper-extremity Fiberglas casts; plaster casts require more layers. Lower-

extremity casts also need more layers, especially if the patient will bear weight on the extremity. Pediatric casts need more reinforcement than adult casts.

▸ Keep the limb in the desired position until the cast hardens. Use bandage scissors to trim excess or rough edges before the material hardens completely. Fiberglas hardens within 5 minutes, allowing for weight bearing within 30 minutes. Plaster of Paris takes up to 24 hours to harden completely.

Complications

▸ Fracture malunion or nonunion (from poor cast positioning or molding)
▸ Functional and ambulation impairment (from joint malpositioning)
▸ Neurologic or vascular compromise (from an excessively tight case)
▸ Skin irritation or breakdown (from insufficient padding)

Special considerations

▸ Keep in mind that Fiberglas is lighter and stronger, hardens more quickly, and is more radiolucent than plaster. Although plaster is cheaper and easier to mold than Fiberglas, it's also heavy, takes a long time to dry, and breaks down if it gets wet or worn down. Use plaster for temporary splints and in areas that require extensive molding to maintain the fracture position, especially in the hand. Applying Fiberglas without wetting it lengthens its drying time, giving you more time to mold or position a limb that's difficult to cast.

▸ When applying a short-arm cast, make sure the distal end doesn't extend past the metacarpophalangeal joint and add extra padding around the base of the thumb. Apply no more than two layers of cast material in the web space between the thumb and index finger, allowing room for the patient to pinch the thumb and index finger together; having the patient pretend to hold a soda can will help him maintain the proper position. Keep the wrist extended at about 35 degrees to promote a grasping movement of the hand.

▸ When applying a thumb spica cast, apply a small tubular stockinette to the thumb and use less padding in the web space than you would for a short-arm cast.

▸ When applying a long-arm cast, add extra padding around the upper arm to prevent skin irritation. Provide a sling to prevent the cast edge from impinging on the underside of the upper arm.

▸ If applying a short-leg cast with the patient sitting on the examination table, take care to prevent ankle plantar flexion; you can use a special metal footrest designed for this purpose. Alternatively, place the patient in a prone position on the table with his knee flexed. Slightly angle the upper edge of the cast from the anterior, just below the tibial tubercle, to the posterior over the proximal calf to prevent the cast from impinging behind the knee when the patient flexes his knee. Make sure you can see all toes at the distal end of the cast. For a walking cast, reinforce the ankle and heel and add a plantar heel wedge to allow the foot to roll forward at heel strike. Apply a cast shoe to protect the toes and reduce wear on the cast.

Patient teaching

▸ Instruct the patient to keep the cast dry; he can use a plastic bag to cover the cast when bathing adjacent areas and in wet weather.
▸ Advise him to elevate the injured limb as much as possible to limit

swelling and to avoid extensive use or weight bearing unless instructed otherwise.

▶ Advise him not to push objects inside the cast to scratch (doing so may cause sores and infection) or to paint or varnish the cast (doing so will prevent air circulation around the skin), although he can have others sign the cast with a felt-tipped marker.

●●● **RED FLAG** *Tell the patient to call his primary care provider if he experiences numbness, tingling, swelling, or pain (signs that the cast may be too tight, pinching nerves or constricting blood flow); irritation; skin breakdown at the cast's edges; and painful or tight areas inside the cast.*

INTRA-ARTICULAR AND BURSA CORTICOSTEROID INJECTION

CPT codes: 20550 injection sites include tendon sheath, ligaments, trigger points; 206000 arthrocentesis, aspiration, and/or injection of joint or bursa (for example, temporomandibular; acromioclavicular; wrist, elbow, or ankle; olecranon bursa); 20610 of major joint or bursa (for shoulder, hip, knee joint, subacromial bursa)

Typically performed simultaneously with arthrocentesis, intra-articular corticosteroid injection can provide immediate relief from pain and swelling in the affected joint. Such injections typically provide only temporary relief, and the underlying cause still needs to be identified. Contraindications include suspected joint infection and recent fracture or known osteoporosis in the area. Corticosteroids used for injection include betamethasone, hydrocortisone, methylprednisolone, and triamcinolone. Because no corticosteroid has proved more effective, the choice lies with the clinician, based on cost and previous injection history.

Equipment

Povidone-iodine solution and alcohol pads • sterile latex gloves (unless the patient is allergic to latex) • drapes • 1% or 2% lidocaine solution without epinephrine, or fluormethane spray, or both, for local anesthesia • sterile syringes (5- and 10-ml) • 25G ⅝″ needle if performing local anesthesia with lidocaine • 18G and 20G 1½″ needles • hemostat • sterile 3″ × 3″ and 4″ × 4″ gauze pads • corticosteroid

Essential steps

▶ Explain the procedure to the patient and address questions or concerns he may have.
▶ Obtain informed consent.
▶ Have all necessary equipment ready.
▶ Place the patient in as comfortable a position as possible to allow performance of the procedure.
▶ Carefully identify landmarks, and mark the exact injection site by indenting the skin with the blunt end of a ballpoint pen or a fingernail. Such a marking won't readily wash away.
▶ Clean the area with povidone-iodine solution and let it dry; repeat this three times.
▶ Before injection, wipe the area with the alcohol pad to avoid getting povidone-iodine in the joint.
▶ Using sterile technique, drape the area and anesthetize it with topical fluoromethane. If appropriate, use the 25G ⅝″ needle to infiltrate the subcutaneous skin with the lidocaine solution (lidocaine may distort landmarks in smaller joints.)
▶ Quickly insert the needle through the skin to minimize patient discomfort. Avoid moving the needle

from side to side as it enters the joint. For smaller joints, use a 22G needle with a 3- to 5-ml syringe. For larger joints, use an 18G needle.

▶ Aspirate as the needle advances into the joint space or bursal sac until fluid flows freely to confirm the intra-articular or bursa location.

▶ Inject the corticosteroid into the joint space.

▶ When performing joint injection with arthrocentesis, use the two-syringe technique. (See *Using the two-syringe technique.*)

▶ To help distribute the cortico-steroid throughout the joint space, perform passive range-of-motion exercises.

▶ Immobilize the joint, and provide adequate analgesia (such as non-steroidal anti-inflammatory drugs) for pain control.

Complications

The most serious complication from intra-articular and bursa cortico-steroid injection is the introduction of infection into the area or the masking of an existing infection; aseptic technique can help reduce this risk. The patient shouldn't receive a corticosteroid injection if infection is suspected.

Repeated injections may also result in necrosis of the joint space and the juxta-articular bone, with subsequent joint destruction and instability. Other complications include tendon rupture, local soft-tissue atrophy, hemarthrosis, and transient nerve palsy.

High-dose or repeated cortico-steroid injections may have long-term systemic effects. The patient may also experience corticosteroid arthropathy, a condition in which relief from symptoms results in the patient overusing the joint, causing further injury.

USING THE TWO-SYRINGE TECHNIQUE

When you're performing joint injection with arthrocentesis, the two-syringe technique can prove valuable. Insert a syringe into the joint and aspirate joint fluid (top illustration).

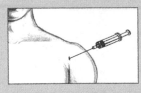

Then attach a hemostat at the needle hub and stabilize the needle while removing the syringe (middle illustration).

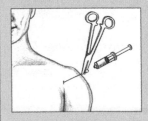

Replace the syringe containing the joint aspirate with a second syringe containing a corticosteroid (bottom illustration), and inject the drug into the joint space.

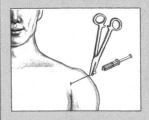

When the injection is finished, remove the needle and apply pressure and a sterile dressing.

Special considerations

▶ You may inject large joints, such as the knee and shoulder, with the equivalent of 80 mg of methylprednisolone acetate with 1 to 2 ml of 1% lidocaine. Smaller joints require only 20 to 40 mg with 0.5 to 1 ml of 1% lidocaine.

▶ The patient shouldn't receive corticosteroid injections more than three times per year; more frequent injections may cause cartilage damage, systemic effects, and avascular necrosis.

▶ For corticosteroid injection, avoid direct contact with the skin or subcutaneous tissue to prevent skin atrophy. For intrabursal injection, inject the corticosteroid around — not into — the tendon or ligament. Because direct injection can lead to tendon or ligament rupture, reposition the needle if it meets resistance.

Patient teaching

▶ Explain to the patient that intra-articular injection is typically done in the office or emergency department and that he can go home after the procedure.

▶ Tell him to apply ice, compress the area with an elastic wrap, and elevate the joint to reduce swelling and pain. He should rest and immobilize the joint for several days after treatment. An immobilization device and crutches may encourage him to avoid overuse and weight-bearing activities on the affected joint. Tell him to follow up within 1 week.

●●● **RED FLAG** *Tell the patient to call his primary care provider for signs of infection, such as increasing redness, swelling, pain, and warmth; cloudy yellow, green, or brown drainage; opening of wound; foul odor; red streak from wound area; fever; and warmth and*

increased pain and stiffness within the joint.

● PAPANICOLAOU TEST

CPT codes: 88142 cytopathology, cervical or vaginal, collected in preservative fluid, automated thin layer preparation; manual screening under physician supervision; 88144 cytopathology, cervical or vaginal, collected in preservative fluid, automated thin layer preparation; with manual screening and computer assisted rescreening under physician supervision; 88147 cytopathology, cervical or vaginal; screening by automated system under physician supervision; 88150 cytopathology, cervical or vaginal; manual screening under physician supervision

The Papanicolaou (Pap) test is most commonly used to detect cervical cancer. The cell sample can be placed on one or two glass slides, or ThinPrep cells can be placed in a supplied bottle of fixative and then placed on slides by the laboratory.

Equipment

One or more slides or bottle ● spatula (wood if using slides, plastic if using ThinPrep) ● cytobrush ● fixative for slide ● appropriate-sized speculum ● sterile gloves ● drape

●●● **RED FLAG** *A cytobrush should always be used for a cervical or endocervical Papanicolaou, even on a pregnant patient.*

Essential steps

Preprocedure, advise the patient to abstain from intercourse, douching or using vaginal medications, spermicidal foams, creams, or gels for 2 days prior to the appointment. These activities may wash away cells or alter test results.

●●● **RED FLAG** *Don't use a lubricant*
●●● *prior to performing a Pap test.*
▶ Determine whether the patient
has allergies, including latex.
▶ Explain the procedure to the patient (if this is her first pelvic examination), and help her into the lithotomy position.
▶ Wash your hands, and put on
gloves.
▶ Examine the vulva as well as
Bartholin's and Skene's glands.
▶ Take the speculum in your dominant hand and moisten it with
warm water to ease insertion. Warn
the patient that you're about to
touch her and advise her to take
several deep breaths. Insert the
speculum into the vagina, making
sure you can see the entire cervix.
If you can't, remove the speculum,
insert your index finger into the
vagina and locate the cervix, and
then reinsert the speculum.

● **CLINICAL PEARL** *If the cervix is*
difficult to visualize, ask the
patient to place her fists under her
sacrum to cause a pelvic tilt. This
works best with females who have a
very posterior cervix.
▶ Insert the cytobrush into the endocervix, turning it 360 degrees. If
you obtain a great deal of mucus,
wipe it away without swabbing the
endocervix.
▶ Take the spatula and lightly
scrape around the ectocervix.
▶ Quickly place the cells on the
slide, first with the spatula and then
the cytobrush. To apply the cells,
roll the brush across the surface of
the slide or stroke both sides of the
broom across the slide, placing the
second stroke directly over the first.
▶ Apply fixative so that the cells
don't dry out.
▶ If you're using ThinPrep, use the
same collection method, except use
a plastic spatula. Once you've obtained the specimen, dip the spatula into the fixative, swish it around

inside the bottle, and scrape off the
cells. Next, take the brush and
move it in a circle in the bottle,
wiping around the inside of the bottle 10 times.
▶ After finishing, remove the speculum from the vagina.

Complications
▶ Bleeding
▶ Discomfort
▶ Flashbacks of trauma or abuse

Special considerations
▶ Look for lesions on the cervix and
in the vaginal area, and include this
area on the Pap smear, making a
note of it on the Pap slip that's sent
to the laboratory. Also note on the
slip if bleeding occurred, and note
"contact bleeding" in the patient's
chart. Don't use the term "friable,"
which can legally be misconstrued
to mean a cancerous lesion, requiring colposcopy and biopsy.
▶ If the patient appears anxious or
upset during the pelvic examination, stop at once, make eye contact, and ask if she wants you to
stop. If she does, stop the examination, but discuss the importance of
having a pelvic examination and
Pap test at the next visit or with another provider. Once the patient has
dressed, discuss your observations
(for example, hands balled into
fists, pallor, tears, and changes in
breathing pattern) and ask if she
wants to discuss anything. Think
about your response in advance;
you don't want to respond with
hesitancy or silence if the patient
discloses trauma or abuse.

Patient teaching
▶ Tell the patient that minor bleeding after the procedure isn't unusual.
▶ Advise her that a Pap smear is a
screening test and that further testing maybe necessary for diagnosis.

● Provide education for prevention of sexually transmitted diseases and the importance of clinical breast examinations and mammography following American Cancer Society guidelines. Also, provide education about breast self-examination.

REMOVAL OF FOREIGN BODY FROM THE EAR

CPT code: 69200 removal of foreign body from external auditory canal without general anesthesia
Cerumen, or earwax, is the substance most commonly found in the external ear canal. Although not a foreign body, copious or hardened earwax may cause pressure or pain and conductive hearing loss in the affected ear and must be removed. Other small objects — including parts of toys, beans, nuts, coins, cotton applicator tips, and insects — may also lodge in the external ear.

LIFE SPAN *Children are at greater risk for foreign bodies in the ear than are adults.*

Equipment

Otoscope ● ear curette, loop, or hook (plastic or wire) ● ear irrigation system (syringe with soft tubing or bulb syringe) ● basin of lukewarm water ● basin to catch irrigation fluid ● protective cover for patient ● viscous lidocaine, topical anesthetics, or mineral oil for ear instillation if foreign object is live insect ● carbamide peroxide or mineral oil for softening impacted wax (if needed) Optional: otic antibiotic or corticosteroid, adjustable light source

Essential steps

● Before beginning, obtain a history of the complaint and related signs and symptoms.

● Explain the procedure to the patient and his parents (in pediatric patients) and answer questions they have.

● Inspect the external ear for signs of infection or injury.

●●● RED FLAG *Refer patients with trauma to the ear to an ear, nose, and throat specialist or the emergency department.*

● Using the otoscope, inspect the external ear canal for edema, erythema, and the presence and type of foreign body; determine the appropriate extraction method.

● Wash your hands, and prepare the equipment.

● Grasping the pinna of the ear, straighten the external ear canal by pulling the ear up and back (in an adult) or down and back (in a child).

● Gently insert the ear curette or loop into the external canal to grasp the object and gradually withdraw it.

● Instill viscous lidocaine, mineral oil, or topical anesthetic into the ear canal before extracting a live insect; the medication immobilizes the insect and reduces discomfort during extraction.

● If these are ineffective, instead try flushing out the object. However, if the object may swell (such as an organic foreign body), don't instill fluid into the ear canal.

●●● RED FLAG *Don't irrigate the ear if tympanic membrane rupture is suspected.*

● Before flushing the ear canal, provide a protective covering for the patient and a drainage basin he can hold below his ear.

● Firmly flush the external ear canal with lukewarm water, using the syringe with soft tubing, bulb syringe, or jet irrigation system (use the jet system cautiously because of the risk of tympanic membrane injury).

▶ Don't force fluid directly at the tympanic membrane or you may injure it; instead, try to direct the flow past the object to flush the canal.

▶ Inspect the external ear canal for patency after extraction; repeat the procedure as needed until the canal is clear.

▶ Dry the external ear canal to reduce the risk of otitis externa.

▶ Instill a topical antibiotic or corticosteroid to control external edema, erythema, and infection.

Complications

▶ Laceration of the external ear canal

▶ Middle ear effusion with ear irrigation (if the tympanic membrane is perforated)

▶ Otitis externa

▶ Tympanic membrane rupture

Special considerations

▶ Don't push the foreign body toward the tympanic membrane during extraction because doing so could cause injury.

▶ Stop trying to extract the object if the patient experiences pain, severe vertigo, or nausea.

▶ Refer the patient to a primary care physician or otolaryngologist if the extraction effort wasn't successful or if the patient has a perforated tympanic membrane, myringotomy tubes, or chronic otitis media.

▶ If the patient has impacted earwax, consider instilling carbamide peroxide or mineral oil three times a day for 3 to 5 days to soften it.

Patient teaching

▶ Advise the patient not to clean the external ear with a cotton-tipped applicator and not to place small objects into the ear canal.

REMOVAL OF FOREIGN BODY FROM THE EYE

CPT code: 65205 removal of foreign body, external eye, conjunctival, superficial; 65210 removal of foreign body, external eye, conjunctival, embedded; 65220 removal of foreign body, external eye, conjunctival, corneal without slit lamp; 99070 eye tray: supplies and material provided by physician over and above what's usually included in office visit

A patient who complains of eye pain, burning, and the feeling that he has something in his eye may have a foreign body in his eye; such objects typically include dust or dirt, or a metal, plastic, or wood particle. If the patient also displays photophobia and a tearing eye, he may have a corneal abrasion. People who take part in such activities as digging, drilling, hammering, welding, and woodworking without appropriate eye protection are at increased risk.

The clinician should evaluate a patient who complains of eye pain for one or more foreign bodies in the eye (some types of injuries can scatter fragments across the cornea). The foreign body typically lodges underneath the upper eyelid or in the superior temporal cul-de-sac where the upper lid attaches to the eyeball; foreign bodies can also lodge in the inferior cul-de-sac below the lower lid.

Equipment

Short-acting ophthalmic anesthetic solution (0.5% proparacaine) • vision-screening device such as a Snellen chart • cotton-tipped applicators or eyelid retractor • gloves • ophthalmoscope • sterile fluorescein stain strips • Wood's light or ophthalmoscope with a blue light • tap water or sterile normal saline solution (for flushing the eye) ● ophthalmic antibiotic solution or ointment (usually broad-spectrum) ● eye patches or eye shield and adhesive tape (if indicated) ● binocular loupe or slit lamp (if available)

Essential steps

▶ Obtain a history of the injury and use of contact lenses and protective eyewear.
▶ Explain the procedure to the patient and address questions or concerns he may have.
▶ Inspect the eye and lid for erythema, drainage, and hemorrhage; if you suspect intraocular perforation or open globe injuries, refer the patient to a primary care physician or ophthalmologist at once.
▶ Perform vision screening.
▶ Examine the pupillary reflex, extraocular movements, anterior and posterior chambers, and fundi.
▶ Wash your hands, and put on gloves.
▶ Open the affected eye, and instill 1 or 2 drops of short-acting ophthalmic anesthetic.
▶ While the patient looks down, evert the upper lid by placing the cotton-tipped applicator on the external upper lid, grasping the lashes, and turning the lid inside out over the applicator to expose the inner surface of the upper lid; you can also use the retractors to expose the conjunctiva.
▶ Examine the entire cornea, including the cul-de-sac, with an ophthalmoscope, slit lamp, or binocular loupe to locate and determine the depth of the foreign object, ascertain whether it's embedded, and choose the best technique for its removal.
▶ If the foreign body is lying on the surface, use an oblique stream of tap water or sterile normal saline solution to flush the eye.

▶ Reexamine the entire conjunctiva to reassess the location and depth of the foreign body.
▶ Use a saline-moistened cotton-tipped applicator to gently remove the foreign body without causing imbedding or scratching of the conjunctiva.
▶ Gently irrigate the eye with saline solution to clean the area.
▶ Stain the conjunctiva with a fluorescein stain strip to assess for corneal abrasion.
▶ Apply ophthalmic antibiotic ointment.
▶ Cover the affected eye with an eye patch to promote patient comfort and protect the eye. Have the patient close both eyes and tightly tape two eye patches over the affected eye.
▶ Administer a tetanus booster, if indicated.

Complications

▶ Conjunctivitis (viral or bacterial)
▶ Corneal ulcer or abrasion
▶ Intraocular foreign body
▶ Uveitis

Special considerations

▶ If you're unable to remove the foreign body or if you suspect intraocular perforation, cover the eye with a patch and protective shielding, have the patient rest the eye and elevate his head, and immediately refer him to an ophthalmologist.
▶ Signs of eye perforation include softness of the orbit on gentle palpation, change in pupillary size or reaction, abnormality of the anterior chamber, and leakage of fluid from the chamber.
▶ Don't apply a topical corticosteroid or pain medications because they may mask changes or interfere with healing.

▶ Use an eye shield to protect the eye without putting pressure on the orbit.

▶ Encourage the patient to wear protective eyewear for occupational and recreational activities.

▶ If the patient complains of increased pain during the procedure, stop at once.

▶ Refer the patient to an ophthalmologist if he has a metallic injury with rust rings, a corneal ulceration that won't heal, signs of uveitis, or vision loss.

Patient teaching

▶ Have the patient schedule a return office visit within 24 hours for reevaluation of the eye and restaining of the cornea as indicated.

▶ Encourage the patient to wear protective eyewear for high-risk occupational and recreational activities, such as arc-welding, mixing chemicals, and lighting fire works.

SKIN LESION BIOPSY AND REMOVAL

CPT code: 11300-303 shaving of epidermal or dermal lesion, single lesion on trunk, arms, or legs; 11305-308 on scalp, neck, hands, feet, or genitalia; 11400-406 excision of benign lesions on trunk, arms, or legs; 11420-426 on scalp, neck, hands, feet, or genitalia; 11600-606 excision of malignant lesions on trunk, arms, or legs; 11620-626 on scalp, neck, hands, feet, or genitalia; 11200 removal of skin tags, multiple fibrocutaneous tags, any area, less than 15 lesions; 11201 each additional 10 lesions

A shave, scissor, or punch biopsy can be either incisional (removing only part of a lesion) or excisional (removing the entire lesion). In general, a clinician should remove the entire lesion, provided doing so allows for proper healing and an esthetically acceptable outcome.

The pathologist should receive an adequate specimen for diagnosis, for instance, a specimen that includes the dermis for a dermal lesion. Sometimes the pathologist also needs a portion of adjacent normal skin if the patient has a more complex skin disease, such as panniculitis; a wedge section can provide the larger and deeper specimen needed. The clinician should also provide as much detail about the site as possible.

A clinician who can't identify or doesn't plan to treat a lesion shouldn't biopsy it; instead, the patient should be referred to a dermatologist. In addition, if a patient has a lesion that looks like skin cancer, he should be referred to a dermatologist.

Types of biopsy

The shave biopsy allows the clinician to take a specimen of a skin lesion that doesn't seem to extend deep into the dermis. It's a quick, easy way to remove superficial lesions and is ideal for raised lesions in the epidermis or superficial dermis, although if necessary, the procedure can extend down to the subcutis. The procedure is faster than a punch biopsy, usually requires only topical aluminum chloride to control bleeding, has a favorable cosmetic outcome, and can provide a relatively large specimen. However, it can leave a depressed scar if the biopsy goes too deep, result in pigment disturbance and, possibly, miss a deeper component of skin cancer. Most clinicians remove lesions with a sterilized razor blade; some prefer a #15 Bard-Parker blade. The inexpensive, sharp, flexible blade allows the clinician to curve the blade to match the surface of the lesion by applying pressure with the index finger and thumb. The clinician can then advance the blade across the base of the lesion with a steady sawing motion.

A variant of the shave biopsy, the scissor biopsy allows removal of small superficial growths, such as skin tags and filiform warts. It usually doesn't require local anesthesia. The clinician uses forceps with teeth to gently grasp and apply traction to the lesion, cuts the lesion at the base with iris scissors, and applies aluminum chloride and pressure to control bleeding.

For a punch biopsy, a specialized instrument is used to remove a cylindrical, full-thickness skin specimen. It's performed to obtain material for pathologic evaluation and to remove small cutaneous lesions quickly and effectively. Punches are available in sizes ranging from 1.5 to 10 mm and can be permanent or disposable; disposable punch biopsy instruments are preferable because they're sterile, inexpensive, and don't dull from repeated use. Because the instrument can only go as deep as the length of the cylinder, a biopsy that may include deeper fat or fascia may require two complete punches. The resulting wound may require suturing.

Punch biopsies generally produce a good cosmetic result, provide a deep specimen, and heal rapidly when sutured. However, they require sterile technique, specimen size is limited by the width and depth of the punch, and the wound may require extra time for suturing.

Equipment

70% isopropyl alcohol, povidone-iodine ● gloves ● local anesthesia ● 25G to 30G ½" to 1" needles and 3- to 5-ml syringe (for injecting the anesthetic) ● razor blade or #15 Bard-Parker blade ● aluminum chloride or electrocautery (to control bleeding) ● cotton-tipped applicators for shave biopsy ● punch, skin hook, or needle ● sharp scissors ● suture equipment ● sterile adhesive strips such as Steri-Strips ● three-layer pressure dressing with antibiotic ointment ● adhesive dressing overlay (for punch biopsy)

Essential steps

▶ Obtain a detailed history and perform a physical examination.
▶ Verify that the patient isn't allergic to iodine preparations or local anesthetics.
▶ Explain the procedure to the patient and address questions or concerns he may have.
▶ Obtain informed consent.
▶ Wash your hands.
▶ After marking the biopsy site, clean the skin with antiseptic solution.
▶ Place a sterile drape over the area, and put on gloves.
▶ Inject the local anesthetic under the lesion, using a 25G or 30G needle to create a wheal.
▶ For a punch biopsy, position the punch vertically over the area. Using your nondominant hand, apply perpendicular tissue traction. This results in an oval rather than a circular defect (a circular defect may result in a redundant cone of skin called a "dog-ear" on closure).
▶ Push the punch against the skin with firm, steady pressure, and simultaneously twist it clockwise. Continue this until you feel some give, indicating the descent of the punch into the fat layer.
▶ Withdraw the punch with the column of tissue. Remove the specimen gently (to avoid histologic artifacts).
▶ Use a skin hook or local anesthesia needle to elevate the plug of tissue, and transect the base with a pair of sharp scissors.

PERFORMING A SHAVE BIOPSY

This illustration of a shave biopsy shows how to position the scalpel so it's almost parallel to the skin surface.

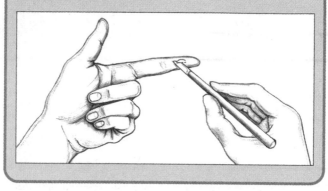

▶ To obtain the best cosmetic result and fastest healing, suture the biopsy site using simple interrupted or vertical mattress sutures. Typically, a 2-mm punch requires one suture, a 4- to 6-mm punch requires two sutures, and a 7- to 10-mm punch requires three to four sutures. Use 4-0 monofilament nylon sutures for wounds on the extremities and trunk and 5-0 and 6-0 monofilament nylon sutures with cutting P3 needles for biopsies taken from the face and anterior neck. (See "Suturing simple lacerations," page 369.) If necessary, reinforce the sutures on a wound under tension with sterile adhesive strips.

▶ Place a three-layer pressure dressing that contains triple antibiotic ointment (Polysporin) on the wound, followed by a nonadherent pad, gauze, and an adhesive dressing overlay.

▶ To perform a shave biopsy, secure the lesion and the surrounding tissue with your nondominant hand while passing the razor blade or scalpel under the lesion. Control the depth of the biopsy with the appropriate angle of entry. (See *Performing a shave biopsy.*)

▶ To control bleeding, apply 20% to 40% aluminum chloride directly to the wound with a cotton-tipped applicator or use electrocautery.

Complications

▶ Infection
▶ Pain
▶ Scarring

Special considerations

▶ Deeper shave biopsies can result in permanent depression at the biopsy site.

●●● RED FLAG *If the patient has an*
●●● *atypical-appearing melanocytic lesion, don't remove it with the shave procedure. Instead, obtain a good specimen for pathology by performing a deep punch biopsy. If unsure of the diagnosis, refer the patient to a dermatologist.*

▶ Don't keep removing the punch from the biopsy site to check your progress or the specimen may have histologic artifacts.

● Refer or consult with a dermatologist for deeper lesions, suspected skin cancer, neoplasms, and facial or penile lesions.

Patient teaching

● Teach the patient how to care for the wound. He should gently clean the biopsy site daily with tap water and soap (with no rubbing or scrubbing) and then apply a little antibiotic ointment, preferably Polysporin rather than an ointment that contains neomycin, which carries a higher risk of allergic reaction. Tell him to continue wound care until the area completely heals.

● Tell him that the wound will appear uniformly pink or red when epithelialization is complete, and explain that keeping the wound covered and occluded promotes rapid healing and decreases the risk of scarring.

● If the punch biopsy site is in an area of tension, advise the patient to minimize activity to prevent bleeding and wound dehiscence.

●●● **RED FLAG** *Tell the patient to call*
●●● *his primary care provider for signs of infection, such as increasing redness, swelling, pain, and warmth; cloudy yellow, green, or brown drainage; opening of wound; foul odor; red streak from wound area; and fever.*

SKIN SCRAPING

CPT code: 87210 specimen smear with interpretation, wet mount with simple stain for infectious agents (potassium hydroxide [KOH] preps); 87220 tissue examination of skin, hair and nails for ecto parasites (KOH slide)

A skin scrape involves the gentle removal of a skin specimen that's then placed on a microscope slide for evaluation. This procedure is commonly used to confirm a diagnosis of a superficial fungal infection or arthropod infestation.

Equipment

#15 Bard-Parker surgical blade (if unavailable, use the edge of a glass microscope slide) ● gloves ● alcohol pad ● microscope slide and coverglass ● 5% to 20% KOH solution

Essential steps

● Explain the procedure to the patient and address questions or concerns he may have.

● Position the patient comfortably with the area to be scraped accessible.

● Wash your hands, and put on gloves.

● Clean the area with an alcohol pad.

● Lightly run the blade perpendicular to the skin; when the blade has collected enough of the superficial layer of the skin, wipe it across the slide. Make sure you use a gentle technique; the patient shouldn't experience pain or bleed.

● Place the coverglass on the slide.

● If you suspect a dermatophyte infection, apply KOH to the edge of the coverglass, allowing capillary action to draw the solution under.

● Gently heat the slide with a match until bubbles begin to expand.

● Blot excess KOH solution with lens paper.

● If you see hyphae (septated, tubelike structures), dermatophytes are present; pseudohyphae (tubelike structures without septa) and budding yeast forms indicate candidiasis.

Complications

No complications are associated with skin scraping.

Special considerations

▶ If KOH results are negative, collect a culture specimen and send it to the microbiology laboratory for growth and species identification.

Patient teaching

▶ Just before scraping, tell the patient that you're about to scrape the skin but that the scraping won't cause pain. Explain that the scraping will help ensure proper diagnosis and treatment.

▶ Instruct the patient to schedule a follow-up appointment based on diagnostic findings.

SOFT-TISSUE ASPIRATION

CPT code: 20600 arthrocentesis, aspiration, and injection: small joint, bursa, or ganglionic cyst (for example, fingers or toes); 20605 intermediate joint, bursa (wrist, elbow, or ankle; olecranon bursa); 20610 major joint or bursa (for example, shoulder, hip, knee joint, subacromial bursa)

Soft-tissue aspiration involves removing fluid or exudate from an area of soft tissue for evaluation and palliative care. Contraindications include severe coagulopathies, swelling on the face, cellulitis, broken skin at the site, and prosthetic joint.

Equipment

Povidone-iodine solution and alcohol pads ● sterile gloves ● drape ● hemostat ● 10-ml syringe with 18G to 20G 1″ needle ● red-topped tube ● elastic bandage sterile 3″ × 3″ or 4″ × 4″ gauze pads ● tape

Essential steps

▶ Explain the procedure to the patient and address questions or concerns he may have.

▶ Obtain informed consent.

▶ Verify that the patient isn't allergic to iodine.

▶ Wash your hands.

▶ Assemble equipment before beginning.

▶ Place the patient in as comfortable a position as possible to allow performance of the procedure. Drape the site.

▶ Clean the site and surrounding area with povidone-iodine solution or with alcohol swabs.

▶ Put on sterile gloves.

▶ Attach an 18G or a 20G 1″ needle to a 10-ml syringe.

▶ Insert the needle, bevel down, into the leading edge of the swelling. Aspirate as you advance the needle.

▶ If the syringe becomes full and needs to be changed, use the two-syringe technique. Attach the hemostat to the needle hub to avoid needle rotation, remove the first syringe, replace it with an empty syringe, and continue aspirating.

▶ Place the aspirated fluid into a red-topped collection tube, and send it to the laboratory for analysis, if indicated.

▶ Apply a pressure dressing and compression device such as an elastic bandage.

Complications

▶ Infection

Patient teaching

▶ Tell the patient to keep the pressure dressing intact for 24 hours and then remove it.

▶ Suggest applying ice or heat for the first 24 hours for some relief from discomfort.

●●● **RED FLAG** *Tell the patient to call* ●●● *his primary care provider for signs of infection, such as increasing redness, swelling, pain, and warmth; cloudy yellow, green, or brown drainage; opening of wound;*

foul odor; red streak from wound area; and fever.

SPLINTING AND TAPING

CPT code: 29125 application short arm splint; 29130 application of finger splint; 29515 application of short leg splint; 29550 strapping: toes

Splinting and taping can stabilize and immobilize acute injuries and provide symptomatic relief of chronic conditions, increasing patient comfort and preventing further injury. Acute injuries — such as sprains, strains, and fractures — typically require immediate joint stabilization; at the scene of the trauma, rigid object can function as a splint. A temporary measure, splinting is initially preferred over circumferential casting for acute injuries because increased swelling within a circumferential cast can lead to vascular compromise, compartment syndrome, and distal swelling.

Inversion injuries with plantar flexion, the most common cause of acute ankle injuries, typically occur in young adults who take part in recreational activities and sports. Fractures are more common in older adults. Chronic conditions such as overuse and repetitive-motion injuries, typically occur in the upper extremities and can usually be managed in a primary care setting or by an orthopedic specialist. Sprains vary based on the level of injury, disability, pain, and swelling. (See *Grading ankle sprains*.)

Chronic injuries typically affect the wrists and hands and usually result from tendosynovitis, as can occur with repetitive-motion injuries (carpal tunnel syndrome and tennis elbow). Splints increase the patient's comfort by keeping the joint in proper alignment.

When taking the patient's history, the clinician should obtain a description of the injury and the joint involved, how and when it occurred, the patient's level of activity right after the injury and at the time of evaluation, and a previous history of injury to the joint. Physical assessment should focus on the joint involved and its physical appearance, including swelling, obvious deformity, bleeding, and ecchymosis, possibly including a comparison with the other, uninjured extremity. The clinician should also assess the patient's neurovascular status and ask the patient if he can move the extremity. Contraindications include neurovascular compromise, soft-tissue compression, and open injury.

●●● **RED FLAG** *Consider referrals for*
●●● *an unstable joint, a fracture, potential limb loss, suspected internal derangement (indicated by clicking, popping, or locking of the joint), persistent pain, or unresolved injury.*

Equipment

Tube stockinette in various diameters ● precast material or casting materials in various widths ● 4″ or 6″ elastic wraps ● 1″ to 2″ adhesive tape ● bucket of water ● soft padding material ● clean scissors ● sling for upper-extremity injuries ● aluminum splints for finger injuries ● wrist and finger splints for wrist or finger injuries ● knee immobilizer for knee injuries

Essential steps

● Explain the procedure to the patient and address questions or concerns he may have.
● Have X-rays performed as appropriate to rule out fracture. (See *Ottawa ankle rules*, page 368.)
● After the X-ray has been read and the extent of the injury is known,

GRADING ANKLE SPRAINS

Grading a sprain injury of the ankle allows uniform assessment and treatment for a wide variety of situations. This chart outlines grades currently used for ankle sprain injuries, the tissue damage involved, signs and symptoms of the injury, and treatment.

Tissue damage	Signs and symptoms	Treatment
GRADE I		
Partial or complete tear of the anterior talofibular ligament	Local tenderness, minimal swelling, but usually able to bear weight with no functional loss or joint instability	▶ Symptomatic treatment with elastic compression support to control swelling ▶ Intermittent removal of immobilization, with active range-of-motion (ROM) exercises, progressing as tolerated ▶ Peroneal strengthening and exercise start at 2 to 3 weeks, depending on patient tolerance
GRADE II		
Partial or complete tear of both the anterior talofibular and calcaneofibular ligaments	Painful weight bearing, minimal ligament function during examination, possible "popping" with injury, moderate to severe swelling (begins within minutes), pain, ecchymosis, and mild joint instability	▶ Same as for grade I, plus immobilization and non-weight-bearing with an air splint or short-leg removable walking cast ▶ Switch to hinged-joint immobilization at 2 weeks
GRADE III		
Grade II injury plus a partial or complete tear of the posterior talofibular ligament	Ligamentous laxity, moderate to severe joint instability, complete interruption in alignment, inability to bear weight and often obvious deformity, diffuse joint swelling (begins within minutes), pain initially but possibly no pain later	▶ Evaluation by an orthopedic surgeon ▶ Short-leg walking cast for 3 weeks ▶ Physical therapy including ROM exercises, peroneal strengthening, and proprioception training after 3 weeks ▶ Possible cast for up to 6 weeks or surgical repair

OTTAWA ANKLE RULES

Use the following Ottawa ankle rules to determine whether X-rays are needed:

▶ If the patient is between ages 18 and 55 and can walk four steps immediately after the injury or when being evaluated, X-rays aren't required.

▶ If the patient feels pain on ambulation immediately after the injury and on evaluation, plus tenderness within 2½″ (6.4 cm) of the posterior edge of the malleoli, order ankle X-rays.

▶ If the patient feels pain on ambulation immediately after the injury and on evaluation, plus tenderness of the fifth metatarsal or navicular, order foot X-rays.

prepare the patient for immobilization. Place him in as comfortable a position as possible that allows splinting or taping.

▶ Measure the splinting material against the patient and then add about 1½″ (4 cm) to the length of the splint to ensure a proper fit. Then fold the material into 10 to 15 overlapping layers.

▶ Apply a soft cotton bandage, such as Webril, to the extremity to protect the skin before applying the cast. Then moisten the plaster or casting material with cool water, apply it to the injured extremity, and mold the plaster to the extremity while maintaining the extremity in the proper position. Secure the splint with an elastic bandage and let it dry.

Complications

A splint that's wrapped too tightly can lead to vascular compromise, ischemia, and compartment syndrome of the affected extremity;

making sure that the elastic bandage is snug but not tight can help prevent this, as can using a linear splint rather than a circular splint.

Exothermic burns can occur when the plaster begins to harden; the plaster should be removed at once if the patient complains of pain from the heat of the drying plaster. Pressure ulcers can result from plaster rubbing against bony prominences; Webril applied directly to the skin beneath the splint can help reduce this complication.

Special considerations

▶ Although several types of finger splints exist, the aluminum finger splint is most commonly used for isolated proximal and distal interphalangeal joint injuries. Place it on the injured finger and secure it with tape; for subsequent injuries, incorporate the splint into a volar arm splint.

▶ Use a volar arm splint for distal radial, ulnar, and carpal fractures and Grades II and III wrist sprains. Have the patient extend his wrist slightly, with the metacarpophalangeal joint flexed 60 to 70 degrees and the fingers flexed 10 to 20 degrees. Maintain this position until the splint hardens, and secure it with an elastic bandage. The splint should extend from the tip of the fingers to about 1¼″ to 1½″ (3 to 4 cm) distal to the elbow joint.

▶ Use an aluminum thumb splint for injuries involving the thumb. Flex the thumb slightly at the distal interphalangeal joint. Measure the splint to fit 1″ to 2″ (2.5 to 5 cm) beyond the wrist. Bend the splint to the position of the thumb, and apply it to the dorsal side of the thumb. Wrap the splint with an elastic wrap; include the thumb in the wrap.

▶ Obtain an ankle fracture brace for injury to the tibias fibular, lateral collateral, or deltoid ligament to limit inversion and eversion. The patient should be in a prone position, with the knee and ankle each flexed 90 degrees. Help him maintain this position as you apply the splint, which should extend from the metatarsal joint to about $1^1/2''$ before the popliteal fossae. Secure with an elastic bandage (usually 4" to 6" [10 to 15 cm] wide.)

▶ For chronic injuries, consider taping to stabilize and support the joint, particularly for an athlete. Taping immobilizes the area and provides supports, allowing the athlete to continue activities with minimal interference. Make sure the tape isn't too tight, and keep in mind that most taping loosens after activity, placing the joint at risk for further injury. Several methods of taping exist; a skilled professional (such as a trainer or sports medicine clinician) should perform such taping.

▶ For a custom-made splint, which may be more comfortable than a standard-sized splint, refer the patient to an orthopedic specialist.

Patient teaching

▶ Teach the patient the RICE regimen — rest, ice, compression, and elevation — (elevate the extremity above the heart for 48 hours).

▶ Tell him to apply ice every 2 to 3 hours for 20 to 30 minutes for the first 24 hours. Then he can switch to moist heat (without wetting the cast) for the next 24 to 48 hours.

▶ Tell him to wear the splint except when sleeping or showering until he's reevaluated and to avoid activities that cause pain.

▶ Have him watch for signs of neurovascular compromise, such as coolness, swelling, and pain in the area around the splint or tape or if the area appears pale or dark in color. If he notes these signs, he

should rest at once with the extremity elevated above his heart. Emphasize that swelling can occur swiftly with activity but will take much longer to subside. If swelling doesn't improve within 30 minutes, he should contact his primary care provider.

▶ Tell him to take acetaminophen or a nonsteroidal anti-inflammatory drug, or both, for pain, as directed.

⦿⦿⦿ **RED FLAG** *Tell the patient to call his primary care provider for signs of neurovascular compromise (peripheral pallor or blue-purple color, pain, coldness, swelling, or numbness and tingling) that don't resolve. The patient should remove the splint or tape and contact his primary care provider.*

SUTURING SIMPLE LACERATIONS

CPT code: 12001-7 simple repair, superficial wounds on scalp, neck, axillae, external genitalia, trunk, and extremities; 12011-18 simple repair, superficial wounds on face, ears, eyelids, nose, lips, and mucous membranes; 12020 superficial dehiscence

Wounds closed with sutures may require the use of both absorbable and nonabsorbable sutures, such as polypropylene (Prolene) and nylon. Usually placed deeper within a wound, absorbable sutures absorb into the body over time; nonabsorbable sutures are used at the surface of the wound and require removal. Sutures are especially important in high-tension areas, where the risk of pulling apart is greatest.

Suturing typically starts with a dermal layer of interrupted absorbable sutures. Nonabsorbable sutures are used on the epidermal layer; these sutures allow for improved approximation and eversion of the wound edges, resulting in optimal cosmetic results. The clinician typically removes these sutures in 1 to 2 weeks, depending on their location.

A simple interrupted suture for the epidermal layer completely closes the wound. This type of suture offers the advantages of properly everting skin edges so that the wound lies flat when it spreads, lining up unequal wound edges, and allowing for regional variations of tension. It takes longer to close a wound with this suture than with a running suture such as a mattress suture.

Wounds closed by approximation of the skin edges heal by primary intention. Wounds heal faster under an occlusive or semiocclusive dressing, which prevents crust formation.

Equipment

20- to 30-ml syringe with a 20G plastic cannula and irrigant ● smooth or multitooth forceps ● needle holder ● scissors ● scalpel, if needed ● appropriate sutures ● needles (round and tapered for mucosa, fascia, and muscle) ● injectable anesthesia (lidocaine or diphenhydramine, as appropriate) ● three-layer pressure dressing

Essential steps

▶ Explain the procedure to the patient and address questions or concerns he may have.
▶ Obtain informed consent.
▶ Position the patient in as comfortable a position as possible and allowing full visualization of the wound.
▶ Wash your hands, and apply gloves.
▶ Clean the wound with povidone-iodine solution in a circular pattern from the wound edges outward.
▶ Infiltrate a local anesthetic by inserting the needle along each side

of the wound and injecting slowly as you withdraw the needle, to ensure uniform distribution.
▶ Examine the wound for foreign bodies or injury to underlying structures, such as a tendon or joint capsule.
▶ Use the syringe and cannula to irrigate the wound with chemical antiseptics or sterile saline irrigant.
▶ Trim and undermine wound edges as needed, to provide effective approximation.
▶ Using your dominant hand, grasp the suture needle securely with the needle holder. Use a toothed forceps in your other hand to stabilize the wound edge in a slightly everted position.
▶ Insert the needle at a right angle through the skin about 0.5 to 1 cm from the wound edge. Grasp the needle from the exterior with the needle holder. Before inserting the needle again, be sure the tissue layers are well approximated with minimal tension.
▶ Repeat the process and then tie the suture, being careful not to pull the suture edges too taut.
▶ Use scissors to trim jagged edges from the wound.
▶ As appropriate, place a vertical mattress suture in the middle of the wound and bisect each half sequentially with vertical mattress sutures. (See *Choosing a suture technique.*)
▶ If the patient has redundant cones of skin, called "dog-ears," after suturing, remove them to optimize the cosmetic result. Excise the residual skin by making a small ellipse that extends the defect or by making an incision that lifts the dog-ear with the skin hook and drapes excess tissue over the side of the wound.
▶ To help equalize tension on wound edges, make a "hockey stick" incision, an angled incision that extends one end of the wound in the shape of a hockey stick. This

CHOOSING A SUTURE TECHNIQUE

The most commonly used suture techniques include the simple continuous, simple interrupted, and horizontal and vertical mattress sutures. The type of suture technique used depends on the site, shape, size, and depth of the wound.

The space left between sutures also varies, according to the wound's location or the amount of tension applied to the wound. For instance, the space between sutures in most wounds is about 0.25 cm, but you should place sutures even closer for facial wounds or those associated with high tension — for example, those on the elbow or knee.

Simple continuous
Simple continuous sutures provide even tension across the incision and are used for quick repair.

Simple interrupted
Simple interrupted sutures allow precise approximation of wound edges.

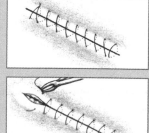

Horizontal mattress
Horizontal mattress sutures reduce dead space within the wound and reinforce subcutaneous tissue.

Vertical mattress
Vertical mattress sutures also reduce dead space within the wound and reinforce subcutaneous tissue. They're used in thick skin, such as in the palms or the soles, and in lax skin. These sutures are difficult to approximate and take more time to place.

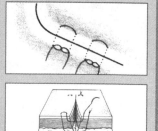

incision creates a curvilinear line that allows for the approximation of skin edges without placing undue tension on specific points along the line.

▶ After suturing the wound, compress the wound gently and look for residual bleeding. Use direct pressure for 5 minutes to minimize swelling and bleeding from the wound edge.

▶ Cover the site with a three-layer pressure dressing for 24 hours.

▶ Splint if necessary.

● Administer antibiotics, such as cephalexin, if the area is infected.
● Administer tetanus prophylaxis if the patient hasn't been or doesn't know if he has been immunized within the past 5 years.

Complications
● Dehiscence
● Infection
● Pain
● Scarring

Special considerations
● Refer the patient to a reconstructive surgeon for debridement or if the wound has a large amount of dead space (expect drain placement). Refer the patient to a physician for complex lacerations or for artery, tendon, ligament, bone, or nerve involvement.
● Scalp sutures should be removed in 5 to 8 days; face sutures, in 3 to 6 days; abdomen, chest, and upper-extremity sutures, in 10 to 12 days; lower-extremity sutures, in 7 to 14 days; and back sutures, in 10 to 14 days.

Patient teaching
● Tell the patient to keep the sutures dry.
● Instruct the patient to remove the initial dressing in 24 hours and then clean the sutured area twice per day with soap and water and cover it with antibiotic ointment.
● Teach the patient how to apply a nonadherent dressing and tape to form a pressure dressing.
● Tell the patient to replace the large dressing with a smaller gauze bandage when drainage no longer appears on the large dressing. Tell him to be careful not to place the gauze itself directly over the wound. Fibers in the gauze can get trapped in the wound edge, become matted, and delay healing.

● For suture removal, have the patient return in 3 to 6 days for face sutures, in 7 to 10 days for ear sutures, and in 5 to 10 days for trunk or extremity sutures.
● Advise the patient to use over-the-counter analgesics, such as acetaminophen or ibuprofen, to manage pain.

RED FLAG *Tell the patient to call his primary care provider for signs of infection, such as increasing redness, swelling, pain, and warmth; cloudy yellow, green, or brown drainage; opening of wound; foul odor; red streak from wound area; and fever.*

WART REMOVAL: CRYOSURGERY

CPT code: 17000 destruction any method (including laser, with or without surgical curettement/local anesthesia) of all benign/premalignant lesions any location, excluding cutaneous vascular proliferative lesions; 17003 multiple lesions; 17110 destruction of < 14 flat warts, molluscum contagiosum, or milia; 17260 destruction of < 0.5-cm malignant lesion from trunk, arms, or legs; 17261-66 indicates increasing lesion diameters; 17270 destruction of < 0.5-cm malignant lesion from scalp, neck, hands, feet, genitalia
Cryosurgery efficiently removes common skin lesions with minimal scar formation, pain, and pigment changes (in light-skinned patients). Cryosurgery uses freezing temperatures to destroy cells. Temperatures of 14° F (−10° C) to −4° F (−20° C) destroy tissue; a temperature of −58° F (−50° C) destroys malignant cells. In the procedure, a blister forms at the dermal-epidermal junction, and the skin superficial to the blister is left essentially bloodless and without sensation. The time needed for freezing varies with the

FREEZE TIME GUIDELINES

Cryosurgery involves use of the appropriate freeze time for the particular type of lesion to be removed. This table shows the times needed to freeze various types of skin lesions.

Keep in mind that if the freeze time noted yields insufficient coverage, allow the area to thaw after being frozen the first time, and then refreeze. Subsequent refreezing obtains deeper penetration of the cold.

Type of lesion	Freeze time (in seconds)
Actinic keratosis	90
Condyloma acuminata	45
Lentigines (freckles)	10 to 15
Molluscum contagiosum	25 to 30
Papular nevi	30 to 45
Sebaceous hyperplasia	30 to 45
Seborrheic keratosis	30
Skin tags and polyps	30 to 45
Verruca plantaris (plantar warts; after debridement)	30 to 40

type of skin lesion. (See *Freeze time guidelines*.)

The procedure is contraindicated in patients with a sensitivity or adverse reaction to cryosurgery, in patients who won't accept the possibility of skin pigment changes, in areas that have compromised circulation or a great deal of hair (cryosurgery destroys hair follicles), and for lesions that require pathologic evaluation. It may also be contraindicated in patients with collagen disorders, ulcerative colitis, glomerulonephritis, high cryoglobulin levels, and for those taking high-dose corticosteroids.

Equipment

Sterile drapes • sterile gloves • tissue freezing kit, nitrous oxide cryosurgery unit or liquid nitrogen • 4″ × 4″ gauze pads soaked with water • antiseptic skin cleaner such as povidone-iodine • cotton-tipped applicators • water-soluble lubricant such as K-Y gel • topical antibiotic such as triple antibiotic ointmen • dry 4″ × 4″ gauze pads • tape

Essential steps

▶ Explain the procedure to the patient and address questions or concerns he may have.
▶ Assess the patient for allergies, particularly to iodine and latex.

▶ Obtain informed consent.
▶ Position the patient comfortably with the lesion easily accessible.
▶ Clean the area with antiseptic skin cleaner.
▶ Drape the lesion, and put on gloves.
▶ Soak a cotton-tipped applicator in the liquid nitrogen.
▶ Apply the liquid to the lesion slowly to avoid splattering. The size of the cotton-tipped applicator and the amount of pressure affect how quickly and how deeply the area will freeze.
▶ Alternatively, you may use a Cryogun with a probe or spray-tipped nozzle to deliver the liquid nitrogen.
▶ Stop freezing when you have an ice ball extending $1/8$″ beyond the lesion's boundaries.
▶ Apply a topical antibiotic.
▶ Cover the area with dry gauze and tape.

Complications

▶ Increased susceptibility to photo-damage
▶ Infection (rare)
▶ Ischemia
▶ Pigment changes

Special considerations

▶ Choose the appropriate cryosurgical tip for the shape and depth of the lesion.
▶ Use caution when treating the palmar surface of the hand because cutaneous sensory nerves run superficially in the hands. If a nerve is affected, the patient usually recovers within 6 weeks. When freezing an area adjacent to a nerve, apply traction and advise the patient that sensory loss may occur.
▶ Refer the patient to a dermatologist for mucosal and periorbital cryosurgery because they require shorter freezing times and may produce excessive swelling that may be esthetically and functionally disabling.

Patient teaching

▶ Advise the patient to keep the skin clean and dry. Explain the role of skin in defending the body against infection. Emphasize hygiene, sparing application of antibiotic ointment to the site, and the importance of keeping the site covered.
▶ Tell him which normal changes to expect, including immediate redness, swelling, and blisters in 16 to 36 hours that decrease within 72 hours. Explain that crusting occurs within 72 hours and resolves within 1 week.
▶ Tell him that in that area, the skin may become lighter or the hair less plentiful but that only minimal scarring should occur. Advise him to wear sunscreen on that area in particular.
▶ If sensory nerves were affected, reassure the patient that recovery typically occurs within 2 months.
▶ Tell him to follow up in 3 to 4 weeks for evaluation and, possibly, retreatment.

●●● RED FLAG *Tell the patient to call* **●●●** *his primary care provider for signs of infection, such as increasing redness, swelling, pain, and warmth; cloudy yellow, green, or brown drainage; opening of wound; foul odor; a red streak from the site; and fever after 24 hours.*

10
Drug hazards
Preventing and treating adverse effects

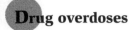rug overdoses

GENERAL GUIDELINES

If your patient has signs of acute drug toxicity, institute advanced life support measures as indicated. Administer the prescribed antidote, if available, and institute measures to block absorption and speed elimination of the drug. Consult with a regional poison control center for additional information about treatment of specific toxins. Early intervention will help prevent serious toxicity. The steps below outline how to manage an acute overdose of ingested systemic drugs.

Starting advanced life support

▶ Establish and maintain an airway. This is usually done by inserting an oropharyngeal or endotracheal airway.
▶ If the patient isn't breathing, start ventilation with a bag-valve mask until a mechanical ventilator is available. Administer oxygen based on readings from pulse oximetry or arterial blood gas levels.
▶ Maintain circulation. Start an I.V. infusion, and obtain laboratory specimens to assess for toxic drug levels, electrolytes, and glucose levels, as indicated.
For hypotension: Administer fluids and vasopressors such as dopamine (Intropin).
For hypertension: Prepare to administer antihypertensive agents (usually beta blockers if catecholamines were ingested). Prepare to treat arrhythmias as indicated for the specific toxin.
▶ Protect the patient from injury, and monitor for seizures. Observe the patient, and provide supportive care. Prepare to administer lorazepam, diazepam, or phenytoin.

Administering the antidote

The antidote is administered as soon as possible. Administer the prescribed antidote according to the class of drugs the patient has taken. (See *Managing poisoning or overdose.*)

Blocking drug absorption

▶ Gastric emptying is effective up to 2 hours after drug ingestion. Two methods are used: syrup of ipecac for a conscious patient who isn't expected to deteriorate and gastric lavage for a comatose patient.
▶ Adsorption with activated charcoal is most effective when administered early, within 30 to 60 minutes of acute poisoning. It's used in place of emesis or lavage if the drug is well adsorbed by activated charcoal or after emesis or lavage to adsorb co-ingestants if the primary toxin isn't well adsorbed by activated charcoal.
▶ A cathartic may be given to speed transit of the poison through the GI tract. Whole-bowel irrigation with a balanced polyethylene glycol and electrolyte solution may be ordered if a sustained-release product was ingested.

Speeding drug elimination

▶ Activated charcoal can be administered in timed doses for 1 to 2 days. The charcoal binds to the drug, thus facilitating its removal in feces.
▶ Diuresis is effective for some drug overdoses. Forced diuresis uses furosemide and osmotic diuretics, alkaline diuresis uses I.V. sodium bicarbonate, and acid diuresis uses oral or I.V. ascorbic acid or ammonium chloride.

(Text continues on page 381.)

MANAGING POISONING OR OVERDOSE

Antidote and indications | **Nursing considerations**

ACETYLCYSTEINE (MUCOMYST, MUCOSIL, PARVOLEX)

▶ Treatment of acetaminophen toxicity

▶ Use cautiously in elderly or debilitated patients and in patients with asthma or severe respiratory insufficiency.
▶ Don't use with activated charcoal.
▶ Don't combine with amphotericin B, ampicillin, chymotrypsin, erythromycin lactobionate, hydrogen peroxide, oxytetracycline, tetracycline, iodized oil, or trypsin. Administer separately.
▶ Don't give to semiconscious or unconscious patients.

ACTIVATED CHARCOAL (ACTIDOSE-AQUA, CHARCOAID, CHARCOCAPS, LIQUI-CHAR)

▶ Treatment of poisoning or overdose with most orally administered drugs, except caustic agents and hydrocarbons

▶ If possible, administer within 30 to 60 minutes of poisoning. Administer larger dose if patient has food in his stomach.
▶ Don't give with syrup of ipecac because charcoal inactivates ipecac. If a patient needs syrup of ipecac, give charcoal after he has finished vomiting.
▶ Don't give in ice cream, milk, or sherbet because they reduce adsorption capacities of charcoal.
▶ Powder form is most effective. Mix with tap water to form a thick syrup. You may add a small amount of fruit juice or flavoring to make the syrup more palatable.
▶ You may need to repeat the dose if the patient vomits shortly after administration.

AMINOCAPROIC ACID (AMICAR)

▶ Antidote for alteplase, anistreplase, streptokinase, or urokinase toxicity

▶ Use cautiously with hormonal contraceptives and estrogens because they may increase the risk of hypercoagulability.
▶ For infusion, dilute solution with sterile water for injection, normal saline solution, dextrose 5% in water (D_5W), or Ringer's solution.
▶ Monitor coagulation studies, heart rhythm, and blood pressure.

AMYL NITRITE

▶ Antidote for cyanide poisoning

▶ Amyl nitrite is effective within 30 seconds, but its effects last only 3 to 5 minutes.
▶ To administer, wrap ampule in cloth and crush. Hold near the patient's nose and mouth so that he can inhale vapor.
▶ Monitor the patient for orthostatic hypotension.
▶ The patient may experience headache after administration.

ATROPINE SULFATE

▶ Antidote for anticholinesterase toxicity

▶ Atropine sulfate is contraindicated for patients with glaucoma, myasthenia gravis, obstructive uropathy, or unstable cardiovascular status.
▶ Monitor intake and output to assess for urine retention.

(continued)

MANAGING POISONING OR OVERDOSE *(continued)*

Antidote and indications	Nursing considerations

BOTULISM ANTITOXIN, TRIVALENT EQUINE

▶ Treatment of botulism

▶ Obtain an accurate patient history of allergies, especially to horses, and of reactions to immunizations.
▶ Test the patient for sensitivity (against a control of normal saline solution in opposing extremity) before administration. Read results after 5 to 30 minutes. A wheal indicates a positive reaction, requiring patient desensitization.
▶ Keep epinephrine 1:1,000 available in case of allergic reaction.

DEFEROXAMINE MESYLATE (DESFERAL)

▶ Adjunctive treatment of acute iron intoxication

▶ Don't administer the drug to patients with severe renal disease or anuria. Use cautiously in patients with impaired renal function.
▶ Keep epinephrine 1:1,000 available in case of allergic reaction.
▶ Use I.M. route if possible. Use I.V. route only when the patient is in shock.
▶ To reconstitute for I.M. administration, add 2 ml of sterile water for injection to each ampule. Make sure the drug dissolves completely. To reconstitute for I.V. administration, dissolve as for I.M. use but in normal saline solution, D_5W, or lactated Ringer's solution.
▶ Monitor intake and output carefully. Warn patient that his urine may turn red.
▶ Reconstituted solution can be stored for up to 1 week at room temperature. Protect from light.

DIGOXIN IMMUNE FAB (OVINE) (DIGIBIND)

▶ Treatment of potentially life-threatening digoxin intoxication

▶ Use cautiously in patients allergic to ovine proteins because the drug is derived from digoxin-specific antibody fragments obtained from immunized sheep. Perform skin test before administering.
▶ Use only in patients in shock or cardiac arrest with ventricular arrhythmias such as ventricular tachycardia or fibrillation; with progressive bradycardia, such as severe sinus bradycardia; or with second- or third-degree atrioventricular block unresponsive to atropine.
▶ Infuse through a 0.22-micron membrane filter, if possible.
▶ Refrigerate powder for reconstitution. If possible, use reconstituted drug immediately, although you may refrigerate it for up to 4 hours.
▶ Drug interferes with digoxin immunoassay measurements, resulting in misleading standard serum digoxin levels until the drug is cleared from the body (about 2 days).
▶ Total serum digoxin levels may rise after administration of this drug, reflecting fat-bound (inactive) digoxin.
▶ Monitor potassium levels closely.

MANAGING POISONING OR OVERDOSE *(continued)*

Antidote and indications	Nursing considerations

EDETATE CALCIUM DISODIUM (CALCIUM DISODIUM VERSENATE, CALCIUM EDTA)

▶ Treatment of lead poisoning in patients with blood levels > 50 mcg/dl	▶ Don't give to patients with severe renal disease or anuria. ▶ Avoid using I.V. route in patients with lead encephalopathy because intracranial pressure may increase; use I.M. route. ▶ Avoid rapid infusion; I.M. route is preferred, especially for children. ▶ If giving a high dose, give with dimercaprol to avoid toxicity. ▶ Force fluids to facilitate lead excretion except in patients with lead encephalopathy. ▶ Before giving, obtain baseline intake and output, urinalysis, blood urea nitrogen, and serum alkaline phosphatase, calcium, creatinine, and phosphorus levels. Then monitor these values on first, third, and fifth days of treatment. Monitor electrocardiogram periodically. ▶ If procaine hydrochloride has been added to I.M. solution to minimize pain, watch for local reaction.

METHYLENE BLUE

▶ Treatment of cyanide poisoning	▶ Don't give to patients with severe renal impairment or hypersensitivity to drug. ▶ Use with caution in glucose-6-phosphate dehydrogenase deficiency; may cause hemolysis. ▶ Avoid extravasation; S.C. injection may cause necrotic abscesses. ▶ Warn the patient that methylene blue will discolor his urine and stools and stain his skin. Hypochlorite solution rubbed on skin will remove stains.

NALOXONE HYDROCHLORIDE (NARCAN)

▶ Treatment of respiratory depression caused by opioid drugs ▶ Treatment of postoperative opioid depression ▶ Treatment of asphyxia neonatorurn caused by administration of opioid analgesics to the mother in late labor	▶ Use cautiously in patients with cardiac irritability or opioid addiction. ▶ Monitor respiratory depth and rate. Be prepared to provide oxygen, ventilation, and other resuscitative measures. ▶ Duration of opioid may exceed that of naloxone, causing the patient to relapse into respiratory depression and requiring repeated administration. ▶ You may administer drug by continuous I.V. infusion to control adverse effects of epidurally administered morphine. ▶ You may see "overshoot" effect—the patient's respiratory rate after receiving drug exceeds his rate before respiratory depression occurred. ▶ Naloxone is the safest drug to use when the cause of respiratory depression is uncertain. ▶ This drug doesn't reverse respiratory depression caused by diazepam. The reversal agent for benzodiazepines is flumazenil. ▶ Although generally believed ineffective in treating respiratory depression caused by nonopioid drugs, naloxone may reverse coma induced by alcohol intoxication.

(continued)

MANAGING POISONING OR OVERDOSE *(continued)*

Antidote and indications **Nursing considerations**

PRALIDOXIME CHLORIDE (PROTOPAM CHLORIDE)

▶ Antidote for organophosphate poisoning and cholinergic drug overdose

▶ Don't give to patients poisoned with carbaryl (Sevin), a carbamate insecticide, because it increases Sevin's toxicity.
▶ Use with caution in patients with renal insufficiency, myasthenia gravis, asthma, or peptic ulcer.
▶ Use in hospitalized patients only; have respiratory and other supportive equipment available.
▶ Administer antidote as soon as possible after poisoning. Treatment is most effective if started within 24 hours of exposure.
▶ Before administering, suction secretions and make sure airway is patent.
▶ Dilute drug with sterile water without preservatives. Give atropine along with pralidoxime.
▶ If the patient's skin was exposed, remove his clothing and wash his skin and hair with sodium bicarbonate, soap, water, and alcohol as soon as possible. He may need a second washing. When washing the patient, wear protective gloves and clothes to avoid exposure.
▶ Observe the patient for 48 to 72 hours after he ingested poison. Delayed absorption may occur. Watch for signs of rapid weakening in the patient with myasthenia gravis being treated for overdose of cholinergic drugs. He may pass quickly from cholinergic crisis to myasthenic crisis and require more cholinergic drugs to treat the myasthenia. Keep edrophonium available.

PROTAMINE SULFATE

▶ Treatment of heparin overdose

▶ Use cautiously after cardiac surgery.
▶ Administer slowly to reduce adverse reactions. Have equipment available to treat shock.
▶ Monitor the patient continuously, and check vital signs frequently.
▶ Watch for spontaneous bleeding (heparin "rebound"), especially in patients undergoing dialysis and in those who have had cardiac surgery.
▶ Protamine sulfate may act as an anticoagulant in extremely high doses.

MANAGING POISONING OR OVERDOSE *(continued)*

Antidote and indications | **Nursing considerations**

SYRUP OF IPECAC (IPECAC SYRUP)

▶ Induction of vomiting in poisoning

▶ Syrup of ipecac is contraindicated for semicomatose, unconscious, and severely inebriated patients and for those with seizures, shock, or absent gag reflex.
▶ Don't give after ingestion of petroleum distillates or volatile oils because of the risk of aspiration pneumonitis. Don't give after ingestion of caustic substances, such as lye, because further injury can result.
▶ Before giving, make sure you have ipecac syrup, not ipecac fluid extract (14 times more concentrated, and deadly).
▶ If two doses don't induce vomiting, consider gastric lavage.
▶ If the patient also needs activated charcoal, give charcoal after he has vomited, or charcoal will neutralize the emetic effect.
▶ The American Academy of Pediatrics (AAP) no longer recommends that parents should keep a bottle of syrup of ipecac in the home because it can be improperly administered and has been abused by persons with eating disorders such as bulimia. AAP recommends that parents keep the universal poison control telephone number (1-800-222-1222) posted by their telephone.

▶ Peritoneal dialysis and hemodialysis are occasionally used in severe overdose.

ANTIDOTES IN POISONING OR OVERDOSE

Institute advanced life support measures as indicated for acute drug toxicity. Consult with a regional poison control center for information on how to treat ingestion of a specific toxin and administer the appropriate antidote.

ACETAMINOPHEN OVERDOSE

In an acute acetaminophen overdose, plasma levels of 300 µg/ml 4 hours after ingestion or 50 µg/ml 12 hours after ingestion are associated with hepatotoxicity. Clinical findings in an overdose include cyanosis, anemia, jaundice, skin eruptions, fever, emesis, central nervous system (CNS) stimulation, delirium, and methemoglobinemia progressing to CNS depression, coma, vascular collapse, seizures, and death. Acetaminophen poisoning develops in stages:
▶ *Stage 1 (12 to 24 hours after ingestion):* nausea, vomiting, diaphoresis, anorexia
▶ *Stage 2 (24 to 48 hours after ingestion):* clinically improved but elevated liver function test results
▶ *Stage 3 (72 to 96 hours after ingestion):* peak hepatotoxicity
▶ *Stage 4 (7 to 8 days after ingestion):* recovery.

To treat acetaminophen toxicity, administer activated charcoal preferably within 1 hour of ingestion. Oral acetylcysteine, a specific antidote for acetaminophen poisoning, is most effective if started within 12 hours after ingestion but can help if started as late as 24 hours after ingestion. Administer an oral loading dose of acetylcysteine, followed by oral maintenance doses every 4 hours for an additional 17 doses. Doses vomited within 1 hour of administration must be repeated. Remove charcoal by lavage before administering acetylcysteine because it may interfere with this antidote's absorption.

Acetylcysteine minimizes hepatic injury by supplying sulfhydryl groups that bind with acetaminophen metabolites. Hemodialysis may be helpful in removing acetaminophen from the body. Syrup of ipecac isn't recommended for acetaminophen overdose. Monitor laboratory parameters and vital signs closely. Provide symptomatic and supportive measures (respiratory support and correction of fluid and electrolyte imbalances). Determine plasma acetaminophen levels at least 4 hours after overdose. If they indicate hepatotoxicity, perform liver function tests every 24 hours for at least 96 hours.

ANALEPTIC OVERDOSE

Individual responses to overdose with analeptic drugs, such as amphetamines or cocaine, vary widely. Toxic doses also vary, depending on the drug and the route of ingestion.

●●● **RED FLAG** *Signs and symptoms*
●●● *of analeptic overdose include restlessness, tremor, hyperreflexia, tachypnea, confusion, aggressiveness, hallucinations, and panic; fatigue and depression usually follow the excitement stage. Other effects may include arrhythmias, shock, altered blood pressure, nausea, vomiting, diarrhea, and abdominal cramps; death is usually preceded by seizures and coma.*

Treat analeptic overdose symptomatically and supportively: If oral ingestion is recent (within 4 hours), use gastric lavage or syrup of ipecac to empty the stomach and reduce further absorption. Follow with activated charcoal. Monitor vital signs and fluid and electrolyte balance. If the drug was smoked or injected, focus on enhancing drug elimination and providing supportive care. Administer sedatives as needed. Urine acidification may enhance excretion. A saline cathartic (magnesium citrate) may hasten GI evacuation of unabsorbed sustained-release drug.

ANTICHOLINERGIC OVERDOSE

●●● **RED FLAG** *Clinical effects of an*
●●● *anticholinergic overdose include such peripheral effects as blurred vision; dilated, nonreactive pupils; decreased or absent bowel sounds; dry mucous membranes; dysphagia; flushed, hot, dry skin; hypertension; hyperthermia; increased respiratory rate; urine retention; and tachycardia.*

Treatment is primarily symptomatic and supportive as needed. If the patient is alert, induce emesis (or use gastric lavage), and follow with a saline cathartic and activated charcoal to prevent further drug absorption. In severe cases, physostigmine may be administered to block central antimuscarinic effects. Give fluids as needed to treat shock. If urine retention occurs, catheterization may be necessary.

ANTICOAGULANT OVERDOSE

●●● **RED FLAG** *Clinical effects of an*
●●● *oral anticoagulant overdose vary with severity. They may include internal or external bleeding or skin necrosis, but the most common sign is hematuria.*

Excessively prolonged prothrombin time or minor bleeding mandates withdrawal of therapy; withholding one or two doses may be adequate in some cases.

Treatment to control bleeding may include oral or I.V. phytonadione (vitamin K_1) and, in severe hemorrhage, fresh frozen plasma or whole blood. Menadione (vitamin K_3) isn't as effective. Use of phytonadione may interfere with subsequent oral anticoagulant therapy.

ANTIHISTAMINE OVERDOSE

●●● **RED FLAG** *Drowsiness is the*
●●● *usual clinical sign of antihistamine overdose. Seizures, coma, and respiratory depression may occur with severe overdose.*

Certain histamine antagonists — such as diphenhydramine — also block cholinergic receptors and produce modest anticholinergic symptoms, such as dry mouth, flushed skin, fixed and dilated pupils, and GI symptoms, especially in children. Phenothiazine-type antihistamines such as promethazine also block dopamine receptors. Movement disorders mimicking Parkinson's disease may be seen.

Treat overdose with gastric lavage followed by activated charcoal. Syrup of ipecac generally isn't recommended because acute dystonic reactions may increase the risk of aspiration. In addition, phenothiazine-type antihistamines may have antiemetic effects. Treat hypotension with fluids or vasopressors, and treat seizures with phenytoin or diazepam. Watch for arrhythmias, and treat accordingly.

BARBITURATE OVERDOSE

●●● **RED FLAG** *A barbiturate over-*
●●● *dose causes unsteady gait,* *slurred speech, sustained nystagmus, somnolence, confusion, respiratory depression, pulmonary edema, areflexia, and coma. Typical shock syndrome with tachycardia and hypo-tension, jaundice, hypothermia followed by fever, and oliguria may occur.*

Maintain and support ventilation and pulmonary function as necessary; support cardiac function and circulation with vasopressors and I.V. fluids as needed. If the patient is conscious and the gag reflex is intact, induce emesis (if ingestion was recent) by administering syrup of ipecac. If emesis is contraindicated, perform gastric lavage while a cuffed endotracheal tube is in place to prevent aspiration. Follow with administration of activated charcoal and saline cathartic. Measure intake and output, vital signs, and laboratory parameters; maintain body temperature. The patient should be rolled from side to side every 30 minutes to avoid pulmonary congestion. Alkalinization of urine may be helpful in removing the drug from the body; hemodialysis may be useful in severe overdose.

BENZODIAZEPINE OVERDOSE

●●● **RED FLAG** *An overdose of benzo-*
●●● *diazepines produces somnolence, confusion, coma, hypoactive reflexes, dyspnea, labored breathing, hypotension, bradycardia, slurred speech, and unsteady gait or impaired coordination.*

Support blood pressure and respiration until drug effects subside; monitor vital signs. Mechanical ventilatory assistance via an endotracheal (ET) tube may be required to maintain a patent airway and support adequate oxygenation. Flumazenil, a specific benzodiazepine antagonist, may be useful. Use I.V. fluids or vasopressors, such as dopamine and phenylephrine, to treat hypotension as needed. If the patient is conscious and his gag reflex is intact, induce emesis (if ingestion was recent) by administering syrup of ipecac.

If emesis is contraindicated, perform gastric lavage while a cuffed ET tube is in place to prevent aspiration. After emesis or lavage, administer activated charcoal with a cathartic as a single dose. Dialysis is of limited value.

CARDIAC GLYCOSIDE OVERDOSE

Clinical effects of a cardiac glycoside overdose are primarily related to the GI, cardiovascular, and central nervous systems.

■■■ **RED FLAG** *Severe cardiac glyco-*
■■■ *side overdose may cause hyper-kalemia, which may develop rapidly and result in life-threatening cardiac effects.*

Cardiac signs of digoxin toxicity may occur with or without other toxicity signs and commonly precede other toxic effects. Because cardiotoxic effects can also occur in heart disease, determining whether these effects result from an underlying heart disease or digoxin toxicity may be difficult. Digoxin has caused almost every kind of arrhythmia; various combinations of arrhythmias may occur in the same patient. Patients with chronic digoxin toxicity commonly have ventricular arrhythmias, atrioventricular (AV) conduction disturbances, or both. Patients with digoxin-induced ventricular tachycardia have a high mortality because ventricular fibrillation or asystole may result.

If toxicity is suspected, the drug should be discontinued and serum drug level measurements obtained. Usually, the drug takes at least 6 hours to be distributed between plasma and tissue and reach equilibrium; plasma levels drawn earlier may show higher digoxin levels than those present after the drug is distributed into the tissues.

Other treatment measures include immediate emesis induction, gastric lavage, and administration of activated charcoal to reduce absorption of the remaining drug. Multiple doses of activated charcoal may help reduce further absorption, especially of a drug undergoing enterohepatic recirculation. Some clinicians advocate cholestyramine administration if digoxin was recently ingested; however, this may not be useful if the ingestion is life-threatening. Interacting drugs probably should be discontinued.

Ventricular arrhythmias may be treated with I.V. potassium (replacement doses; but not in patients with significant AV block), I.V. phenytoin, I.V. lidocaine, or I.V. propranolol. Refractory ventricular tachyarrhythmias may be controlled with overdrive pacing. Procainamide may be used for ventricular arrhythmias that don't respond to the above treatments. In severe AV block, asystole, and hemodynamically significant sinus bradycardia, atropine restores a normal rate.

Administration of digoxin-specific antibody fragments (digoxin immune Fab [Digibind]) treats life-threatening digoxin toxicity. Each 40 mg of digoxin immune Fab binds about 0.6 mg of digoxin in the bloodstream. The complex is then excreted in the urine, rapidly decreasing serum levels and therefore cardiac drug concentrations.

CNS DEPRESSANT OVERDOSE

■■■ **RED FLAG** *Signs of central ner-*
■■■ *vous system (CNS) depressant*

overdose include prolonged coma, hypotension, hypothermia followed by fever, and inadequate ventilation even without significant respiratory depression. Absence of pupillary reflexes, dilated pupils, loss of deep tendon reflexes, tonic muscle spasms, and apnea may occur.

Treatment of CNS depressant overdose involves support of respiratory and cardiovascular function; mechanical ventilation may be necessary. Maintain adequate urine output with adequate hydration while avoiding pulmonary edema. Empty gastric contents by inducing emesis. For lipid-soluble drugs such as glutethimide, charcoal and resin hemoperfusion are effective in removing the drug; hemodialysis and peritoneal dialysis are of minimal value. Because of the significant storage of glutethimide in fat tissue, blood levels commonly show large fluctuations with worsening of symptoms.

IRON SUPPLEMENT OVERDOSE

RED FLAG *Symptoms of poisoning result from iron's acute corrosive effects on the GI mucosa as well as the adverse metabolic effects caused by iron overload.*

LIFE SPAN *Iron supplements represent a major source of poisoning, especially in small children. In fact, as little as 1 g of ferrous sulfate can kill an infant.*

Four stages of acute iron poisoning have been identified, and signs and symptoms may occur within the first 10 to 60 minutes of ingestion or may be delayed several hours.

The *first* findings reflect acute GI irritation and include epigastric pain, nausea, and vomiting. Diarrhea may present as green, followed by tarry stools, and then as melena.

Hematemesis may be accompanied by drowsiness, lassitude, shock, and coma. Local erosion of the stomach and small intestine may further enhance the absorption of iron. If death doesn't occur in the first phase, a *second* phase of apparent recovery may last 24 hours.

A *third* phase, which can occur 4 to 48 hours after ingestion, is marked by central nervous system abnormalities, metabolic acidosis, hepatic dysfunction, renal failure, and bleeding diathesis. This may progress to circulatory failure, coma, and death.

If the patient survives, the *fourth* phase consists of late complications of acute iron intoxication and may occur 2 to 6 weeks after overdose. Pyloric and duodenal stenosis may cause gastric outlet obstruction resulting in persistent vomiting.

Patients who develop vomiting, diarrhea, leukocytosis, or hyperglycemia and have an abdominal X-ray positive for iron within 6 hours of ingestion are likely to be at risk for serious toxicity. Empty the stomach by inducing emesis with syrup of ipecac, and perform gastric lavage.

If patients have had multiple episodes of vomiting or the vomitus contains blood, avoid ipecac and perform lavage. Some clinicians add sodium bicarbonate to the lavage solution to convert ferrous iron to ferrous carbonate, which is poorly absorbed. Disodium phosphate has also been used; however, some children may develop life-threatening hyperphosphatemia or hypercalcemia. Other possible treatments include lavage with normal saline solution, administration of a saline cathartic, surgical removal of tablets, and chelation therapy with deferoxamine mesylate. Hemodialysis is of little value. Supportive treatment includes monitoring acid-base balance, maintaining a patent airway, and controlling shock and dehydration with appropriate I.V. therapy.

NONSTEROIDAL ANTI-INFLAMMATORY DRUG OVERDOSE

●●● **RED FLAG** *Clinical manifesta-*
●●● *tions of overdose with non-steroidal anti-inflammatory drugs include dizziness, drowsiness, pares-thesia, vomiting, nausea, abdomi-nal pain, headache, sweating, nys-tagmus, apnea, and cyanosis.*

To treat an ibuprofen overdose, empty the stomach at once by in-ducing emesis with syrup of ipecac or gastric lavage. Administer acti-vated charcoal by nasogastric tube. Provide symptomatic and support-ive measures, including respiratory support and correction of fluid and electrolyte imbalances. Monitor lab-oratory tests and vital signs closely. Alkaline diuresis may enhance renal excretion. Dialysis is of minimal value because ibuprofen is strongly protein-bound.

OPIATE OVERDOSE

Rapid I.V. administration of opiates may result in overdose because of the delay in maximum central ner-vous system (CNS) effect (30 min-utes).

●●● **RED FLAG** *The most common*
●●● *signs of morphine overdose are respiratory depression with or with-out CNS depression and miosis (pin-point pupils). Other acute toxic effects include hypotension, brady-cardia, hypothermia, shock, apnea, cardiopulmonary arrest, circulatory collapse, pulmonary edema, and seizures.*

To treat acute overdose: First, es-tablish adequate respiratory ex-change via a patent airway and

ventilation as needed; then admin-ister an opioid antagonist (nalox-one) to reverse respiratory depres-sion. (Because the duration of ac-tion of morphine is longer than that of naloxone, repeated doses of naloxone are necessary.) Naloxone shouldn't be given unless clinically significant respiratory or cardiovas-cular depression is present. Monitor vital signs closely.

If the patient presents within 2 hours of an oral overdose, empty the stomach immediately by induc-ing emesis (with syrup of ipecac) or using gastric lavage. Use caution to avoid risk of aspiration. Administer activated charcoal via a nasogastric tube for further removal of the drug in an oral overdose.

Provide symptomatic and support-ive treatment (continued respiratory support and correction of fluid or electrolyte imbalance). Monitor lab-oratory parameters, vital signs, and neurologic status closely.

PHENOTHIAZINE OVERDOSE

●●● **RED FLAG** *Central nervous sys-*
●●● *tem depression due to phenoth-iazine overdose is characterized by deep, unarousable sleep and possible coma, hypotension or hypertension, extrapyramidal symptoms, abnormal involuntary muscle movements, agi-tation, seizures, arrhythmias, electro-cardiogram changes, hypothermia or hyperthermia, and autonomic ner-vous system dysfunction.*

Treatment is symptomatic and supportive, including maintaining vital signs, a patent airway, stable body temperature, and fluid and electrolyte balance. Don't induce vomiting; phenothiazines inhibit the cough reflex, so aspiration may oc-cur. Use gastric lavage and then ac-tivated charcoal and saline cathar-tics. Dialysis doesn't help. Regulate body temperature as needed. Treat hypotension with I.V. fluids; don't give epinephrine. Treat seizures with parenteral diazepam or barbiturates, arrhythmias with parenteral phenytoin, and extrapyramidal reactions with benztropine or parenteral diphenhydramine.

SALICYLATE OVERDOSE

RED FLAG *Clinical effects of salicylate overdose include metabolic acidosis with respiratory alkalosis, hyperpnea, tachypnea, seizures, tetany and cardiovascular, respiratory, and renal collapse.*

To treat aspirin overdose, empty the patient's stomach immediately by inducing emesis with syrup of ipecac if the patient is conscious, or by gastric lavage. Administer activated charcoal via a nasogastric tube. Provide symptomatic and supportive measures (respiratory support and correction of fluid and electrolyte imbalances). Closely monitor laboratory values and vital signs. Enhance renal excretion by administering sodium bicarbonate to alkalinize urine. Use a cooling blanket or sponging if the patient's rectal temperature is above 104° F (40° C). Hemodialysis is effective in removing aspirin but is used only in severe poisoning or in those at risk for pulmonary edema.

TRICYCLIC ANTIDEPRESSANT OVERDOSE

RED FLAG *An overdose of tricyclic antidepressants is commonly life-threatening, particularly when combined with alcohol.*

The first 12 hours after ingestion are a stimulatory phase characterized by excessive anticholinergic activity (agitation, irritation, confusion, hallucinations, hyperthermia, parkinsonian symptoms, seizures,

urine retention, dry mucous membranes, pupillary dilation, constipation, and ileus). This phase precedes central nervous system (CNS) depressant effects, including hypothermia, decreased or absent reflexes, sedation, hypotension, cyanosis, and cardiac irregularities, including tachycardia, conduction disturbances, and quinidine-like effects on the electrocardiogram.

The severity of an overdose is best indicated by a widening of the QRS complex, which usually represents severe toxicity; obtaining serum measurements usually isn't helpful. Metabolic acidosis may follow hypotension, hypoventilation, and seizures.

Treatment is symptomatic and supportive, including maintaining a patent airway, stable body temperature, and fluid and electrolyte balance. Induce emesis if the patient is conscious; follow with gastric lavage and activated charcoal to prevent further absorption. Dialysis is of little use. Treat seizures with parenteral diazepam or phenytoin, arrhythmias with parenteral phenytoin or lidocaine, and acidosis with sodium bicarbonate. Don't give barbiturates; they may enhance CNS and respiratory depressant effects.

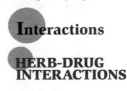

Interactions

HERB-DRUG INTERACTIONS

Herbs can interact with drugs and produce undesirable — even hazardous — effects. Such interactions can decrease therapeutic efficacy or cause toxicity. (See *Effects of herb-drug interactions*, pages 388 to 396.)

(Text continues on page 396.)

EFFECTS OF HERB-DRUG INTERACTIONS

Herb	Drug	Possible effects
Aloe (dried juice from leaf)	Antiarrhythmics, cardiac glycosides	Ingestion of aloe juice may lead to hypokalemia, which may potentiate cardiac glycosides and antiarrhythmics.
	Licorice, thiazide diuretics, other potassium-wasting drugs such as corticosteroids	May cause additive effect of potassium wasting with thiazide diuretics and other potassium-wasting drugs.
	Orally administered drugs	May decrease absorption of drugs because of more rapid GI transit time.
	Stimulant laxatives	May increase risk of potassium loss.
Bilberry	Anticoagulants, antiplatelets	Decreases platelet aggregation.
	Hypoglycemics, insulin	May increase serum insulin levels, causing hypoglycemia; additive effect with diabetes drugs.
Capsicum	Angiotensin-converting enzyme (ACE) inhibitors	May cause cough.
	Anticoagulants, antiplatelets	Decreases platelet aggregation and increases fibrinolytic activity, prolonging bleeding time.
	Antihypertensives	May interfere with antihypertensives by increasing catecholamine secretion.
	Aspirin, other nonsteroidal anti-inflammatory drugs (NSAIDs)	Stimulates GI secretions to help protect against NSAID-induced GI irritation.
	Central nervous system (CNS) depressants, such as barbiturates, benzodiazepines, opioids	Increases sedative effect.
	Cocaine	Concomitant use (including exposure to capsicum in pepper spray) may increase effects of cocaine and risk of adverse reactions, including death.
	Histamine-2 (H_2) blockers, proton-pump inhibitors	Decreases effects resulting from the increased catecholamine secretion by capsicum.

EFFECTS OF HERB-DRUG INTERACTIONS *(continued)*

Herb	Drug	Possible effects
Capsicum *(continued)*	Hepatically metabolized drugs	May increase hepatic metabolism of drugs by increasing glucose-6-phosphate dehydrogenase and adipose lipase activity.
	Monoamine oxidase inhibitors (MAOIs)	May decrease effectiveness because of increased acid secretion by capsicum.
	Theophylline	Increases absorption of theophylline, possibly leading to higher serum levels or toxicity.
Chamomile	Anticoagulants	Warfarin constituents may enhance anticoagulant therapy and prolong bleeding time.
	Drugs requiring GI absorption	May delay drug absorption.
	Drugs with sedative properties such as benzodiazepines	May cause additive effects and adverse reactions.
	Iron	Tannic acid content may reduce iron absorption.
Echinacea	Hepatotoxics	Hepatotoxicity may increase with drugs known to elevate liver enzyme levels.
	Immunosuppressants	Echinacea may counteract immunosuppressant drugs.
	Warfarin	Increases bleeding time without increased International Normalized Ratio (INR).
Evening primrose	Anticonvulsants	Lowers seizure threshold.
	Antiplatelets, anticoagulants	Increases risk of bleeding and bruising.
Feverfew	Anticoagulants, antiplatelets	May decrease platelet aggregation and increase fibrinolytic activity.

(continued)

EFFECTS OF HERB-DRUG INTERACTIONS *(continued)*

Herb	Drug	Possible effects
Garlic	Anticoagulants, antiplatelets	Enhances platelet inhibition, leading to increased anticoagulation.
	Antihyperlipidemics	May have additive lipid-lowering properties.
	Antihypertensives	May cause additive hypotension.
	Cyclosporine	May decrease effectiveness of cyclosporine. May induce metabolism and decrease cyclosporine to subtherapeutic levels; may cause rejection.
	Hormonal contraceptives	May decrease efficacy of contraceptives.
	Insulin, other drugs causing hypoglycemia	May increase serum insulin levels, causing hypoglycemia, an additive effect with antidiabetics.
	Nonnucleotide reverse transcriptase inhibitors	May affect metabolism of these drugs.
	Saquinavir	Decreases saquinavir levels, causing therapeutic failure and increased viral resistance.
Ginger	Anticoagulants, antiplatelets	Inhibits platelet aggregation by antagonizing thromboxane synthetase and enhancing prostacyclin, leading to prolonged bleeding time.
	Antidiabetics	May interfere with diabetes therapy because of hypoglycemic effects.
	Antihypertensives	May antagonize antihypertensive effect.
	Barbiturates	May enhance barbiturate effects.
	Calcium channel blockers	May increase calcium uptake by myocardium, leading to altered drug effects.
	Chemotherapy	May reduce nausea associated with chemotherapy.

EFFECTS OF HERB-DRUG INTERACTIONS *(continued)*

Herb	Drug	Possible effects
Ginger *(continued)*	H_2-blockers, proton-pump inhibitors	May decrease effectiveness because of increased acid secretion by ginger.
Ginkgo	Anticoagulants, antiplatelets	May enhance platelet inhibition, leading to increased anticoagulation.
	Anticonvulsants	May decrease effectiveness of anticonvulsants.
	Drugs known to lower seizure threshold	May further reduce seizure threshold.
	Insulin	Ginkgo leaf extract can alter insulin secretion and metabolism, affecting blood glucose levels.
	Thiazide diuretics	Ginkgo leaf may increase blood pressure.
Ginseng	Alcohol	Increases alcohol clearance, possibly by increasing activity of alcohol dehydrogenase.
	Anabolic steroids, hormones	May potentiate effects of hormone and anabolic steroid therapies. Estrogenic effects of ginseng may cause vaginal bleeding and breast nodules.
	Antibiotics	Siberian ginseng may enhance effects of some antibiotics.
	Anticoagulants, antiplatelets	Decreases platelet adhesiveness.
	Antidiabetics	May enhance blood glucose–lowering effects.
	Antipsychotics	Because of CNS stimulant activity, avoid use with antipsychotics.
	Digoxin	May falsely elevate digoxin levels.
	Furosemide	May decrease diuretic effect with furosemide.
	Immunosuppressants	May interfere with immunosuppressive therapy.

(continued)

EFFECTS OF HERB-DRUG INTERACTIONS *(continued)*

Herb	Drug	Possible effects
Ginseng *(continued)*	MAOIs	Potentiates action of MAOIs. May cause insomnia, headache, tremors, and hypomania.
	Stimulants	May potentiate stimulant effects.
	Warfarin	Causes antagonism of warfarin, resulting in a decreased INR.
Goldenseal	Antihypertensives	Large amounts of goldenseal may interfere with blood pressure control.
	CNS depressants, such as barbiturates, benzodiazepines, opioids	Increases sedative effect.
	Diuretics	Causes additive diuretic effect.
	General anesthetics	May potentiate hypotensive action of general anesthetics.
	Heparin	May counteract anticoagulant effect of heparin.
	H_2-blockers, proton-pump inhibitors	May decrease effectiveness because of increased acid secretion by goldenseal.
Grapeseed	Warfarin	Increases effects and INR because of tocopherol content of grapeseed.
Green tea	Acetaminophen, aspirin	May increase effectiveness of these drugs by as much as 40%.
	Adenosine	May inhibit hemodynamic effects of adenosine.
	Beta-adrenergic agonists (albuterol, isoproterenol, metaproterenol, terbutaline)	May increase the cardiac inotropic effect of these drugs.
	Clozapine	May cause acute exacerbation of psychotic symptoms.
	Disulfiram	Increases risk of adverse effects of caffeine; decreases clearance and increases half-life of caffeine.

EFFECTS OF HERB-DRUG INTERACTIONS *(continued)*

Herb	Drug	Possible effects
Green tea *(continued)*	Hormonal contraceptives	Decreases clearance by 40% to 65%. Increases effects and adverse effects.
	Lithium	Abrupt caffeine withdrawal increases lithium levels; may cause lithium tremor.
	MAOIs	Large amounts of green tea may precipitate hypertensive crisis.
	Mexiletine	Decreases caffeine elimination by 50%. Increases effects and adverse effects.
	Verapamil	Increases plasma caffeine levels by 25%. Increases effects and adverse effects.
	Warfarin	Causes antagonism resulting from vitamin content of green tea.
Kava	Alcohol	Potentiates depressant effect of alcohol and other CNS depressants.
	Benzodiazepines	Use with benzodiazepines has resulted in comalike states.
	CNS stimulants or depressants	May hinder therapy with CNS stimulants.
	Hepatotoxic drugs	May increase risk of liver damage.
	Levodopa	Decreases effectiveness because of dopamine antagonism by kava.
Licorice	Antihypertensives	Decreases effect of antihypertensive therapy. Large amounts of licorice cause sodium and water retention and hypertension.
	Aspirin and other NSAIDs	May provide protection against damage to GI mucosa induced by aspirin or other NSAIDs.
	Corticosteroids	Causes additive and enhanced effects of the corticosteroids.

(continued)

EFFECTS OF HERB-DRUG INTERACTIONS *(continued)*

Herb	Drug	Possible effects
Licorice *(continued)*	Digoxin	Licorice causes hypokalemia, which predisposes to digoxin toxicity.
	Hormonal contraceptives	Increases fluid retention and potential for increased blood pressure resulting from fluid overload.
	Hormones	Interferes with estrogen or antiestrogen therapy.
	Insulin	Causes hypokalemia and sodium retention when used together.
	Spironolactone	Decreases effects of spironolactone.
Melatonin	CNS depressants, such as barbiturates, benzodiazepines, opioids	Increases sedative effect.
	Fluoxetine	Improves sleep in some patients with major depressive disorder.
	Fluvoxamine	May significantly increase melatonin levels; may decrease melatonin metabolism.
	Immunosuppressants	May stimulate immune function and interfere with immunosuppressive therapy.
	Isoniazid	May enhance effects of isoniazid against some *Mycobacterium* species.
	Nifedipine	May decrease effectiveness of nifedipine; increases heart rate.
	Verapamil	Increases melatonin excretion.
Milk thistle	Drugs causing diarrhea	Increases bile secretion; commonly causes loose stools. May increase effect of other drugs commonly causing diarrhea. May have liver membrane-stabilization and antioxidant effects, leading to protection from liver damage from various hepatotoxic drugs, such as acetaminophen, phenytoin, ethanol, phenothiazines, and butyrophenones.

EFFECTS OF HERB-DRUG INTERACTIONS *(continued)*

Herb	Drug	Possible effects
Nettle	Anticonvulsants	May increase sedative adverse effects; may increase risk of seizure.
	Anxiolytics, hypnotics, opioids	May increase sedative adverse effects.
	Iron	Tannic acid content may reduce iron absorption.
	Warfarin	Antagonism resulting from vitamin K content of aerial parts of nettle.
Passion flower	CNS depressants, such as barbiturates, benzodiazepines, opioids	Increases sedative effect.
St. John's wort	5-hydroxytryptamine agonists (triptans)	Increases risk of serotonin syndrome.
	Alcohol, opioids	Enhances the sedative effect of opioids and alcohol.
	Anesthetics	May prolong effect of anesthesia drugs.
	Barbiturates	Decreases barbiturate-induced sleep time.
	Cyclosporine	Decreases cyclosporine levels below therapeutic levels, threatening transplanted organ rejection.
	Digoxin	May reduce serum digoxin concentrations, decreasing therapeutic effects.
	Human immunodeficiency virus protease inhibitors (PIs); indinavir; nonnucleoside reverse transcriptase inhibitors (NNRTIs)	Induces cytochrome P-450 metabolic pathway, which may decrease therapeutic effects of drugs using this pathway for metabolism. Use of St. John's wort and PIs or NNRTIs should be avoided because of the potential for subtherapeutic antiretroviral levels and insufficient virologic response that could lead to resistance or class cross-resistance.

(continued)

EFFECTS OF HERB-DRUG INTERACTIONS *(continued)*

Herb	Drug	Possible effects
St. John's wort *(continued)*	Hormonal contraceptives	Increases breakthrough bleeding when taken with hormonal contraceptives; decreases serum levels and effectiveness of contraceptives.
	Irinotecan	Decreases serum irinotecan levels by 50%.
	Iron	Tannic acid content may reduce iron absorption.
	MAOIs, nefazodone, selective serotonin reuptake inhibitors (SSRIs), trazodone	Causes additive effects with SSRIs, MAOIs, and other antidepressants, potentially leading to serotonin syndrome, especially when combined with SSRIs.
	Photosensitizing drugs	Increases photosensitivity.
	Reserpine	Antagonizes effects of reserpine.
	Sympathomimetic amines such as pseudoephedrine	Causes additive effects.
	Theophylline	May decrease serum theophylline levels, making the drug less effective.
	Warfarin	May alter INR. Reduces effectiveness of anticoagulant, requiring increased dosage of drug.
Valerian	Alcohol	Claims no risk for increased sedation with alcohol, although debated.
	CNS depressants, sedative hypnotics	Enhances effects of sedative hypnotic drugs.
	Iron	Tannic acid content may reduce iron absorption.

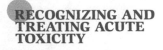

RECOGNIZING AND TREATING ACUTE TOXICITY

Treatment of substance abuse is a long-term process commonly beset with relapses. You need to understand the signs and symptoms of toxicity before you can take steps to help the patient recover from his addiction. (See *Managing acute toxicity.*)

(Text continues on page 403.)

MANAGING ACUTE TOXICITY

Substance	Signs and symptoms	Interventions

ALCOHOL (ETHANOL)

▶ Beer and wine ▶ Distilled spirits ▶ Other preparations, such as cough syrup, aftershave, mouthwash	▶ Alcohol breath odor ▶ Ataxia ▶ Bradycardia ▶ Coma ▶ Hypotension ▶ Hypothermia ▶ Nausea and vomiting ▶ Respiratory depression ▶ Seizures	▶ Induce vomiting or perform gastric lavage if ingestion occurred in the previous 4 hours. Give activated charcoal and a saline cathartic. ▶ Start I.V. fluid replacement and administer dextrose 5% in water, thiamine, B-complex vitamins, and vitamin C to prevent dehydration and hypoglycemia and to correct nutritional deficiencies. ▶ Institute safety measures to protect the patient from injury. ▶ Give an anticonvulsant such as diazepam to control seizures. ▶ Watch the patient for signs and symptoms of withdrawal, such as hallucinations and alcohol withdrawal delirium. If these occur, consider giving chlordiazepoxide, chloral hydrate, or paraldehyde. (Be sure to administer paraldehyde with a glass syringe or glass cup to avoid a chemical reaction with plastic.) ▶ Auscultate the patient's lungs frequently to detect crackles or rhonchi, possibly indicating aspiration pneumonia. If you note these breath sounds, consider antibiotics. ▶ Monitor the patient's neurologic status and vital signs every 15 minutes until he is stable. Assist with dialysis if his vital functions are severely depressed.

AMPHETAMINES

▶ Amphetamine sulfate (Benzedrine): bennies, greenies, cartwheels ▶ Dextroamphetamine sulfate (Dexedrine): dexies, hearts, oranges ▶ Methamphetamine: speed, meth, crystal	▶ Altered mental status (from confusion to paranoia) ▶ Coma ▶ Diaphoresis ▶ Dilated reactive pupils ▶ Dry mouth ▶ Exhaustion ▶ Hallucinations ▶ Hyperactive deep tendon reflexes ▶ Hypertension	▶ If the drug was taken orally, induce vomiting or perform gastric lavage; give activated charcoal and a sodium or magnesium sulfate cathartic. ▶ Lower the patient's urine pH to 5 by adding ammonium chloride or ascorbic acid to his I.V. solution. ▶ Force diuresis by giving the patient mannitol. ▶ Give a short-acting barbiturate such as pentobarbital to control stimulant-induced seizures.

(continued)

MANAGING ACUTE TOXICITY *(continued)*

Substance	Signs and symptoms	Interventions

AMPHETAMINES (continued)

| | ▶ Hyperthermia
▶ Shallow respirations
▶ Tachycardia
▶ Tremors and seizure activity | ▶ Institute safety measures to protect the patient from injury, especially if he's paranoid or hallucinating.
▶ Give haloperidol I.M. to treat agitation or assaultive behavior.
▶ Give an alpha-adrenergic blocker such as phentolamine for hypertension.
▶ Watch for cardiac arrhythmias. If these develop, consider propranolol to treat tachyarrhythmias or lidocaine to treat ventricular arrhythmias.
▶ Treat hyperthermia with tepid sponge baths or a hypothermia blanket.
▶ Provide a quiet environment to avoid overstimulation.
▶ Be alert for signs and symptoms of withdrawal, such as abdominal tenderness, muscle aches, and long periods of sleep.
▶ Observe suicide precautions, especially if the patient shows signs of withdrawal. |

ANTIPSYCHOTICS

| ▶ Chlorpromazine (Thorazine)
▶ Phenothiazines
▶ Thioridazine (Mellaril) | ▶ Constricted pupils
▶ Decreased deep tendon reflexes
▶ Decreased level of consciousness (LOC)
▶ Dry mouth
▶ Dysphagia
▶ Extrapyramidal effects (dyskinesia, opisthotonos, muscle rigidity, ocular deviation)
▶ Hypotension
▶ Hypothermia or hyperthermia
▶ Photosensitivity
▶ Respiratory depression
▶ Seizures
▶ Tachycardia | ▶ Expect to perform gastric lavage if the patient ingested the drug within the past 6 hours. (Don't induce vomiting because phenothiazines have an antiemetic effect.) Consider activated charcoal and a cathartic.
▶ Give diphenhydramine to treat extrapyramidal effects.
▶ Give physostigmine to reverse anticholinergic effects in severe cases.
▶ Replace fluids I.V. to correct hypotension; monitor the patient's vital signs frequently.
▶ Monitor his respiratory rate, and give supplemental oxygen to treat respiratory depression.
▶ Give an anticonvulsant such as diazepam or a short-acting barbiturate such as pentobarbital sodium to control seizures.
▶ Keep the patient's room dark to avoid exacerbating his photosensitivity. |

MANAGING ACUTE TOXICITY *(continued)*

Substance	Signs and symptoms	Interventions

ANXIOLYTIC SEDATIVE-HYPNOTICS

▶ Benzodiazepines (Valium, Librium)	▶ Coma ▶ Confusion ▶ Decreased reflexes ▶ Drowsiness ▶ Hypotension ▶ Seizures ▶ Shallow respirations ▶ Stupor	▶ Induce vomiting or perform gastric lavage; consider activated charcoal and a cathartic. ▶ Give supplemental oxygen to correct hypoxia-induced seizures. ▶ Replace fluids I.V. to correct hypotension; monitor the patient's vital signs frequently. ▶ For benzodiazepine overdose, or to reverse the effect of benzodiazepine-induced sedation or respiratory depression, give flumazenil (Romazicon).

BARBITURATE SEDATIVE-HYPNOTICS

▶ Amobarbital sodium (Amytal sodium): blue angels, blue devils, blue birds ▶ Phenobarbital (Luminal): phennies, purple hearts, goofballs ▶ Secobarbital sodium (Seconal): reds, red devils	▶ Blisters or bullous lesions ▶ Cyanosis ▶ Depressed LOC (from confusion to coma) ▶ Flaccid muscles and absent reflexes ▶ Hyperthermia or hypothermia ▶ Hypotension ▶ Nystagmus ▶ Poor pupil reaction to light ▶ Respiratory depression	▶ Induce vomiting or perform gastric lavage if the patient ingested the drug within 4 hours; consider activated charcoal and a saline cathartic. ▶ Maintain his blood pressure with I.V. fluid challenges and vasopressors. ▶ If the patient has taken a phenobarbital overdose, give sodium bicarbonate I.V. to alkalinize his urine and speed the drug's elimination. ▶ Apply a hyperthermia or hypothermia blanket to help return the patient's temperature to normal. ▶ Prepare your patient for hemodialysis if toxicity is severe. ▶ Perform frequent neurologic assessments, and check your patient's pulse rate, temperature, skin color, and reflexes frequently. ▶ Notify the physician if you see signs of respiratory distress or pulmonary edema. ▶ Watch for signs and symptoms of withdrawal, such as hyperreflexia, tonic-clonic seizures, and hallucinations. Provide symptomatic relief of withdrawal symptoms. ▶ Institute safety measures to protect the patient from injury.

(continued)

MANAGING ACUTE TOXICITY *(continued)*

Substance	Signs and symptoms	Interventions

COCAINE

▶ Cocaine hydrochloride: crack, freebase	▶ Abdominal pain ▶ Alternating euphoria and apprehension ▶ Coma ▶ Confusion ▶ Dilated pupils ▶ Fever ▶ Hyperexcitability ▶ Hyperpnea ▶ Hypertension or hypotension ▶ Nausea and vomiting ▶ Pallor or cyanosis ▶ Perforated nasal septum or mouth sores ▶ Respiratory arrest ▶ Spasms and seizures ▶ Tachycardia ▶ Tachypnea ▶ Visual, auditory, and olfactory hallucinations	▶ Calm the patient by talking to him in a quiet room. ▶ If cocaine was ingested, induce vomiting or perform gastric lavage; give activated charcoal. ▶ Give the patient a tepid sponge bath, and administer an antipyretic to reduce fever. ▶ Monitor his blood pressure and heart rate. Expect to give propranolol for symptomatic tachycardia. ▶ Administer an anticonvulsant such as diazepam to control seizures. ▶ Scrape the inside of his nose to remove residual amounts of the drug. ▶ Monitor his cardiac rate and rhythm — ventricular fibrillation and cardiac standstill can occur as a direct cardiotoxic result of cocaine ingestion. Defibrillate the patient, and initiate cardiopulmonary resuscitation, if indicated.

GLUTETHIMIDE

▶ Doriden: Ciba, CB (street names for drug)	▶ Apnea ▶ Central nervous system depression (from unresponsiveness to deep coma) ▶ Drowsiness ▶ Hypotension ▶ Hypothermia ▶ Impaired thought processes (memory, judgment, attention span) ▶ Irritability ▶ Nystagmus ▶ Paralytic ileus	▶ If the drug was taken orally, induce vomiting or perform gastric lavage; give activated charcoal and a cathartic. ▶ Maintain the patient's blood pressure with I.V. fluid challenges and vasopressors. ▶ Assist with hemodialysis or hemoperfusion if the patient has hepatic or renal failure or is in a prolonged coma. ▶ Administer an anticonvulsant, such as diazepam, for seizures. ▶ Perform hourly neurologic assessments: Coma may recur because of the drug's slow release from fat deposits.

MANAGING ACUTE TOXICITY *(continued)*

Substance	Signs and symptoms	Interventions

GLUTETHIMIDE (continued)

	‣ Poor bladder control ‣ Respiratory depression ‣ Small, reactive pupils ‣ Twitching, spasms, and seizures	‣ Be alert for signs of increased intracranial pressure, such as decreasing LOC and widening pulse pressure. Consider mannitol I.V. ‣ Watch for signs and symptoms of withdrawal, such as hyperreflexia, tonic-clonic seizures, and hallucinations, and provide symptomatic relief of withdrawal symptoms. ‣ Institute safety measures to protect the patient from injury.

HALLUCINOGENS

‣ Lysergic acid diethylamide (LSD): hawk, acid, sunshine ‣ Mescaline (peyote): mese, cactus, big chief	‣ Agitation and anxiety ‣ Depersonalization ‣ Dilated pupils ‣ Fever ‣ Flashback experiences ‣ Hallucinations ‣ Hyperactive movement ‣ Impaired judgment ‣ Increased heart rate ‣ Intensified perceptions ‣ Moderately increased blood pressure ‣ Synesthesia	‣ Reorient the patient repeatedly to time, place, and person. ‣ Institute safety measures to protect the patient from injury. ‣ Calm the patient by talking to him in a quiet room. ‣ If the drug was taken orally, induce vomiting or perform gastric lavage; give activated charcoal and a cathartic. ‣ Give diazepam I.V. to control seizures.

OPIOIDS

‣ Codeine ‣ Heroin: junk, smack, H, snow ‣ Hydromorphone hydrochloride (Dilaudid): D, lords ‣ Morphine: Mort, M, monkey, Emma	‣ Bradycardia ‣ Constricted pupils ‣ Depressed LOC (but the patient is usually responsive to persistent verbal or tactile stimuli)	‣ Give naloxone until the drug's CNS depressant effects are reversed. ‣ Replace fluids I.M. to increase circulatory volume. ‣ Correct hypothermia by applying extra blankets; if the patient's body temperature doesn't increase, use a hyperthermia blanket.

(continued)

MANAGING ACUTE TOXICITY *(continued)*

Substance	Signs and symptoms	Interventions

OPIOIDS (continued)

| | ▸ Hypotension
▸ Hypothermia
▸ Seizures
▸ Skin changes (pruritus, urticaria, flushed skin)
▸ Slow, deep respirations | ▸ Reorient the patient frequently.
▸ Auscultate the lungs frequently for crackles, possibly indicating pulmonary edema. (Onset may be delayed.)
▸ Administer oxygen via nasal cannula, mask, or mechanical ventilation to correct hypoxemia from hypoventilation.
▸ Monitor cardiac rate and rhythm, being alert for atrial fibrillation. (This should resolve when hypoxemia is corrected.)
▸ Be alert for signs of withdrawal, such as piloerection (goose flesh), diaphoresis, and hyperactive bowel sounds.
▸ Institute safety measures to protect the patient from injury. |

PHENCYCLIDINE (PCP)

| ▸ Angel dust, peace pill, hog | ▸ Amnesia
▸ Blank stare
▸ Cardiac arrest
▸ Decreased awareness of surroundings
▸ Drooling
▸ Gait ataxia
▸ Hyperactivity
▸ Hypertensive crisis
▸ Hyperthermia
▸ Muscle rigidity
▸ Nystagmus
▸ Recurrent coma
▸ Seizures
▸ Violent behavior | ▸ If the drug was taken orally, induce vomiting or perform gastric lavage; instill and remove activated charcoal repeatedly.
▸ Acidify the patient's urine with ascorbic acid to increase drug excretion.
▸ Expect to continue to acidify urine for 2 weeks because signs and symptoms may recur when fat cells release PCP stores.
▸ Give diazepam and haloperidol to control agitation or psychotic behavior.
▸ Institute safety measures to protect the patient from injury.
▸ Administer diazepam to control seizures.
▸ Institute seizure precautions.
▸ Provide a quiet environment and dimmed light.
▸ Give propranolol for hypertension and tachycardia, and give nitroprusside for severe hypertension.
▸ Closely monitor urine output and serial renal function tests. Rhabdomyolysis, myoglobinuria, and renal failure may occur in severe intoxication.
▸ If renal failure develops, prepare the patient for hemodialysis. |

Monitoring

THERAPEUTIC DRUG MONITOR- ING GUIDELINES

It's important to consider many is-sues when monitoring a patient on drug therapy, such as the drug's half-life; the patient's age, height, and weight; time required to estab-lish a steady-state dose; and the level of the drug in the patient's blood. The level of drug in a pa-tient's blood may help indicate whether the dosing regimen has achieved its therapeutic goals. Most drugs are metabolized in the liver and excreted in the kidneys. Some patients metabolize drugs quickly and their blood levels are inade-quate to produce the intended ther-apeutic effect. Others metabolize drugs slowly, and even ordinary doses can have toxic results.

Even with the optimum drug dosage, the patient is still at risk for adverse drug reactions, especially patients with cardiovascular, hepat-ic, and renal disease. It's important to monitor therapeutic drug levels and laboratory tests that may indi-cate potential adverse effects of the drug therapy. (See *Therapeutic drug monitoring guidelines*, pages 404 to 407.)

ADVERSE REACTIONS VS. AGE-RELATED CHANGES

The physiologic changes of aging make older adults more susceptible to drug-induced illnesses and ad-verse drug reactions than individu-als in other age-groups. The most serious reactions experienced by older adults result from such drugs as antiarrhythmics, anticholinergics, antihypertensives, benzodiazepines, cardiac glycosides, corticosteroids, diuretics, hypnotics and sedatives, and nonprescription drugs.

In older adults with chronic disor-ders, drug therapy can help extend and enhance the quality of life. Drugs are used to successfully man-age such disorders as arthritis, dia-betes mellitus, glaucoma, heart dis-ease, hypertension, and osteoporo-sis. However, the danger lies in concurrent use of multiple medica-tions to manage multiple disorders. It's important that adverse drug re-actions are identified and that the clinical findings aren't attributed to physiologic changes of aging. (See *Adverse reactions misinterpreted as age-related changes*, pages 408 and 409.)

THERAPEUTIC DRUG MONITORING GUIDELINES

Drug	Laboratory test monitored	Therapeutic ranges of test
Biguanides (metformin)	Creatinine	Men: 0.8 to 1.2 mg/dl (SI, 62 to 115 µmol/L) Women: 0.6 to 0.9 mg/dl (SI, 53 to 97 µmol/L)
	Fasting glucose	< 110 mg/dl (SI, < 6.1 mmol/L)
	Glycosylated he-moglobin (Hb)	4% to 6% of total Hb (SI, 0.04 to 0.06)
	Complete blood count (CBC)	*****
Digoxin	Digoxin	0.8 to 2 ng/ml (SI, 1.0 to 2.6 nmol/L)
	Electrolytes (especially potassium, magnesium, and calcium)	Potassium: 3.5 to 5 mEq/L (SI, 3.5 to 5 mmol/L) Magnesium: 1.3 to 2.1 mg/dl (SI, 0.65 to 1.05 mmol/L) Sodium: 135 to 145 mEq/L (SI, 135 to 145 mmol/L) Chloride: 100 to 108 mEq/L (SI, 100 to 108 mmol/L) Calcium: 8.2 to 10.2 mg/dl (SI, 2.05 to 2.54 mmol/L)
	Creatinine	0.8 to 1.2 mg/dl (SI, 62 to 115 µmol/L)
Erythropoietin	Hematocrit (HCT)	Women: 36% to 48% (SI, 0.36 to 0.48) Men: 42% to 52% (SI, 0.42 to 0.52)
Ethosuximide	Ethosuximide	40 to 100 mcg/ml (SI, 283 to 708 µmol/L)
Gemfibrozil	Lipids	Total cholesterol: < 200 mg/dl (SI, < 5.18 mmol/L) LDL (optimal): < 100 mg/dl (SI, < 2.59 mmol/L) HDL (desirable): ≥ 60 mg/dl (SI, ≥ 1.55 mmol/L) Triglycerides: < 150 mg/dl (SI, < 1.70 mmol/L)
Heparin	Partial thrombo-plastin time (PTT)	1.5 to 2 times control

Note: *** For those areas marked with five asterisks, these values can be used:**
Hemoglobin: women: 12 to16 g/dl (SI, 120 to 160 g/L); men: 14 to 17.4 g/dl (SI, 140 to 174 g/L)
Hematocrit: women: 36% to 48% (SI, 0.36 to 0.48); men: 42% to 52% (SI, 0.42 to 0.52)
Red blood cells (RBCs): 4.5 to 5.5 million/µl (SI, 4.5 to 5.5 × 10^{12}/L)
White blood cells: 4,000 to 10,000/µl (SI, 4 to 10 × 10^9/L)
Differential: neutrophils: 54% to 75% (SI, 0.54 to 0.75); eosinophils: 1% to 4% (SI, 0.01 to 0.04); basophils: 0% to 1% (SI, 0 to 0.01); monocytes: 2% to 8% (SI, 0.02 to 0.08); lymphocytes: 25% to 40% (SI, 0.25 to 0.4)

Monitoring guidelines

Check renal function and hematologic parameters before initiating therapy and at least annually thereafter. If the patient has impaired renal function, don't use metformin because it may cause lactic acidosis. Monitor the patient's response to therapy by periodically evaluating fasting glucose and glycosylated Hb levels. A patient's home monitoring of glucose levels helps monitor compliance and response.

Check digoxin levels at least 12 hours, but preferably 24 hours, after the last dose is administered. To monitor maintenance therapy, check drug levels at least 1 to 2 weeks after therapy is initiated or changed. Make adjustments in therapy based on the entire clinical picture, not solely on drug levels. Also, check electrolyte levels and renal function periodically during therapy.

After therapy is initiated or changed, monitor the HCT twice weekly for 2 to 6 weeks until stabilized in the target range and a maintenance dose is determined. Monitor HCT regularly thereafter.

Check drug level 8 to 10 days after therapy is initiated or changed.

Therapy is usually withdrawn after 3 months if the response is inadequate. The patient must be fasting to measure triglyceride levels.

When drug is given by continuous I.V. infusion, check PTT every 4 hours in the early stages of therapy. When drug is given by deep S.C. injection, check PTT 4 to 6 hours after injection.

---

* For those areas marked with one asterisk, these values can be used:
Alanine aminotransferase: 8 to 50 U/L (SI, 0.14 to 0.85 µkat/L)
Aspartate aminotransferase: men: 8 to 46 U/L (SI, 0.14 to 0.78 µkat/L); women: 7 to 34 U/L (SI, 0.12 to 0.58 µkat/L)
Lactate dehydrogenase: 60 to 220 U/L (SI, 1.9 to 3.6 µkat/L)
Gamma-glutamyl tranpeptidase: < 40 U/L (SI, < 0.51 µkat/L)
Total bilirubin: 0.2 to 1 mg/dl (SI, 3 to 22 µmol/L)

(continued)

THERAPEUTIC DRUG MONITORING GUIDELINES *(continued)*

Drug	Laboratory test monitored	Therapeutic ranges of test
HMG-CoA reductase inhibitors (fluvastatin, lovastatin, pravastatin, simvastatin)	Lipids Liver function tests	Total cholesterol: < 200 mg/dl (SI, < 5.18 mmol/L) LDL (optimal): < 100 mg/dl (SI, < 2.59 mmol/L) HDL (desirable): ≥ 60 mg/dl (SI, ≥ 1.55 mmol/L) Triglycerides: < 150 mg/dl (SI, < 1.7 mmol/L) *
Insulin	Fasting glucose Glycosylated Hb	< 110 mg/dl (SI, < 6.1 mmol/L) 4% to 6% of total Hb (SI, 0.04 to 0.06)
Phenytoin	Phenytoin CBC	10 to 20 mcg/ml (SI, 40 to 79 µmol/L) *****
Potassium chloride	Potassium	3.5 to 5 mEq/L (SI, 3.5 to 5 mmol/L)
Procainamide	Procainamide N-acetylpro-cainamide (NAPA) CBC	4 to 8 mcg/ml (SI, 17 to 42 µmol/L) (procainamide) 5 to 30 mcg/ml (combined procainamide and NAPA) *****
Theophylline	Theophylline	10 to 20 mcg/ml (SI, 44 to 111 µmol/L)
Thyroid hormone	Thyroid function tests	Thyroid-stimulating hormone: 0.3 to 5 mIU/L (SI, 0.3 to 5 mIU/L) T_3: 80 to 200 ng/dl (SI, 1.2 to 3 nmol/L) T_4: 5 to 13.5 mcg/dl (SI, 64.3 to 173.7 nmol/L)
Warfarin	International Normalized Ratio (INR)	For an acute myocardial infarction, atrial fibrillation, treatment of pulmonary embolism, prevention of systemic embolism, tissue heart valves, valvular heart disease, or prophylaxis or treatment of venous thrombosis: 2 to 3 (SI, 2 to 3) For mechanical prosthetic valves or recurrent systemic embolism: 2.5 to 3.5 (SI, 2.5 to 3.5)

Note: ***** For those areas marked with five asterisks, these values can be used:
Hemoglobin: women: 12 to16 g/dl (SI, 120 to 160 g/L); men: 14 to 17.4 g/dl (SI, 140 to 174 g/L)
Hematocrit: women: 36% to 48% (SI, 0.36 to 0.48); men: 42% to 52% (SI, 0.42 to 0.52)
Red blood cells (RBCs): 4.5 to 5.5 million/µl (SI, 4.5 to 5.5 × 10^{12}/L)
White blood cells: 4,000 to 10,000/µl (SI, 4 to 10 × 10^9/L)
Differential: neutrophils: 54% to 75% (SI, 0.54 to 0.75); eosinophils: 1% to 4% (SI, 0.01 to 0.04);
basophils: 0% to 1% (SI, 0 to 0.01); monocytes: 2% to 8% (SI, 0.02 to 0.08); lymphocytes: 25% to 40% (SI, 0.25 to 0.4)

Monitoring guidelines

Perform liver function tests at baseline, 6 to 12 weeks after therapy is initiated or changed, and periodically thereafter. If adequate response isn't achieved within 6 weeks, consider changing the therapy.

Monitor the patient's response to therapy by evaluating glucose and glycosylated Hb levels. Glycosylated Hb level is a good measure of long-term control. A patient's home monitoring of glucose levels helps measure compliance and response.

Monitor phenytoin levels immediately before the next dose and 2 to 4 weeks after therapy is initiated or changed. Obtain a CBC at baseline and monthly early in therapy. Watch for toxic effects at therapeutic levels. Adjust the measured level for hypoalbuminemia or renal impairment, which can increase free drug levels.

Check the level weekly after oral replacement therapy is initiated until stable and every 3 to 6 months thereafter.

Measure procainamide levels 6 to 12 hours after a continuous infusion is started or immediately before the next oral dose. Combined (procainamide and NAPA) levels can be used as an index of toxicity when renal impairment exists. Obtain CBC periodically during longer-term therapy.

Obtain theophylline levels immediately before the next dose of a sustained-release oral product and at least 2 days after therapy is initiated or changed.

Monitor thyroid function test results every 2 to 3 weeks until an appropriate maintenance dose is determined.

Check INR daily, beginning 3 days after therapy is initiated. Continue checking it until the therapeutic goal is achieved, and monitor it periodically thereafter. Also check the levels 7 days after a change in warfarin dose or concomitant, potentially interacting therapy.

---

* For those areas marked with one asterisk, these values can be used:
Alanine aminotransferase: 8 to 50 U/L (SI, 0.14 to 0.85 μkat/L)
Aspartate aminotransferase: men: 8 to 46 U/L (SI, 0.14 to 0.78 μkat/L); women: 7 to 34 U/L
  (SI, 0.12 to 0.58 μkat/L)
Lactate dehydrogenase: 60 to 220 U/L (SI, 1.9 to 3.6 μkat/L)
Gamma-glutamyl tranpeptidase: < 40 U/L (SI, < 0.51 μkat/L)
Total bilirubin: 0.2 to 1 mg/dl (SI, 3 to 22 μmol/L)

ADVERSE REACTIONS MISINTERPRETED AS AGE-RELATED CHANGES

In elderly patients, adverse drug reactions can easily be misinterpreted as the typical signs and symptoms of aging. The table below, which shows common adverse reactions for common drug classifications, can help you avoid such misinterpretations.

Drug classifications	Agitation	Anxiety	Arrhythmias	Ataxia	Changes in appetite	Confusion	Constipation	Depression	Difficulty breathing	
ACE inhibitors						●	●	●		
Alpha₁-adrenergic blockers		●					●	●		
Antianginals	●	●	●			●				
Antiarrhythmics			●				●		●	
Anticholinergics	●	●	●			●	●	●		
Anticonvulsants	●		●	●	●	●	●		●	
Antidepressants, tricyclic	●	●	●	●	●	●	●		●	
Antidiabetics, oral										
Antihistamines					●	●	●			
Antilipemics							●			
Antiparkinsonians	●	●		●		●	●	●		
Antipsychotics	●	●	●	●	●	●	●	●		
Barbiturates	●	●	●			●			●	
Benzodiazepines	●			●		●	●	●	●	
Beta-adrenergic blockers		●	●					●	●	
Calcium channel blockers		●	●				●		●	
Corticosteroids	●					●		●		
Diuretics						●				
NSAIDs		●				●	●	●		
Opioids	●	●				●	●	●	●	
Skeletal muscle relaxants	●	●		●		●		●		
Thyroid hormones			●		●					

	Disorientation	Dizziness	Drowsiness	Edema	Fatigue	Hypotension	Insomnia	Memory loss	Muscle weakness	Restlessness	Sexual dysfunction	Tremors	Urinary dysfunction	Visual changes
		●			●	●	●				●			●
		●	●	●	●	●	●				●		●	●
		●		●	●	●	●			●	●		●	●
		●		●	●									
	●	●	●		●	●		●	●	●			●	●
		●	●	●	●	●	●					●		●
	●	●	●		●	●	●			●	●		●	●
		●			●									
	●	●	●		●							●	●	●
		●			●		●		●		●		●	●
	●	●	●		●	●	●		●			●	●	●
		●	●		●	●	●			●	●	●	●	●
	●		●		●	●				●				
	●	●			●		●	●	●			●	●	●
		●			●	●	●	●				●	●	●
		●		●	●	●	●				●		●	●
				●	●		●		●					●
		●			●	●			●				●	
		●	●		●		●		●					●
	●	●	●		●	●	●	●		●	●		●	●
		●	●		●	●	●					●		
							●					●		

11

Health promotion

Maintaining health over the life span

Current atmosphere

PERFECT TIMING

In recent years, public interest in maintaining a healthy lifestyle has grown dramatically. More and more people are recognizing that their lifestyle directly affects their health. In fact, up to 50% of the deaths from the 10 leading causes of mortality in the United States can be linked to modifiable behaviors such as smoking. As a nurse practitioner, you can help your patients achieve a healthier lifestyle by promoting preventive care.

Guidelines by age

MATERNAL-NEONATAL HEALTH

Good antepartum care plays a key role in maternal and infant health. It can help decrease the risk of a patient delivering preterm or having a low-birth-weight baby, two predictors of infant morbidity and mortality. Ideally, a comprehensive prenatal program begins before conception and continues throughout the antepartum period — for example, prenatal vitamins should be started 3 months before conception. Initiating a comprehensive prenatal program gives you the chance to encourage healthy behaviors and prevent disease, such as teaching expectant mothers about proper nutrition and weight gain and the dangers of smoking, alcohol, caffeine, and illicit drugs. In addition, this kind of preparation allows early detection and treatment of problems.

⣿ RED FLAG *If the patient has a prior history of neural tube*
defects, the dose of the prenatal folic acid supplement is increased until the end of the first trimester.

Routine prenatal care should focus on the medical, psychosocial, educational, and nutritional needs of the patient and her family. During the initial prenatal visit, take a complete history and perform a comprehensive physical examination. Make sure the patient receives appropriate laboratory and diagnostic studies as well as comprehensive risk assessment. A patient with an uncomplicated pregnancy should generally visit your office every 4 weeks until 28 weeks' gestation, every 2 to 3 weeks until 36 weeks, and weekly thereafter until delivery. However, timing and the specific content of prenatal visits will vary depending on the risk status of the mother and fetus.

Nutrition

The pregnant patient needs to understand the crucial role of nutrition in maintaining a healthy pregnancy. Your assessment and counseling can help her deal with such common complaints as nausea and vomiting, pica (a craving for nonfood substances), lactose intolerance, and constipation. You can also help her understand the risks of high caffeine and sodium intake, alcohol and substance abuse, and inappropriate weight gain. Specifically, you can suggest that she:
▶ eat a well-balanced diet with sufficient protein, carbohydrates, vegetables, fresh fruits (she should wash and dry fruits before eating), and dairy products
▶ take daily vitamin and mineral supplements (ferrous iron and folic acid)
▶ restrict caffeine intake to no more than one cup of coffee, tea, or cola per day

● avoid eating raw or rare meat during pregnancy and practice good hand-washing technique when handling raw meat

● avoid soft cheeses, unpasteurized milk products, and deli meats that may potentially cause the foodborne illness listeriosis

● try to maintain an ideal weight gain during pregnancy (depending on body mass index, ideal weight gain can vary from 15 to 40 lb) by avoiding dieting, fasting, and skipping meals and refraining from overeating

● avoid excess salt intake, particularly during pregnancy, as it can elevate blood pressure.

Exercise

Although the pregnant patient shouldn't take part in rigorous exercise that causes extreme fatigue, such as prolonged jogging or skiing, she can safely take part in a program geared toward improving muscle strength and flexibility. Such a program may improve muscle tone and posture, which can help reduce some of the discomforts of pregnancy. If she has never exercised, she shouldn't begin a demanding exercise program during pregnancy.

Alcohol, tobacco, and drug use

One of your most important roles is offering the patient education and counseling about the dangers of alcohol, tobacco, and drugs.

Alcohol

Except for genetic factors, alcohol use during pregnancy ranks as the most common cause of mental retardation. Alcohol acts as a potent central nervous system depressant, and the effects of alcohol on the fetus include prenatal and postnatal growth deficiency, mental retardation, behavioral disturbances, and congenital defects such as craniofacial anomalies (fetal alcohol syndrome). Because it isn't known what level of alcohol can cause fetal malformations, tell the patient — whether pregnant or considering pregnancy — to avoid all alcohol.

Tobacco

Tobacco use in all forms during pregnancy — even breathing second-hand smoke — can result in a low-birth-weight infant. Using tobacco while breast-feeding an infant results in nicotine in breast milk. Suggest that your patient stop using tobacco immediately to avoid its adverse effects, including significant maternal and fetal morbidity.

Drugs

Marijuana is the third most commonly used recreational drug in pregnancy, following alcohol and tobacco. The active component of marijuana is a highly active psychotropic compound that's teratogenic in animal models. Although data about the drug's effects on pregnancy outcomes aren't conclusive, some studies suggest it may cause intrauterine growth retardation (IUGR) and increased prematurity. Most current data don't suggest an increased risk of major fetal anomalies, but you should still warn your patients against using marijuana during pregnancy.

Heroin and methadone, which are both addictive drugs, increase the risk of premature labor and delivery, IUGR, fetal distress, low birth weight, neonatal infection, and passage of meconium stool in utero when used during pregnancy. If your patient is taking either drug, refer her to a drug treatment program and an obstetrician experienced in managing pregnancies of patients with addictive disorders.

INFANT AND CHILD HEALTH

Infants and children need a comprehensive primary care program to help them grow into healthy adulthood. Each child in such a program should receive ongoing assessment of his growth and development, preventive care, well-child visits, and scheduled immunizations. (See *Immunization schedule for infants and children,* page 414.) The child's parents should also be taught about nutrition and exercise and guidelines on how to prevent injuries during the accident-prone childhood years.

Nutrition

To develop and grow normally, a child must have proper nutrition. A child grows very rapidly during the first 6 to 12 months and requires high-calorie, high-protein nutrition. Breast milk meets this need the best, but infant formula enriched with vitamins and minerals can also meet the infant's nutritional needs.

Breast-feeding

A healthy, well-nourished mother's breast milk can provide complete nutrition — including vitamins and micronutrients — for her infant during his first 4 to 6 months. For the first 1 to 2 months, the infant usually takes 2 to 3 oz of breast milk every 2 hours (10 to 15 minutes on each breast). After age 3 months, he may take 4 to 5 oz per feeding every 4 to 5 hours. At age 4 to 6 months, the child starts solid foods, but the mother can still breast-feed him.

Formula feeding

If the parents plan to bottle-feed their infant, they can choose from several commercially available iron-fortified infant formulas. Most are made from cow's milk or soy protein. For infants older than 6 months, the parents can choose a weaning formula, but these formulas don't seem to have an advantage over breast-feeding or iron-fortified infant formulas.

Tell the parents to follow the manufacturer's preparation and storage instructions. To prevent dental cavities, remind the parents not to prop the bottle.

Solid foods

Children can begin eating solid foods when they show normal development, usually between ages 4 and 6 months. When the child starts solid foods, suggest to the parents that they limit formula to no more than 32 oz (1 L) per day or slowly decrease the frequency of breast-feeding to supplement solid foods.

Suggest they start the child with one or two feedings per day, beginning with rice cereal and progressing to fruits, vegetables, and meats. They can gradually adjust the schedule so that it eventually matches the family's mealtimes. Tell them to introduce only one new solid food at a time and to wait from 3 to 5 days before adding another food; this allows the parents to note adverse reactions the child may have. Suggest they offer one-item foods instead of combination foods. Tell them to wait to introduce egg whites, wheat, and fish until the child is much older.

● ● ● **RED FLAG** *Caution parents not*
● ● ● *to feed grapes, peanuts, popcorn, hot dogs, raisins, hard candy, and pieces of raw carrots to children younger than age 4 because these foods are associated with choking in younger children.*

Exercise

Along with proper nutrition, children need healthy physical activity. Exercise can help children resist temptations, such as eating junk

IMMUNIZATION SCHEDULE FOR INFANTS AND CHILDREN

Before immunization, ask the parents if the child is receiving corticosteroids or other drugs that suppress the immune response or if he had a recent febrile illness. Obtain a history of allergic responses, especially to antibiotics, eggs, feathers, and past immunizations. Keep in mind that a child who's at risk for acquired immunodeficiency syndrome or who tests positive for human immunodeficiency virus infection may need special consideration.

After immunization, tell the parents to watch for and report reactions other than local swelling and pain and mild temperature elevation. Give them the child's immunization record. The following general vaccine recommendations for 2003 were approved by the Advisory Committee on Immunization Practices, the American Academy of Pediatrics, and the American Academy of Family Physicians for use in healthy infants and children.

Age	Immunization
Birth	Hepatitis B
1 to 4 months	Hepatitis B
2 months	Diphtheria, tetanus, and acelluler pertussis vaccine (DTaP), *Haemophilus influenzae* type B (HIB), inactivated poliovirus (IPV), pneumococcal
4 months	DTaP, HIB, IPV, pneumococcal
6 months	DTaP, HIB, pneumococcal
6 to 18 months	Hepatitis B, IPV
12 to 15 months	HIB, measles, mumps, and rubella (MMR), pneumococcal
12 to 18 months	Varicella
15 to 18 months	DTaP
4 to 6 years	DTaP, IPV, MMR
11 to 18 years	Tetanus and diphtheria toxoids

food, taking drugs, and taking part in illegal activities with peers. Suggest to parents that they help their children fill empty time with after-school activities, volunteerism, sports, and spending time with friends and family.

Suggest family walks after dinner or games, such as tag or basketball; even small changes in regular physical activity burn up calories. As the child gains muscle tone, loses baby fat, and becomes fit, he'll find such exercise less tiring.

Injury prevention

One of the greatest risks children face is the risk of accidental injury or death. The most common cause of accidental death is motor vehicle accidents followed, in order, by drowning, fires, and all burns. Falls, poisoning, aspiration, suffocation, and firearm accidents account for most of the remaining unintentional injuries or deaths in children.

In recent years, the emphasis has shifted from changing individual behaviors to changing the surroundings — for instance, requiring the use of seat belts for children — to make children safer. You can teach parents the importance of creating a safe environment for their children. Suggest that parents use the following guidelines from the American Academy of Pediatrics to help keep their children safe. Where appropriate, teach children how to keep themselves safe and healthy.

For infants and preschoolers

◗ Use infant and child car seats.
◗ Use home smoke detectors (change batteries twice yearly).
◗ Keep hot tap water temperatures at a safe level. Set your water heater no higher than 120° F (49° C).
◗ Install window screens and stairway guards or gates to prevent falls.
◗ Erect sturdy fences and safety guards around swimming pools.
◗ Don't use an infant walker.
◗ Use a crib with slats 2″ apart, with a firm, snug-fitting mattress; keep the sides of the crib raised.
◗ Empty water out of all buckets, tubs, and wading pools.
◗ Keep all drugs and household products marked poisonous out of reach of children.
◗ Keep up-to-date on immunizations.
◗ Place infants on their back to sleep.

◗ Use flame-resistant sleepwear.
◗ Never leave infants unattended in the care of young siblings.
◗ Don't drink hot liquids or smoke while holding an infant.
◗ Feed children age-appropriate foods, and offer age-appropriate toys for play.
◗ Watch infants at mealtimes and while they're in the bathtub or pool.
◗ Put sunscreen on children, and don't expose them to too much sun.
◗ Learn cardiopulmonary resuscitation (CPR).

For school-age children

◗ Use booster seats or seatbelts, depending on a child's age.
◗ Make sure children wear bicycle helmets.
◗ Insist on protective equipment for in-line skating and skateboarding.
◗ Install home smoke detectors.
◗ Follow pedestrian safety rules.
◗ Remove firearms from the home, or unload all guns and keep guns and ammunition locked in separate cabinets.
◗ Put sunscreen on children, and don't expose them to too much sun.
◗ Learn CPR.
◗ Teach children how and when to call 911.
◗ Assess the child's readiness for sexual development counseling by keeping lines of communication open.
◗ Discuss home safety rules about visitors, telephone use, and responses to fires and other emergencies.

ADOLESCENT HEALTH

Adolescents and adults are less likely to schedule wellness visits, so it's important to assess immunization status at each encounter (See *Immunization schedule for infants and children*). Tetanus and diphtheria toxoids (Td) is recommended for the adolescent as well as measles, mumps, and rubella vaccine (MMR), for those who didn't receive the second dose by age 6 years.

By the time they reach adolescence, many young people already have risk factors for chronic diseases that increase the risk of morbidity and mortality in adults. Obesity, for instance, is at an all-time high in children and adolescents. However, adolescents still have a chance to develop healthy habits that can carry into adulthood. School and after-school activities can still shape habits, and even the adolescent's keen awareness of body image can help. Obsession with body image can cause problems; dysfunctional body image is common by fifth grade, especially in girls. Parents, teachers, and health care providers can also use body image awareness to steer adolescents to healthier lifestyle choices.

Nutrition

Nutrition can pose a particular problem in adolescence, when eating disorders may become a problem. Recognizing and treating such disorders early on can prevent them from becoming critical. Here are some steps you can take.

▶ Encourage parents to make healthy foods readily available to their teenager, and to discourage foods high in sodium and added sugars.
▶ Teach the adolescent how to identify foods high and low in fat, saturated fat, and cholesterol. Teach him how to read food labels and evaluate diet claims.
▶ Teach the adolescent the importance of balancing food intake and physical activity; suggest three

meals per day and at least three half-hour exercise periods each week.
▶ Teach the adolescent the dangers of unsafe weight-loss methods (weight-cycling, decreased metabolism, electrolyte imbalance, and energy loss) and the benefits of a safe weight-loss program that includes three meals per day, nutritious snacks, and regular exercise.
▶ Help the adolescent examine what motivates good and bad eating habits. If he has an eating disorder, suggest keeping a food diary and recording the cues that affect eating behavior (for instance, mood, hunger, stress, or other persons). Refer him to counseling to develop alternative coping mechanisms.

Exercise

Healthy exercise patterns established in adolescence can carry into adulthood, resulting in a lower risk of such chronic diseases as hypertension and cardiovascular disease and lower mortality. Unfortunately, while more physically active than adults, many young people still don't engage in moderate or vigorous physical activity at least 3 days per week, and physical activity tends to decline steadily during adolescence.

You can take several steps to encourage adolescent patients to get the exercise they need. Suggest that they take part in activities with peers and friends. Remind parents that they can act as role models by keeping fit themselves and by arranging family activities that encourage fitness. Also, suggest that they provide appropriate sports equipment, take their children to sports and fitness programs, and make sure children have access to play areas; all of these actions help promote physical activity.

Education and counseling

Adolescents face many challenges and risks, from the risk of violence, to the temptation to smoke or take drugs, to the dangers of high-risk sexual behaviors. They need education and counseling to learn how to deal with these risks. You can start such teaching by offering some basic guidelines that all adolescents can follow.

▶ Listen to good friends and valued adults, and trust their feelings.

▶ Seek help if you frequently feel angry, depressed, or hopeless.

▶ Set reasonable but challenging goals for yourself.

▶ Learn how to handle peer pressure and how to say no.

▶ Respect the rights and needs of others, and be sure that yours are also respected.

Injury and violence prevention

Unintentional and intentional injuries are the leading cause of death for children and adolescents. Violence — particularly homicide — is the second leading cause of death in 15- to 24-year-olds. For every violence-related death, at least 100 people suffer nonfatal injuries. Young people who experience violence as victims, witnesses, or perpetrators suffer serious short-term and long-term consequences — cognitively, emotionally, and developmentally. Adolescents also face the risk of suicide — a risk that increases with age. Suicide ranks as one of the leading causes of death in 15- to 24-year-olds.

Suggest that adolescents use the following safety guidelines from the American Academy of Pediatrics:

▶ Use seat belts and follow speed limits.

▶ Avoid alcohol, especially while driving or participating in water-related sports.

▶ Wear motorcycle or bicycle helmets; use mouth guards and protective sports gear.

▶ Use protective equipment for in-line skating and skateboarding.

▶ Use personal flotation devices when boating.

▶ Use sunscreen and minimize exposure to the sun; avoid tanning salons.

▶ Learn cardiopulmonary resuscitation.

▶ Seek counseling from parents or other trusted adults for help with puberty issues and sexual development and behavior.

▶ Discuss home safety rules about visitors, telephone use, and responses to fires and other emergencies.

Smoking and substance use

Every year, 757,000 people younger than age 18 become regular smokers even though it's clear that using tobacco causes harm. If the current use of tobacco continues, it's estimated that 6.4 million children will die prematurely from tobacco use. You can help adolescents resist tobacco and drug use, using their interest in body image to help you.

▶ Remind teenagers that smoking causes yellow teeth, bad breath, wrinkles, and a stale smoke odor that clings to clothes and hair.

▶ State firmly that smoking, chewing tobacco, and use of alcohol, drugs, diet pills, or steroids will damage their health.

▶ Advise adolescents to avoid situations where drugs or alcohol are present.

High-risk sexual behaviors

Adolescents face danger from high-risk sexual behaviors. Consequences include adolescent pregnancy, sexually transmitted diseases, and human immunodeficiency virus infection. You can help adolescents prevent risk from sexual behaviors by encouraging

ADULT IMMUNIZATION SCHEDULE

The immunization schedule that appears below is recommended for adult patients older than age 18.

Vaccine	Timing and considerations
Hepatitis A for those at risk	Two doses 6 to 12 months apart to provide long-term protection; first dose 4 weeks before departure to endemic countries
Hepatitis B if never had initial series	Three doses: second dose at least 1 month after first; third dose 5 months after first dose
Measles, mumps, and rubella	Two doses 1 month apart if born after 1957 and immunity can't be proved
Tetanus-diphtheria if never had initial series	Three doses: second dose after 1 month, third dose 6 to 12 months after second; booster for all patients every 10 years
Varicella-zoster	Two doses for susceptible adults who haven't had chickenpox; second dose 1 month after first dose
Influenza (Flu)	Annually before flu season (September to December in the United States), especially for those ages 65 and older and those with heart or lung disease, diabetes, chronic conditions and those who work or live with high-risk individuals
Pneumococcal	One dose at age 65; also recommended for persons with chronic disease (see indications for influenza) and those with kidney disorders and sickle cell anemia; possibly a repeat dose 5 years later for those at highest risk; may be given anytime of the year

Adapted from the U.S. Department of Health and Human Services, U.S. Preventative Services Task Force (2003).

parents to talk openly with adolescent children and by counseling your adolescent patients about responsible sexual decision making.

ADULT HEALTH

Adult patients also need support to maintain health. As adults age, they face chronic diseases that can lead to earlier death, such as stroke and heart disease. They also face changes that decrease quality of life, such as chronic pain or decreased vision and hearing. You can help adult patients make lifestyle choices to improve their quality of life. Through proper nutrition and exercise, up-to-date immunizations and testing, and education and counseling, adults can continue to maintain a healthy lifestyle. (See *Adult immunization schedule* and *Adult health maintenance schedule*.)

ADULT HEALTH MAINTENANCE SCHEDULE

The health maintenance schedule that appears below is recommended for adult patients older than age 18.

Evaluations	Recommendations
SCREENINGS	
Blood pressure	‣ Each visit
Height, weight, skin assessment	‣ Annually
Cholesterol	‣ Men: every 5 years beginning at age 35 ‣ Women: every 5 years beginning at age 45 ‣ Begin at age 20 if cardiovascular risk is present (diabetes, family history of cardiovascular disease)
Fasting blood glucose (diabetes screening)	‣ Every 3 years; shorter intervals for high-risk persons, such as those with hypertension or hyperlipidemia
Hearing and vision	‣ Every 5 years and annually after age 50
Osteoporosis	‣ Annually, beginning at age 65; annually, beginning at age 60 for women at increased risk for osteoporotic fractures
CANCER DETECTION	
Breast ‣ Clinical breast examination	‣ Every year for women ages 40 and older ‣ Every 3 years for women ages 20 to 39
‣ Mammogram	‣ Every year for women ages 40 and older
‣ Breast self-examination	‣ Monthly for women ages 20 and older (optional)
Cervix ‣ Papanicolaou (Pap) test	‣ All women should begin cervical cancer screening 3 years after they begin to have vaginal intercourse, but no later then age 21 ‣ Annually for women beginning at age 21 ‣ Beginning at age 30, every 2 to 3 years after three or more consecutive satisfactory examinations with normal findings ‣ May stop in women age 70 and older with three or more consecutive examinations and no abnormal Pap test in the past 10 years

(continued)

ADULT HEALTH MAINTENANCE SCHEDULE *(continued)*

Evaluations	Recommendations

CANCER DETECTION *(continued)*

Endometrium
For all women at risk for hereditary nonpolyposis colon cancer

▶ Tissue sampling	▶ Annually, beginning at age 35

Colon and rectum (one of the examinations below)
For men and women ages 50 and older

▶ Fecal occult blood test (FOBT)	▶ Every year
▶ Flexible sigmoidoscopy	▶ Every 5 years
▶ FOBT plus flexible sigmoidoscopy	▶ FOBT every year plus flexible sigmoidoscopy every 5 years (preferred by clinicians over either of two alone)
▶ Colonoscopy	▶ Every 10 years
▶ Double-contrast barium enema	▶ Every 5 years

Prostate
For men ages 50 and older with life expectancy of at least 10 years and younger men at high risk at age 45

▶ Prostate-specific antigen	▶ Annually
▶ Digital rectal examination	▶ Annually

Testicular
▶ Testicular examination	▶ Annually
▶ Testicular self-examination	▶ Monthly, particularly for men between ages 15 and 40, who are at higher risk

COUNSELING

▶ Physical activity ▶ Nutrition (includes calcium intake and folic acid for women) ▶ Sun exposure ▶ Oral health ▶ Sexually transmitted diseases and human immunodeficiency virus infection ▶ Injury prevention and polypharmacy ▶ Chemoprevention (cardiovascular disease risk and aspirin therapy)	▶ Annually
▶ Smoking cessation, drug and alcohol use and abuse	▶ Every visit

Nutrition

To maintain proper nutrition, adult patients need to choose healthy foods to fit their needs. Teach patients how decreasing metabolism, a more sedentary lifestyle, and fat redistribution (all common with advancing age) affect the body. Emphasize the importance of nutritious food (including foods rich in antioxidants) in proper portions.

Exercise

Proper exercise plays a key role in weight control, muscle tone, physical endurance, glucose metabolism, and energy levels. Suggest to your adult patients that they exercise for at least 30 minutes three or more times per week. If they haven't exercised much before, suggest starting slowly to increase enjoyment and compliance and decrease discomfort. Recommend activities that also offer other rewards, such as biking with a friend, walking the dog, or joining a health club; studies show that physical activities that offer secondary rewards are more likely to become habits.

Education and counseling

Like younger patients, adults also need education and counseling. Specific areas include stress reduction, smoking and substance abuse, and sexual practices.

Stress reduction

Stress plays a significant role in many disorders, including hypertension, cardiac disease, GI upset, and constipation. Many adults try to relieve stress with methods that actually cause long-term harm — smoking, alcohol consumption, overeating, taking pills, or taking out their aggressions on someone else. You can help your patient by teaching him how the body and mind work together so that relaxing one helps relax the other.

Smoking and substance abuse

If your patient is a smoker, discuss the importance of smoking cessation at each visit. Discuss the different pharmacotherapy treatment options and refer the patient to a smoking cessation program.

Provide counseling for alcohol and substance abuse problems. Refer the patient and family to self-help groups such as Alcoholics Anonymous or Al-Anon. Treatment of substance abuse may require detoxification, and short- and long-term rehabilitation after follow-up care.

Sexual practices

Adults, like adolescents, are at risk for contracting sexually transmitted diseases (STDs). Although human immunodeficiency virus (HIV) infection occurs predominantly in persons ages 17 to 55, the incidence is rapidly increasing in people over age 50. This group may not have benefited from HIV-prevention education, which is mainly targeted at younger people. It's important to take a sexual history from older patients or to inquire about sexual activity. If the patient is sexually active, provide education and counseling related to prevention of STDs and HIV infection.

12
Complementary therapies
Enhancing and healing techniques

AROMATHERAPY

In aromatherapy, essential oils distilled from various plants are either inhaled or instilled to achieve various therapeutic effects. Aromatherapy is said to be effective in reducing stress, preventing disease, and even treating certain illnesses — physical as well as psychological.

Aromatherapy is popular in Europe, where essential oils are inhaled, massaged into the skin, or placed in bathwater to create pleasant sensations, promote relaxation, or treat specific ailments. Aromatherapy can be used — either alone or with such therapies as massage or herbal therapy — to treat bacterial and viral infections, anxiety, pain, muscle disorders, arthritis, herpes simplex, herpes zoster, skin disorders, premenstrual syndrome, headaches, and indigestion. When absorbed by body tissues, these oils are thought to interact with hormones and enzymes to produce changes in blood pressure, pulse rate, and other physiologic functions. (See *Therapeutic effects of essential oils,* page 424.)

Aromatherapy may be administered by a trained aromatherapist or self-administered. In the United States, where interest in aromatherapy has skyrocketed, several organizations train and certify people to self-administer and administer aromatherapy. These organizations can also provide information to interested laypeople and health care providers, referrals to aromatherapists, and sources for obtaining essential oils.

Although there's no scientific evidence indicating that aromatherapy prevents or cures disease, nurses trained in aromatherapy may recommend specific oils as adjuncts to conventional therapies, teach patients how to use them, and administer treatment themselves.

Equipment

Essential oil (or oils) • optional: carrier oil, massage table, towel, bowel of hot water, bathtub, diffuser, candle, ceramic ring

The optional supplies will vary according to the manner in which the oil is being administered — for example, by massage, inhalation, bath, or diffusion.

Implementation

▶ Massage requires a carrier oil and, for a full body massage, a massage table. Massage involves diluting the essential oil in the appropriate carrier oil and applying it to the exposed body part or the entire body using massage techniques.
▶ Inhalation requires a bowl of hot water and a large towel. The patient leans over a bowl of steaming water that contains a few drops of the essential oil. With the towel draped over his head and the bowl to concentrate the steam, the patient inhales the vapors for a few minutes.
▶ A bath requires a tub filled with warm water. The patient adds a few drops of essential oil to the surface of the bath water and then soaks in the tub for 10 to 20 minutes, inhaling the vapors as he soaks.
▶ Diffusion requires a micromist or candle diffuser or a ceramic ring that can be placed on a light bulb. This method involves placing a few drops of the essential oil in the diffuser and turning on the heat source to diffuse microparticles of the oil into the air. The average treatment is 30 minutes.

Special considerations

▶ Be aware that certain oils — such as basil, fennel, lemon grass, rosemary, and verbena — may cause irritation if the patient has sensitive

> ### CLINICAL PEARL
> # THERAPEUTIC EFFECTS OF ESSENTIAL OILS
>
> This chart lists some popular essential oils and the traditional indications for which practitioners use them.
>
> | Essential oil | Traditional therapeutic uses |
> | --- | --- |
> | **Chamomile**
(Anthemis nobilis) | ▶ Anti-inflammatory, antifungal, and antibacterial effects
▶ Relieving mental or physical stress
▶ Balancing body and mind |
> | **Eucalyptus**
(Eucalyptus radiata) | ▶ Antiviral and expectorant effects
▶ Relieving nausea and motion sickness
▶ Clearing the sinuses
▶ Soothing irritable bowel
▶ Stimulant effect |
> | **Geranium**
(Pelargonium x asperum) | ▶ Antiviral and antifungal effects
▶ Stimulating metabolism in the skin
▶ Improving cell regeneration
▶ Improving circulation
▶ Relieving pain
▶ Improving vital organ function |
> | **Lavender**
(Lavandula augustifolia) | ▶ Anti-inflammatory and antibacterial effects
▶ Treating burns, insect bites, and minor injuries
▶ Soothing stomachache and colic
▶ Relieving toothache and teething pain
▶ Relieving mental or physical stress |
> | **Peppermint**
(Mentha piperita) | ▶ Antibacterial and antiviral effects
▶ Decongestant and expectorant effects
▶ Relieving nausea and motion sickness
▶ Soothing irritable bowel
▶ Stimulant effect |
> | **Rosemary**
(Rosmarinus officinalis) | ▶ Antibacterial, antifungal, and antiviral effects
▶ Restoring energy and alleviating stress
▶ Improving cell regeneration |
> | **Tea tree**
(Melaleuca alternifolia) | ▶ Anti-inflammatory, antibacterial, and antiviral effects
▶ Treating burns, insect bites, and minor injuries
▶ Providing calmness and sedation |

skin. If such irritation develops, advise him to stop using these oils.

●●● **RED FLAG** *Excessive exposure to certain oils, such as wintergreen, sage, aniseed, thyme, lemon, fennel, clove, cinnamon, camphor, and cedar wood, can result in poisoning.*

▶ Different administration methods require specific safety precautions. When using inhalation therapy, the patient should keep his face far enough from the water's surface to avoid a burn injury. When using the diffusion method, he should be at least 3′ (1 m) away from the diffuser.

LIFE SPAN *Aromatherapy is contraindicated during pregnancy because it poses a toxic risk to the mother and fetus. It should be used with caution in infants and children younger than age 5 because many essential oils are toxic to patients in this age-group.*

Patient teaching

▸ Caution the patient to keep essential oils away from the eyes and mucous membranes to avoid irritation. If contact occurs, he should flush with plenty of water; if flushing doesn't relieve the pain, he should seek medical attention.
▸ Inform the patient not to apply citrus oils before exposure to the sun.
▸ Advise the patient to avoid applying cinnamon or clove oil to the skin.

ART THERAPY

Art therapy is the creative use of various expressive media to help a patient deal with thoughts, emotions, life changes, personal issues, and conflicts buried deep within his subconscious. The concept behind art therapy is that if the patient can externalize his feelings for examination and reflection, he can discover meaning and insight, which supports growth, change, healing, and integration of the whole person.

Creative activities include drawing, painting, sculpting, collaging, and puppetry. Mask making is another powerful and popular form of expression commonly used within groups and in individual healing rituals. Photography, videography, and computer-generated art are newer forms of art therapy.

Art therapy is useful in patients with posttraumatic stress disorder, substance abuse, addictions, catastrophic illness (for example, cancer or acquired immunodeficiency syndrome), chronic pain or disease, prolonged hospitalization or treatment, or extensive surgery. This therapy may also help patients who have lost their voice (through surgery, tracheostomy, or intubation), who are aging and experiencing a decrease in function, or who have chronic fatigue or immune dysfunction syndrome.

Equipment

The art form used, and the equipment required to use it, should be chosen according to the patient's age and level of ability, and according to safety guidelines.

Implementation

▸ Make sure the patient is physically capable of carrying out the artistic activity. Medications, a weakened condition, inflamed or painful joints in hands or fingers, or neurologic damage can impair a patient's ability to engage in certain activities.
▸ Someone who's physically unable to manipulate media may still participate in collaging — for example, by choosing pictures, words, or materials for someone else to cut and paste or by indicating the position of cutouts and colors. Likewise, computer programs may be available to create art with adapted controls.
▸ Explain the creative procedure to the patient, and make sure he's willing to participate.
▸ Assess the patient's need for special equipment or other accommodations.

▶ Collect and prepare all necessary materials.

▶ Provide a quiet and comfortable environment and arrange a clean, flat surface on which the patient can work.

▶ Reassure the patient that he need not have previous knowledge or training in art. For example, if drawing is the activity of choice, stick figures can get his message across effectively.

▶ Allow the patient time to complete the project to his satisfaction. Sometimes it's important for the patient to attend to every small detail and search for just the right color.

▶ When the project is complete, allow the patient to show it to you and tell you about it.

▶ Be supportive of the patient's efforts, and summarize the experience for him.

▶ If a patient is especially proud of his artwork, arrange to have it displayed so that others may admire it, thereby adding a source of acknowledgment for the patient.

Special considerations

▶ Some patients may not be open to participating in art therapy, either because they're shy and self-conscious or because they just aren't interested. Don't insist: Instead, work on building a trusting therapeutic relationship. The patient may be willing to participate in the future.

▶ Praise all of the patient's efforts, and be careful not to make suggestions about colors or forms. Remain nonjudgmental and supportive.

▶ When appropriate, encourage the patient to draw a picture representing himself in relation to his illness. You may suggest that the patient draw himself before the disease, with the disease, and after treatment.

▶ Listen attentively. There may be a healing story involved, or perhaps the patient will come up with new insights. You may want to point out certain details.

▶ Repeat back to the patient what he has said to validate the meaning.

●●● **RED FLAG** *Strong emotions may*
●●● *surface as a patient explores and connects with underlying emotions. If the patient shows signs of agitation or uncontrolled emotion, end the session and reassure him that it's normal to have strong feelings and appropriate to express them.*

▶ Notice how the patient represents his size in relation to other figures or objects. Is the entire body drawn? What are the dominant colors and shapes? Is there a smile or frown drawn on the face? What's the overall mood?

▶ After the session, document the type of activity and the patient's response.

▶ Refer the patient to other health care professionals as appropriate.

BIOFEEDBACK

Biofeedback measures and immediately reports information about a patient's physiologic processes, such as heart rate or blood pressure. In biofeedback, electrodes are attached to pertinent areas of his body to monitor such physiologic processes as skeletal muscle activity, heart or brain wave activity, body temperature, or blood pressure. The electrodes feed information into a small monitoring box that reports the results by a sound or light that varies in pitch or brightness as the body function increases or decreases (the "feedback"). A biofeedback therapist leads the patient in mental exercises to help him regulate these and other functions, such as bladder control or muscle tension, to achieve the desired result. The patient eventually learns to control his body's inner mechanisms through conscious mental processes, thereby improving his overall health.

The most common forms of biofeedback involve measuring muscle tension, skin temperature, electrical conductance or resistance within the skin, brain waves, and respiration. As advances in technology have made measurement devices more sophisticated, the applications of biofeedback have expanded. Sensors can now measure the activity of the internal and external rectal sphincters, the activity of the bladder's detrusor muscle, esophageal motility, and stomach acidity.

Biofeedback has a vast range of preventive and restorative applications. It's most successful in cases where psychological factors play a role in the patient's health disturbance, such as sleep disorders and stress-related disorders. Patients with disorders arising from poor muscle control, such as incontinence, postural problems, back pain, and temporomandibular joint syndrome, also benefit. Biofeedback training has also been shown to benefit patients who have lost control of function due to brain or nerve damage or chronic pain disorders.

Improvement has also been seen in patients with heart dysfunctions, GI disorders, swallowing difficulties, esophageal dysfunction, tinnitus, eyelid twitching, fatigue, and cerebral palsy.

●●● RED FLAG *Biofeedback isn't rec-*
●●● *ommended for severe structural problems, such as fractured bones or slipped discs.*

● CLINICAL PEARL *Some biofeed-*
back treatments are accepted in traditional medicine. The American

Medical Association, for instance, has endorsed electromyogram biofeedback training for the treatment of muscle contraction headaches.

Equipment

Biofeedback machine and electrodes • soap and water to clean skin for electrode placement • goggles (optional)

Implementation

▶ Provide the patient with a private environment that's free from noise or other distractions.
▶ Gather the necessary equipment, and wash your hands.
▶ Explain the procedure to the patient, and answer questions he may have. If relaxation techniques or imagery will be used at the same time, review them with the patient.
▶ Depending on the body function that will be monitored, clean and prepare the skin and attach the electrodes according to the manufacturer's instructions.
▶ Set the monitor where both you and the patient can easily see the results.
▶ Set a goal for the session with the patient, and review the information he'll be seeing on the monitor.
▶ Turn on the monitor, and establish a baseline for the targeted body function.
▶ If goggles will be used, help the patient place them comfortably over his eyes.
▶ When the patient is ready, begin the session by starting the relaxation tapes or imagery sequence.
▶ At the close of the session, disconnect the monitor and remove the electrodes.
▶ Clean the patient's skin as needed.

Special considerations

▶ You'll probably work with a trained biofeedback practitioner when conducting the session.
▶ The patient may experience local skin irritation from the electrodes used in the biofeedback monitoring. Wash the skin well with soap and water to remove leftover irritants, and pat it dry.

Patient teaching

▶ Reassure the patient that biofeedback isn't a diagnostic test or a test he needs to pass, but a learning experience.

DANCE THERAPY

Also known as dance movement therapy, dance therapy capitalizes on the direct relationship between body movement and the mind. Specific aspects of dance therapy — such as music, rhythm, and synchronous movement — alter mood states, reawaken old memories and feelings, and reduce isolation. Dance therapy also organizes thoughts and actions and helps the patient establish relationships. In addition, it provides touch, socialization, and a sense of connectedness. Used in a group setting, dance therapy is believed to create the emotional intensity necessary for behavioral change.

● **CLINICAL PEARL** *In addition to its emotional benefits, dance therapy promotes flexibility, strengthens muscles, and improves both cardiovascular and pulmonary function.*

Dance therapy is used to help emotionally disturbed patients express their feelings, gain insight, and develop relationships. It's also used to help physically disabled people increase movement and self-esteem while providing an enjoyable, creative outlet. For older people, dance therapy is used to maintain physical function, enhance self-worth, develop relationships, and help them express fear and grief.

A wide variety of disorders and disabilities, such as depression, brain injury, developmental disabilities, and addictions, can be treated using dance therapy. Typically, the target patient has social, emotional, cognitive, or physical problems. Caregivers and patients with cancer, acquired immunodeficiency syndrome, and Alzheimer's disease use it to reduce stress.

● **CLINICAL PEARL** *Dance therapy can be used to prevent disease and promote health among healthy patients.*

Group dance, probably the most common form of dance therapy, allows people of different physical abilities to participate. By simply tapping their toes or patting their thighs in time to the music, patients can feel a part of the session. Dance routines range from simple clapping and swaying to intricate aerobic sessions.

Equipment

A room with sufficient space to provide a dance floor ● CD player and CDs, radio tuned to a music station, or participants with musical instruments ● chairs for participants to sit in if they grow tired

The music should be appropriate to the group, in its pace and its aesthetic appeal. Fast-moving rock music is probably less enjoyable for a group of agile senior citizens than a fast polka would be. Use faster music to stimulate group members and slower music to calm them.

Implementation

▶ Arrange furniture in the space so that participants can move freely.
▶ Arrange chairs around the periphery for those who can't stand or

who may become tired during the session.

● ● ● **RED FLAG** *Prior to starting*
● ● ● *dance therapy, assess the group
for risk factors. The presence of one
or more risk factors doesn't preclude
group members from participating
but may influence the type of dance
and the length of the session. Risk
factors to consider include poor cardiovascular status, a history of
chronic obstructive pulmonary disease, and degenerative musculoskeletal problems.*

▶ Explain the purpose of the session, and encourage everyone to
participate to the degree they feel
able.
▶ When the group is ready, start the
music and position yourself so
you're facing the group.
▶ If a structured routine is being
used, demonstrate the movements
you're seeking and encourage the
group to mimic your movements.
▶ If free expression is the goal, circulate through the group, providing
encouragement and motivation to
those who are hesitant.
▶ Praise the participants' efforts,
and encourage them to discuss the
feelings they experienced while
dancing.
▶ After the session, document the
type of activity and the group's response.

Special considerations

▶ Rapid motion may result in dizziness.
▶ Help a patient who becomes
dizzy to a seat as needed, and
check his vital signs.
● ● ● **RED FLAG** *Because dancing is
● ● ● an aerobic activity, watch for
signs of cardiovascular compromise,
such as dizziness, flushing, profuse
sweating, and disorientation.*

● IMAGERY

Imagery is a mind-body technique
in which a patient uses his imagina-
tion to promote relaxation and to
help relieve symptoms or better
cope with them. It's successfully
used to control pain and to enhance
immune function, and it's also used
as an adjunctive therapy for several
diseases. Imagery is widely used in
cancer patients to help mobilize the
immune system, to alleviate the
nausea and vomiting associated
with chemotherapy, to relieve pain
and stress, and to promote weight
gain. It's also used in many cardiac
rehabilitation programs and centers
specializing in chronic pain. Imagery can also be effective in helping patients tolerate medical procedures. People with strong imagina-
tions — those who can literally
"worry themselves sick" — are excellent candidates for using imagery
to positively affect their health.

Palming and guided imagery are
two popular imagery techniques.
▶ In *palming,* the patient places his
palms over his closed eyes and tries
to fill his entire field of vision with
only the color black. He then tries
to picture the black changing to a
color he associates with stress such
as red and then mentally replaces
that color with one he finds soothing such as pale blue.
▶ In *guided imagery,* the patient is
asked to visualize a goal he wants
to achieve and then picture himself
taking action to achieve it. This
type of therapy is intended to complement traditional medical treatments (such as cancer treatment)
rather than replace them.

As an active means of relaxation,
imagery is a central part of almost
all stress-reduction techniques. It's
also a useful self-care tool. With
proper instruction, the patient can
use imagery to relieve stress, en-

hance immune function (for example, to fight a cold virus), and improve his sense of well-being.

Implementation

▶ Provide the patient with a private, quiet environment that's free from distractions, and a comfortable place in which to lie down.

CLINICAL PEARL *Some types of imagery require the use of prerecorded instructions to guide the patient through the steps to visualize the desired result.*

▶ If using a taped imagery sequence, make sure the tape player is working and that the room has an electrical outlet.

▶ Help the patient into a comfortable position and explain the exercise. Answer questions the patient may have.

▶ When the patient is comfortable, instruct him to close his eyes, and lower the lights if possible.

▶ Use a steady, soothing, low voice throughout the exercise.

▶ Instruct the patient to take a few deep breaths and to imagine that with each breath he's taking in calmness and peacefulness and releasing tension, discomfort, and worry. Tell him to let his breath find its own rate and rhythm, and to continue to breathe in calmness and peacefulness and breathe out tension and worry.

▶ Help the patient relax his body. Instruct him to imagine that he's breathing calmness into his feet and legs and releasing tension with each exhalation. Continue this sequence moving from feet to head, having him breathe calmness into each successive body part.

▶ As you complete this portion of the exercise, remind the patient to let his whole body sink into a peaceful, relaxed state.

▶ Tell the patient to imagine himself in a place that's peaceful and beautiful, perhaps somewhere he has visited or a special place where he would like to be. Encourage him to notice the details in this place, such as colors, shapes, and living things found there. Have him think about the sounds and smells of the place and pay attention to feelings of peacefulness and relaxation.

▶ While remaining quiet, allow the patient to spend as long as he wants in this place; tell him that when he's ready, he should allow the images to fade and slowly bring himself back to the outer world.

▶ If the patient is willing, discuss the experience with him, concentrating on the positive feelings of relaxation and peace.

▶ Document the length of the session, the imagery path used, and the patient's response.

Special considerations

▶ To enhance the effects of imagery, consider adding a smell to trigger the image that the patient is trying to experience.

RED FLAG *Imagery is contraindicated in psychotic patients.*

▶ Occasionally, an imagery session may lead a person to remember an unpleasant period or event in his life. If this occurs, stop the session and encourage the patient to tell you what he was seeing and feeling. If the patient becomes upset, stay with him. When possible, notify the physician.

▶ Be aware that patients with breathing problems may have difficulty controlling their breathing.

MEDITATION

The ancient art of meditation — focusing one's attention on a single sound or image or on the rhythm of one's own breathing — has been found to have positive effects on health. By directing attention away from worries about the future or preoccupation with the past, meditation reduces stress, a major contributing factor in many health problems. Stress reduction in turn results in a wide range of physiologic and mental health benefits, from decreased oxygen consumption, heart rate, and respiratory rate to improved mood, spiritual calm, and heightened awareness.

Most meditation approaches fall into one of two techniques: concentrative meditation or mindful meditation. *Concentrative meditation* involves focusing on an image, a sound (called a mantra), or one's own breathing to achieve a state of calm and heightened awareness. Transcendental meditation is a form of concentrative meditation in which the individual repeats a mantra over and over again while sitting in a comfortable position. When other thoughts enter his mind, he's instructed to notice them — and then return to the mantra. Concentrating on the mantra prevents distracting thoughts.

Mindful meditation takes the opposite approach. Instead of focusing on a single sensation or sound, the individual is aware of all sensations, feelings, images, thoughts, sounds, and smells that pass through his mind without actually thinking about them. The goal is a calmer, clearer, nonreactive state of mind.

Meditation has a wide variety of indications. It's used to enhance immune function in patients with cancer, acquired immunodeficiency syndrome, and autoimmune disorders, and has been successful in treating drug and alcohol addiction as well as posttraumatic stress disorder. Anxiety disorders, pain, and stress are also commonly treated with meditation. Meditation can also be used with dietary and lifestyle changes for patients with hypertension or heart disease.

Implementation

▶ To assist your patient with meditation, you'll need a private, quiet environment that's free from distractions and offers a comfortable place for him to sit or recline.
▶ If you'll be helping a patient with meditation, begin by explaining the procedure and answering questions. Tell the patient that he can stop the exercise if he becomes uncomfortable. Help him into a comfortable position. If he's in a sitting position, ask him to keep his back straight and let his shoulders droop.
▶ Using a calm, soothing, low voice, instruct the patient to close his eyes, if doing so feels comfortable. Tell him to focus on his abdomen, feeling it rise each time he inhales and fall each time he exhales. Tell him to concentrate on his breathing. Explain that if his mind wanders off his breathing, he should simply bring it back, regardless of the thought that distracted him.
▶ Have the patient practice the exercise for 15 minutes every day for a week; then evaluate its benefits with him.
▶ Document the session, the instructions you gave the patient, and his response.

Special considerations

▶ Meditation may elicit negative emotions, disorientation, or memories of early childhood abuses or other traumas. If this occurs, try to determine the source of the patient's upsetting feeling or memory, and direct him to a safer, more pleasant thought or memory. If this isn't possible, stop the session, notify the physician, and stay with the patient until he's calm and controlled.

● Be aware that patients with respiratory problems may have difficulty with meditation techniques that focus on breathing.

●●● **RED FLAG** *Meditation should be used cautiously in schizophrenic patients and those with attention deficit hyperactivity disorder.*

Patient teaching

● Remind the patient that meditation isn't a substitute for medical treatment. If he's taking a prescribed medication, such as an antihypertensive, tell him to keep taking it.

MUSIC THERAPY

Music therapy uses the universal appeal of rhythmic sound to communicate, explore, and heal. It can take the form of creating music, singing, moving to music, or just listening to music. Music therapy benefits patients with developmental disabilities, mental health disorders, substance addictions, and chronic pain. Studies have demonstrated the positive effects of music in reducing pain and procedural anxiety as well as in dental anesthesia.

Patients who listen to classical music before surgery and then again in the postanesthesia care unit report minimal postoperative disorientation. Music has also been successfully used to communicate with Alzheimer's patients and head trauma victims when other approaches have failed. In a study on the effects of music on Alzheimer's patients, those who listened to big band music during their days were more alert and happier and had better long-term recollection than the control group. Throughout the illness, music can reorient confused patients. In the final stages of the disease, it provides psychological comfort.

Equipment

CD player and CDs, radio, or musical instrument

Choose music that's appropriate to the patient or patients and the session objectives. The music should be meaningful to the participants. For sessions that involve making music, collect instruments appropriate for the individual or group. For sessions that involve singing, choose music recognizable to the individual or group members. Provide words for the songs, either in writing or by repeating them.

Implementation

● Arrange a comfortable environment.

● If the session includes more than one participant, introduce them to one another. Explain the purpose of the session, and encourage everyone to participate as he feels able.

● When the individual or group is ready, start the music and position yourself so that you're facing the listeners.

● If the individual or group will be listening to music, watch the reactions. If the music is being made by the participants, offer support.

● Encourage the participants to discuss the feelings that arose while listening to or making the music. Offer praise and support.

● After the session, document the type of activity and the individual or group's response.

Special considerations

Music is especially effective as a means of reminiscence therapy for older people. For many of them, the music they enjoyed in their youth hasn't been part of their lives for decades.

PET THERAPY

A pet can help the patient combat loneliness and help bridge the gap between the patient and the health care provider. Commonly used in long-term care facilities, pet therapy helps patients break through apathy and depression and improves interaction with others. Some facilities adopt a pet as a mascot and let the residents share responsibility for caring for it, thus helping to build a sense of community.

Equipment

Pet that's well-behaved and has a good temperament

Pets that have gone through obedience training are ideal. Make sure the pet has been checked by a veterinarian and is up-to-date on his immunizations.

Implementation

▶ Allow the patient to play with and hold the pet.
▶ Encourage him to talk to the animal and reminisce about pets he once had.
▶ Provide as much time as the patient needs, if possible.

Special considerations

▶ Make sure the environment is appropriate for pet therapy. The facility should have an area where the pet can retreat and be kept out of the way of patients who are allergic to animals, have no interest in pets, or are afraid of them.
▶ If the pet is chosen as a mascot for the facility, have a responsible person make a schedule for residents who are interested in caring for the animal.
▶ If the pet isn't a permanent resident of the facility, arrange for a volunteer from an animal shelter to accompany the pet to ensure the safety of the animal and the patients.

PRAYER AND MENTAL HEALING

Humans have used prayer and mental healing throughout the ages to seek assistance from a higher being for a wide range of problems. The underlying beliefs of those who use prayer for healing are the same for all religions, including belief that a higher power exists, that humans can communicate with this higher being through prayer, and that this deity can hear human prayers and intervene in human affairs, including healing the sick. In prayer, the person communicates directly with the divine being, asking the being to intervene to heal the patient. In mental healing, the power of the divine being is channeled through a healer.

The two main categories of mental healing are type 1 and type 2. In type 1 healing, the healer enters into a spiritual level of consciousness wherein he views himself and the patient as a single being. No physical contact with the patient is necessary. Type 2 mental healing requires the healer to touch the patient in an attempt to transfer energy from the healer's hands to the diseased parts of the patient's body. Most people who use prayer or mental healing view these practices as adjuncts to conventional medical treatment.

Although the therapeutic uses of prayer and mental healing are limitless, the reliability of these practices still needs to be established. Proponents of prayer argue that even if prayer can't cure disease, it can at least relieve some of its effects, enhance the effectiveness of conventional medical treatments, and provide meaning and comfort to the patient.

Implementation

▶ Facilitate the use of prayer and mental healing by asking the patient such questions as "Is religion important to you?" and "Is it important in how you cope with your illness?"

▶ If religion is important to the patient, explore his religious practices with him to identify ways to incorporate them into his present situation.

▶ Determine whether the patient would like to discuss his faith with the facility chaplain or another clergy member.

▶ Provide the patient with privacy in a quiet, distraction-free environment in which to practice his preferred form of prayer or mental healing.

Special considerations

▶ One of the benefits of prayer and mental healing is the lack of complications.

▶ Patients who have attempted prayer and haven't seen the results they expected may express a sense of disappointment when the topic of spirituality is discussed. If this occurs and if it's possible, arrange for a clergy member to explore the patient's feelings with him.

▶ Remain nonjudgmental when implementing the exercise.

▶ Some prayer rituals may be more than your health care facility can handle. Rites involving incense, large groups, or loud music and dance can stress even the most tolerant facility. Although you should be sensitive to the patient's religious beliefs, sometimes a compromise is in order. For example, you could suggest that the patient be wheeled to an outside area of the facility if incense is involved or to a conference room off the unit during off-hours if noise is an issue or a prayer vigil involves a large number of people.

▶ Be aware that ethical questions arise if prayer and mental healing are used without the patient's knowledge. Some people may express concern that prayer and mental healing may be used to harm an individual instead of healing him.

▶ Advise your patient to consider prayer a complementary therapy, not a substitute for conventional medical care. If you have a patient whose religion advocates the use of prayer as the sole form of treatment, make sure he understands the consequences of forgoing conventional medical treatment so he can make an informed decision.

REFLEXOLOGY

Reflexology is a widely practiced form of manual therapy involving the application of pressure to specific parts of the body, usually the soles of the feet (but sometimes the palms of the hands). It's based on the theory that these parts of the body correspond to and can therapeutically affect various organs and glands. For example, the top of the big toe is said to connect to the brain, and the arch area to the solar plexus. Some practitioners believe that these points follow the same meridians used in acupuncture.

The roots of reflexology can be traced back 3,000 years to folk medicine traditions in China, India, and Egypt. The current revival of interest in this technique began in the early 1900s with an American ear, nose, and throat specialist, William Fitzgerald, who discovered that his patients felt less pain when he applied pressure to specific points on their soles or palms before surgery. In the 1930s, Eunice Ingham, a physical therapist, expanded on Fitzgerald's work. Ingham believed that applying varying levels of pressure to certain areas could not only decrease pain but also provide other health benefits. She mapped the specific reflex zones on the feet that reflexologists use today. (See *Right foot reflex zones,* page 436.)

Reflexologists, most of whom are masseurs, physical therapists, or nurses with special training, say that their technique works by reducing the amount of lactic acid in the feet and breaking up calcium crystals that accumulate in the nerve endings, blocking the flow of energy. Many health clubs and spas offer reflexology treatments. No specific license or certification is needed to practice reflexology.

Like full body massage, reflexology relieves stress and muscle tension and produces relaxation. Reflexologists claim that they can also treat numerous conditions, including skin disorders (eczema and acne), GI disorders (diarrhea and constipation), hypertension, migraines, anxiety, and asthma.

Implementation

▶ Reflexology requires only a treatment table or chair or a stool to elevate the feet. A quiet environment is preferred.
▶ The patient is either seated comfortably in a reclining chair or placed in a supine position on a treatment table, with feet raised and supported. The therapist is seated facing the patient's soles.
▶ After an initial assessment of the patient's feet for alterations in skin thickness and abnormalities in foot structure, the therapist feels for tender areas and signs of tension or thickening on the sole.
▶ A treatment session typically begins with relaxation techniques designed to release tension and make

the patient comfortable with the manipulation of his feet.
▶ The therapist uses thumbs and fingers to apply gentle but firm pressure to the reflex zones of the foot, paying more attention to zones that are tender to the touch. Working systematically, the therapist begins with the toes and proceeds in small, creeping movements proximally toward the heel. (For therapy using the hand, the therapist starts with the fingers and moves proximally toward the wrist.) A typical session lasts 20 to 60 minutes.

Special considerations

▶ Advise your patient to postpone reflexology treatments if he has cuts, boils, bruises, or other injuries on his feet.

RED FLAG *If the patient has diabetes, peripheral vascular disease, or another vascular problem in his legs, such as thrombosis or phlebitis, instruct him to check with his physician before trying reflexology.*

LIFE SPAN *If the patient is pregnant, advise her to get her physician's consent before trying this therapy.*

▶ Many people who claim to perform reflexology are actually providing a simple foot massage. If your patient wants treatment for a specific symptom, he should make sure the practitioner has been trained in reflexology.

REIKI

Reiki is a Japanese healing therapy that utilizes emotional, spiritual, and universal energy. While its origins trace back to ancient Buddhist practices, Reiki as a modern healing method was introduced in the late 19th century by Dr. Mikao Usui, a Japanese Buddhist monk. The word

RIGHT FOOT REFLEX ZONES

The illustration below, showing the organs and body parts associated with specific regions of the right foot, serves as a map that guides reflexologists in performing therapy.

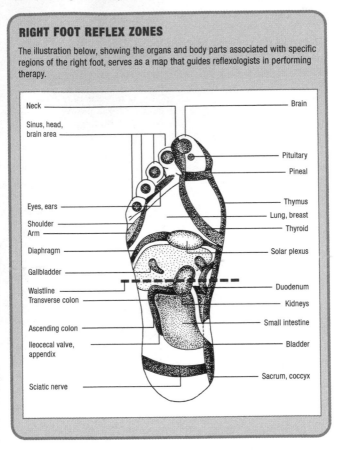

Reiki refers to the universal life energy, and is derived from the Japanese words *rei*, which means spirit, and *ki*, meaning energy life force.

Reiki therapy is the transference of energy through the practitioner to the patient; this healing therapy isn't a passive practice. The Reiki practitioner utilizes specific healing techniques for restoring and balancing the natural life force energy within the body. The Reiki practitioner places her hands on or above the patient and the patient draws energy from the practitioner as needed. The patient becomes an active agent in his or her healing by identifying body, mind, and spirit needs and using energy for restoration and balance. Reiki therapy may bring deep relaxation, and help relieve pain; the goal of therapy is to help restore the body's energy balance and enhance the body's natural ability to heal itself.

Reiki has been studied in primary pain management treatment as well as adjuvant therapy with opioids. When used with terminally ill patients, Reiki therapy has been associated with an increased quality-of-life with relief from pain, anxiety, dyspnea and edema. Reiki has also been documented to benefit patients with autoimmune illness, including multiple sclerosis, lupus, and rheumatoid arthritis. Reiki has also been used in patients with pancreatitis, fibromyalgia, heart failure, emphysema, and cancer.

Implementation

Reiki treatments vary from a full body treatment, which may last about 45 minutes, to treatment of an isolated body area (such as a shoulder or knee), which could last about 10 minutes.

After an initial consultation, the patient (who remains fully clothed) is positioned on a table, mat, or couch. The Reiki practitioner places her hands on or above the patient and the energy is then channeled through the practitioner to the patient in a series of hand positions over the main energy centers of the body (chakras), starting at the head and moving down the body. During Reiki treatments, patients may feel the flow of energy in various ways. They may report a feeling of warmth or heat from the practitioner's hands. Sometimes patients may experience a tingling sensation.

Patients have reported a feeling of deep meditation a sense colors, and some patients recall past experiences. Sometimes there's spontaneous emotional release from areas that have been blocked off. Some patients don't feel a physical sensation at all but describe mental or emotional changes such as a sense of calmness or peace. Nearly every-

one experiences a treatment as deeply relaxing.

Special considerations

▶ Only trained Reiki practitioners should perform the treatment. Training involves three degrees of learning and attainment of Reiki skills and may take several years to complete.

▶ Reiki practitioners don't diagnosis illness or prescribe treatment. If the patient wasn't referred by his primary care practitioner for the treatment, the Reiki practitioner should advise the patient to follow up with his primary care provider.

▶ The Reiki practitioner should relax prior to the treatment and make the patient as comfortable as possible during the treatment.

▶ The Reiki practitioner should allow the patient to express his emotions during and after treatment, and provide support as needed.

THERAPEUTIC MASSAGE

Massage, the process of stroking, rubbing, and kneading the body, has played an important role in traditional medical systems through the centuries. It's used primarily for stress reduction and relaxation, but can serve as a complementary therapy for a wide range of conditions, including chronic pain, digestive disorders, inflammation, intestinal disorders, joint mobility disorders, and muscle tension.

The primary physiologic effect of therapeutic massage is improved blood circulation. As the muscles are kneaded and stretched, blood returning to the heart increases and toxins, such as lactic acid, are carried out of the muscle tissue to be excreted from the body. Improved circulation results in increased perfusion and oxygenation of tissues.

Improved oxygenation of the brain helps us think more clearly and feel more alive; improved perfusion and oxygenation of other organ systems leads to improved digestion and elimination as well as quicker wound healing. Massage also appears to trigger the release of endorphins, the body's natural pain relievers.

Most practitioners use a combination of one or all of the five basic techniques of massage:

▶ In *effleurage,* the therapist performs a long, gliding stroke using the whole hand or the thumb. This is a warm-up technique. The gliding stroke, which should always move toward the heart, improves circulation.

▶ *Petrissage* is a kneading and compressing motion in which the muscles are grabbed and lifted. This motion relieves sore muscles by clearing away lactic acid and increasing circulation to the muscle tissue.

▶ In *friction,* the therapist uses the thumbs and fingertips to work around the joints and the thickest part of the muscles. Circular motions break down adhesions and may also help make soft tissues and joints more flexible. For larger muscles, the palm or heel of the hand may be used.

▶ In *tapotement,* the therapist uses the sides of the hands, fingertips, cupped palms, or slightly closed fists to make chopping, tapping, and beating motions. These motions invigorate and stimulate the muscles, resulting in a burst of energy. However, when the muscles are cramped, strained, or spastic, tapotement can exacerbate the problem if performed for a longer period.

▶ In *vibration,* the therapist presses her fingers or flattened hands firmly into the muscle then "vibrates"

(transmits a trembling motion) the area rapidly for a few seconds. This motion is repeated until the entire muscle has been vibrated. This helps stimulate the nervous system and may increase circulation and improve gland function.

Equipment

Sturdy massage table ● lubricating oil ● quiet room ● sheet or towel ● music

Implementation

▶ Have the patient undress in private and cover himself with a sheet or towel.

▶ With the patient on the massage table, play soothing music to induce relaxation.

▶ To respect the patient's modesty, the body is kept fully draped, exposing only the area being worked on at the moment.

▶ A scented oil is usually used to prevent friction between the therapist's hands and the patient's skin while he kneads various muscle groups in a systematic way from head to toe.

Special considerations

▶ A trained massage therapist pays close attention to body language as well as the patient's comments, to avoid causing pain or discomfort.

●●● **RED FLAG** *Massage is con-*
●●● *traindicated in those with diabetes, varicose veins, phlebitis, or other blood vessel problems because massaging damaged tissue may dislodge a blood clot. Also, massage shouldn't be performed on patients with pitting edema.*

▶ Advise your patients who are seeking a massage therapist to get recommendations from people who have been satisfied with their treatment. They should also make sure the therapist is properly trained and licensed and belongs to a professional organization.

🔵 **CLINICAL PEARL** *The therapist performing the massage should take these precautions:*

▸ *Avoid massaging the abdomen of a patient with hypertension or gastric or duodenal ulcers.*

▸ *Don't massage within 6″ (15 cm) of bruises, cysts, fractured bones, or breaks in skin integrity.*

🔵 THERAPEUTIC TOUCH

Developed in the 1970s, therapeutic touch is a widely used complementary therapy, developed by nurses for nurses, to bring a more humane and holistic approach to their practice. This technique focuses on "healing" rather than "curing" and is built on the belief that all healing is basically self-healing.

Central to therapeutic touch is the concept of a universal life force that practitioners believe permeates space and sustains all living organisms. In healthy people, this vital energy flows freely in and through the body in a balanced way that nourishes all body organs. When people get sick, it's because this energy field is out of equilibrium. By using their hands to manipulate the energy field above the patient's skin, practitioners of therapeutic touch say they can restore equilibrium, thereby reactivating the mind-body-spirit connection and empowering the patient to participate in his own healing. Although the existence of a human energy field hasn't been proved scientifically, nurses claim that they can actually feel something best described as energy when performing this technique.

Despite its name, therapeutic touch doesn't require actual physical contact during a treatment. In most case, the nurse's hands remain several inches above the patient's body.

Therapeutic touch is widely used by practitioners of holistic nursing and other health professionals and is practiced in many hospitals, hospices, long-term care facilities, and other settings. Although most practitioners are nurses, other health care professionals (such as massage therapists, physical therapists, dentists, and medical physicians) and nonprofessionals have incorporated this therapy in their practices. According to practitioners, anyone can study this technique and apply it to himself.

Therapeutic touch is used as a complementary therapy for virtually all medical and nursing diagnoses as well as surgical procedures. Practitioners say it's especially helpful for patients with wounds or infections because it eases discomfort and speeds the healing process. However, the technique is best known for its ability to relieve pain and anxiety. Because of this characteristic, therapeutic touch is helpful in treating stress-related disorders, such as tension headaches, hypertension, ulcers, and emotional problems. It's also used in Lamaze classes and delivery rooms to induce relaxation and in neonatal intensive care units to help speed the growth of premature infants.

Implementation

▸ Select an environment that will enable the patient to relax and the nurse to concentrate. This may include a comfortable chair, bed, or massage table for the patient and, possibly, soothing music to help create a relaxing atmosphere.

▸ The nurse achieves a calm, meditative state that allows her to be sensitive to the patient's signs and symptoms. This heightened sensitivity is also necessary for perceiving subtle changes in the patient's energy field.

▶ After becoming centered, the nurse begins her assessment by slowly moving her hands over the patient's body, 2″ to 4″ (5 to 10 cm) away from the skin surface, to detect alterations in the energy field, such as feelings of cold or heat, vibration, or blockages.

▶ Depending on the assessment findings, the nurse then performs interventions aimed at balancing the energy field and removing obstructions. Possible interventions include unruffling a chaotic and tangled field, eliminating "congestion," and acting as a conduit to direct the "life energy" from the environment into the patient.

▶ Throughout the treatment, the patient remains quiet and relaxed. According to practitioners, it isn't necessary for the patient to consciously believe in the power of the procedure.

▶ To be effective in channeling energy into the patient, the nurse must have "conscious intent" — that is, the intent to become a calm, focused instrument of healing, enabling the patient's body to ultimately heal itself.

Special considerations

✿ **LIFE SPAN** *Care must be taken to moderate the length and strength of the treatment for small children and elderly people because their bodies are more fragile. A common sign of overtreatment in these patients is restlessness during or after the treatment.*

▶ Patients who warrant extra sensitivity and shorter treatment periods include pregnant women, patients with head injuries or psychosis, emaciated patients, and patients in shock.

▶ Respect the personal preferences of those being treated. People have different tolerances for touch, and some regard this type of energy work as an invasion of their personal space.

YOGA THERAPY

Among the oldest known health practices, yoga (meaning "union" in Sanskrit) is the integration of physical, mental, and spiritual energies to promote health and wellness. It can be practiced by the young and old alike, either individually or within groups, and can be started at any age.

Based on the idea that a chronically restless or agitated mind causes poor health and decreased mental strength and clarity, yoga outlines specific regimens for lifestyle, hygiene, detoxification, physical activity, and psychological practices. By integrating these practices, yoga aims to raise the individual's physical vitality and spiritual awareness.

Types of yoga

Of the several styles of yoga developed over the centuries, the most common in the West is hatha yoga. It combines physical postures and exercises (called *asanas*), breathing techniques (called *pranayamas*), relaxation, diet, and "proper thinking." Asanas fall into two categories: meditative and therapeutic. *Meditative asanas* promote proper blood flow through the body by bringing the spine and body into perfect alignment. The mind and body are brought into a state of relaxation and stillness, which facilitates concentration during meditation. These asanas also keep the heart, glands, and lungs properly energized. *Therapeutic asanas* are commonly prescribed for joint pain. The "cobra," "locust spinal twist," and "shoulder stand" are examples of therapeutic asanas.

The goal of a properly executed asana is to create a balance between movement and stillness, which is the state of a healthy body. Very little movement is needed. Instead, the mind provides discipline, awareness, and a relaxed openness to maintain the posture and properly execute the asana. Using these asanas, the individual learns to regulate such autonomic functions as heartbeat and respirations while relaxing physical tensions.

Pranayamas focus on disciplined breathing. Pranayama exercises regulate the flow of *prana* (breath and electromagnetic force), keeping the individual healthy. Pranayama has been shown to aid digestion, regulate cardiac function, and alleviate various physical ailments. It can be especially effective at reducing the frequency of asthma attacks.

Breathing and consciousness

The goal of breathing in yoga is to make the process as smooth and regular as possible. The assumption is that the rhythm of the mind is mirrored in the rhythm of breathing. By keeping respirations steady and rhythmic, the mind will remain calm and focused.

Samadhi, or spiritual realization, is an additional component of Eastern yoga. Yoga practitioners compare samadhi to a fourth state of consciousness, separate from the normal states of waking, dream, and sleep. The technique called *HongSau* uses meditation to develop the powers of concentration. Thought and energy are withdrawn from outer distractions and focused on a goal or problem the individual chooses. The *Aum* technique expands the individual's awareness

beyond the limitations of the body and mind, allowing the user to experience what is called the "Divine Consciousness," which is believed to underlie and uphold all life. *Aum* is the sound that exists with every inhaled breath. The sounds of inhalation are "a" through the mouth and "um" through the nose. Taken together, these sounds of attraction form the sound *Aum.* To achieve "Divine Consciousness," the user alters his breathing and focuses on sounding out the "a" and the "um" sounds.

Benefits of yoga

Among yoga's measured benefits are improvement in the individual's health, vitality, and peace of mind. Yoga is successfully used to alleviate stress and anxiety, lower blood pressure, relieve pain, improve motor skills, treat addictions, increase auditory and visual perception, and improve metabolic and respiratory function. Yoga has also been effective in treating lung ailments because it can increase lung capacity and lower respiratory rates.

Yoga has been credited with decreasing serum cholesterol and increasing histamine levels to fight allergies. Its ability to help the user regulate blood flow is being studied in cancer therapy. Scientists are eager to see whether restricted blood flow to the tumor region will slow growth.

Implementation

▶ Provide a private, quiet environment that's free from distractions.
▶ Participants should have enough room to move without touching or distracting other members.
▶ Each participant will need a small blanket, large towel, or mat to use in some of the postures.

● Explain the purpose of the session, and describe the planned exercises and their benefits.
● Answer questions, and remind the participants that they don't have to engage in postures that may be uncomfortable.
● When the group is ready, talk them through the positions or breathing techniques, demonstrating each one.
● After they've all assumed the position, begin the breathing pattern, and circulate among the students to assess and adjust their technique, as needed.
● Praise their efforts.
● After you've led them through all of the planned exercises, close the session by having everyone take slow, deep breaths.
● Document the session, the techniques used, and the patients' responses.

Special considerations

● Some of the more physical aspects of yoga can cause muscle injury if they aren't properly performed, or if an older adult tries to force his body into position.
● Caution patients to attempt the various techniques and postures cautiously, and remind them that very few people are able to perform all of the techniques in the beginning.
● Yoga techniques exist to fit the needs of all people, regardless of their physical condition. Individuals who can't perform some of the more physically demanding postures can still benefit from the breathing or meditation techniques.

Appendices
Selected references
Index

Crisis values of laboratory tests

Test	Low value	Common causes and effects	High value	Common causes and effects
Calcium, serum	< 6 mg/dl (SI, < 1.5 mmol/L)	Vitamin D or para-thyroid hormone deficiency: tetany, seizures	> 13 mg/dl (SI, > 3.2 mmol/L)	Hyperparathyroid-ism: coma
Carbon dioxide	< 10 mEq/L (SI, < 10 mmol/L)	Complex pattern of metabolic and res-piratory factors	> 40 mEq/L (SI, > 40 mmol/L)	Complex pattern of metabolic and res-piratory factors
Creatinine, serum	—	—	> 4 mg/dl (SI, > 353.6 µmol/L)	Renal failure: coma
Glucose, blood	< 40 mg/dl (SI, 2.2 mmol/L)	Excess insulin ad-ministration: brain damage	> 300 mg/dl (SI, > 16.6 mmol/L)	Diabetes: diabetic ketoacidosis
Hemoglobin	< 8 g/dl (SI, < 80 g/L)	Hemorrhage, vita-min B_{12} or iron de-ficiency: heart fail-ure	> 18 g/dl (SI, > 180 g/L)	Chronic obstructive pulmonary disease: thrombosis, poly-cythemia vera
International Normalized Ratio	—	—	> 3.0	Disseminated intra-vascular coagula-tion: uncontrolled oral anticoagulation
Partial pres-sure of arter-ial carbon dioxide	< 20 mm Hg (SI, < 2.7 kPa)	Complex pattern of metabolic and res-piratory factors	> 70 mm Hg (SI, > 9.3 kPa)	Complex pattern of metabolic and res-piratory factors
Partial pres-sure of arter-ial oxygen	< 50 mm Hg (SI, < 6.7 kPa)	Complex pattern of metabolic and res-piratory factors	—	—
Partial thrombo-plastin time	—	—	> 40 sec (SI, > 40 s) > 70 sec (SI, > 70 s) (for patient on heparin)	Anticoagulation fac-tor deficiency: hem-orrhage

Test	Low value	Common causes and effects	High value	Common causes and effects
pH, blood	< 7.2 (SI, < 7.2)	Complex pattern of metabolic and respiratory factors	> 7.6 (SI, > 7.6)	Complex patterns of metabolic and respiratory factors
Platelet count	< 50,000/µl	Bone marrow suppression: hemorrhage	> 500,000/µl	Leukemia, reaction to acute bleeding: hemorrhage
Potassium, serum	< 3 mEq/L (SI, < 3 mmol/L)	Vomiting and diarrhea, diuretic therapy: cardiotoxicity, arrhythmia, cardiac arrest	> 6 mEq/L (SI, > 6 mmol/L)	Renal disease diuretic therapy: cardiotoxicity, arrhythmia
Prothrombin time	—	—	> 14 sec (SI, > 14 s) > 20 sec (SI, > 20 s) (for patient on warfarin)	Anticoagulant therapy, anticoagulation factor deficiency: hemorrhage
Sodium, serum	< 120 mEq/L (SI, < 120 mmol/L)	Diuretic therapy: profuse sweating, GI suctioning, diarrhea, vomiting, burns	> 160 mEq/L (SI, > 160 mmol/L)	Dehydration: vascular collapse
White blood cell count	< 2,000/µl (SI, < 2 × 10^9/L)	Bone marrow suppression: infection	> 20,000/µl (SI, > 20 × 10^9/L)	Leukemia: infection

Laboratory value changes in elderly patients

Standard normal laboratory values reflect the physiology of adults ages 20 to 40. However, normal values for older patients usually differ because of age-related physiologic changes.

Certain test results, however, remain unaffected by age. These include partial thromboplastin time, prothrombin time, serum acid phosphatase, serum carbon dioxide, serum chloride, aspartate aminotransferase, and total serum protein. You can use this chart to interpret other changeable test values in your elderly patients.

Test values ages 20 to 40	Age-related changes	Considerations
Serum		
Albumin 3.5 to 5 g/dl (SI, 35 to 50 g/L)	Younger than age 65: Higher in males Older than age 65: Equal levels that then decrease at same rate	Increased dietary protein intake needed in older patients if liver function is normal; edema: a sign of low albumin level
Alkaline phosphatase 30 to 85 IU/L (SI, 42 to 128 U/L)	Increases 8 to 10 IU/L	May reflect liver function decline or vitamin D malabsorption and bone demineralization
Beta globulin 0.7 to 1.1 g/dl (SI, 7 to 11 g/L)	Increases slightly	Increases in response to decrease in albumin if liver function is normal; increased dietary protein intake needed
Blood urea nitrogen 8 to 20 mg/dl (SI, 2.9 to 7.5 mmol/L)	Increases, possibly to 69 mg/dl (SI, 25.8 mmol/L)	Slight increase acceptable in absence of stressors, such as infection or surgery
Cholesterol Desirable: < 200 mg/dl (SI, < 5.18 mmol/L)	Men: Increases to age 50, then decreases Women: Lower than men until age 50, increases to age 70, then decreases	Rise in cholesterol level (and increased cardiovascular risk) in women as a result of postmenopausal estrogen decline; dietary changes, weight loss, and exercise needed

Test values ages 20 to 40	Age-related changes	Considerations
Serum *(continued)*		
Creatine kinase 55 to 170 U/L (SI, 0.94 to 2.89 µkat/L)	Increases slightly	May reflect decreasing muscle mass and liver function
Creatinine Men: 0.8 to 1.2 mg/dl (SI, 62 to 115 µmol/L) Women: 0.6 to 0.9 mg/dl (SI, 53 to 97 µmol/L)	Increases, possibly to 1.9 mg/dl in men (SI, 168 µmol/L)	Important factor to prevent toxicity when giving drugs excreted in urine
Creatinine clearance Men: 94 to 140 ml/min/1.73 m² (SI, 0.91 to 1.35 ml/s/m²) Women: 72 to 110 ml/min/1.73 m² (SI, 0.69 to 1.06 ml/s/m²)	Men: Decreases; formula: $([140 - \text{age}]) \times$ kg body weight)/$(72 \times$ serum creatinine) Women: 85% of men's rate	Reflects reduced glomerular filtration rate; important factor to prevent toxicity when giving drugs excreted in urine
Hematocrit Men: 45% to 52% (SI, 0.45 to 0.52) Women: 36% to 48% (SI, 0.36 to 0.48)	May decrease slightly (unproven)	Reflects decreased bone marrow and hematopoiesis
Hemoglobin Men: 14 to 17.4 g/dl (SI, 140 to 174 g/L) Women: 12 to 16 g/dl (SI, 120 to 160 g/L)	Men: Decreases by 1 to 2 g/dl Women: Unknown	Reflects decreased bone marrow, hematopoiesis, and (for men) androgen levels
High-density lipoprotein Desirable: ≥ 60 mg/dl (SI, ≥ 1.55 mmol/L)	Levels higher in women than in men but equalize with age	Compliance with dietary restrictions required for accurate interpretation of test results
Lactate dehydrogenase 71 to 207 U/L (SI, 1.2 to 3.52 µkat/L)	Increases slightly	May reflect declining muscle mass and liver function
Leukocyte count 4,000 to 10,000/µl (SI, 4 to 10 × 10⁹/L)	Decreases to 3,100 to 9,000/µl (SI, 3.1 to 9 × 10⁹/L)	Decrease proportionate to lymphocyte count
Lymphocyte count 25% to 40% (SI, 0.25 to 0.4)	Decreases	Decrease proportionate to leukocyte count

Test values ages 20 to 40	Age-related changes	Considerations
Serum *(continued)*		
Platelet count 140,000 to 400,000/µl (SI, 140 to 400 × 10⁹/L)	Change in characteristics: decreased granular constituents, increased platelet-release factors	May reflect diminished bone marrow and increased fibrinogen levels
Potassium 3.5 to 5 mEq/L (SI, 3.5 to 5 mmol/L)	Increases slightly	Requires avoidance of salt substitutes containing potassium, vigilance in reading food labels, and knowledge of the signs and symptoms of hyperkalemia
Thyroid-stimulating hormone 0.3 to 5 mIU/ml (SI, 0.3 to 5 mU/L)	Increases slightly	Suggests primary hypothyroidism or endemic goiter at much higher levels
Thyroxine 5 to 13.5 mcg/dl (SI, 64.3 to 173.7 nmol/L)	Decreases 25%	Reflects declining thyroid function
Triglycerides < 150 mg/dl (SI, < 1.7 mmol/L)	Increases slightly	Suggests abnormalities at any other levels, requiring additional tests such as serum cholesterol
Triiodothyronine 80 to 220 ng/dl (SI, 1.2 to 3 nmol/L)	Decreases 25%	Reflects declining thyroid function
Urine		
Glucose 0 to 15 mg/dl (SI, 0 to 8 mmol/L)	Decreases slightly	May reflect renal disease or urinary tract infection (UTI); unreliable check for older people with diabetes because glucosuria may not occur until plasma glucose level exceeds 300 mg/dl
Protein 50 to 80 mg/24 hours (SI, 50 to 80 mg/d)	Increases slightly	May reflect renal disease or UTI
Specific gravity 1.032 (SI, 1.032)	Decreases to 1.024 (SI, 1.024) by age 80	Reflects 30% to 50% decrease in number of nephrons available to concentrate urine

Understanding HIPAA

The goal of the Health Insurance Portability and Accountability Act (HIPAA) is to provide safeguards against the inappropriate use and release of personal medical information, including all medical records and identifiable health information in any form (electronic, paper, or oral). Under the privacy standards, any health information that's individually identifiable, such as the patient's medical record, verbal and telephone conversations, and computer and financial records, must be protected. Other examples of protected information include the patient's:

▶ name
▶ date of birth
▶ Social Security number
▶ addresses (including e-mail address)
▶ telephone and fax numbers
▶ insurance identification numbers
▶ health beneficiary information.

In addition to the above-protected information, HIPAA also provides patients with these six rights:

▶ the right to give consent before information is released for treatment, payment, or health care operations
▶ the right to be educated about the provider's policy on privacy protection
▶ the right to access their medical records
▶ the right to request that their medical records be amended for accuracy
▶ the right to access the history of nonroutine disclosures (those disclosures that didn't occur in the course of treatment, payment, or health care operations, or those not specifically authorized by the patient)
▶ the right to request that the provider restrict the use and routine disclosure of information he has (providers aren't required to grant this request, especially if they think the information is important to the quality of care for the patient, such as disclosing human immunodeficiency virus status to another medical provider who's providing treatment).

Enforcement of HIPAA

Enforcement of HIPAA regulations resides with the U.S. Department of Health and Human Services (HHS) and is based primarily on significant financial fines. HHS can impose civil penalties up to $25,000 per year per plan for unintentional violations. With hundreds of requirements, fines could quickly add up. Criminal penalties can also be imposed for intentional violations, including fines up to $250,000, 10 years of imprisonment, or both.

Impact on health care practice

Keep in mind that HIPAA regulations aren't intended to prohibit health care providers from talking to one another or patients. Instead, they exist to help ease the communication process. The regulations require organizations to make "reasonable" accommodations to protect patient privacy and to employ "reasonable" safeguards to prevent inappropriate disclosure. Changes in health care practice will likely be needed to meet these reasonable accommodations and safeguards.

Employers must provide education and guidance to employees regarding the policies and procedures to be followed at their individual institutions. Responsibilities include:

▶ establishing policies and procedures for protecting confidentiality of patient information

▶ providing employee training related to the new regulations and designating employees who will be responsible for ensuring regulation compliance

▶ developing a patient medical record security system so that only those who need the patient records to treat the patient, operate the medical practice, or obtain payment will have access to the records.

Health care providers should be aware of how infractions will be handled because they, as well as the institution, face penalties for violations. Some safeguards health care providers can enact in their everyday practice include:

▶ ensuring that computer passwords are protected

▶ making sure computer screens aren't in public view

▶ keeping patient charts closed when not in use

▶ immediately filing loose patient records

▶ not leaving faxes and computer printouts unattended

▶ properly disposing of unneeded patient information in accordance with the facility's procedure.

Food and Drug Administration's list of toxic herbs

These herbs have been declared unsafe by the Food and Drug Administration because the plants contain poisonous components.

Common name	Botanical name
arnica	*Arnica montana*
belladonna	*Atropa belladonna*
bittersweet	*Solanum dulcamara*
bloodroot	*Sanguinaris canadensis*
broom-tops	*Cytisus scoparius*
buckeye	*Aesculus hippocastanum*
heliotrope	*Heliotropium eropaeum*
hemlock	*Conium maculatum*
henbane	*Hyoscyamus niger*
jimsonweed	*Datura stramonium*
lily of the valley	*Convallaria majalis*
lobelia	*Lobelia inflata*
mandrake	*Mandragora officinarum*
mayapple	*Podophyllum peltatum*
mistletoe	*Phoradendron flavescens*
periwinkle	*Vinca major, Vinca minor*
snakeroot	*Eupatorium rugosum*
tonka bean	*Dipteryx odorata, Coumarouna odorata*
wahoo bark	*Euonymus atropurpureus*
wormwood	*Artemisia absinthium*
yohimbe	*Corynanthe yohimbe*

Potential agents of bioterrorism

Listed below are examples of biological agents that may be used as biological weapons and the major signs and symptoms for each.

Potential agents	Major associated signs and symptoms														
	Abdominal pain	Back pain	Blood pressure, decreased	Chest pain	Chills	Cough	Diarrhea, bloody	Diarrhea, watery	Diplopia	Dysarthria	Dysphagia	Dyspnea	Fever	Headache	
Anthrax (cutaneous)													●	●	
Anthrax (GI)	●						●						●		
Anthrax (inhalation)			●	●	●	●						●	●		
Botulism									●	●	●	●			
Cholera			●					●							
Plague (bubonic and septicemic)					●								●		
Plague (pneumonic)				●	●	●						●	●	●	
Smallpox	●	●											●	●	
Tularemia				●	●	●						●	●	●	

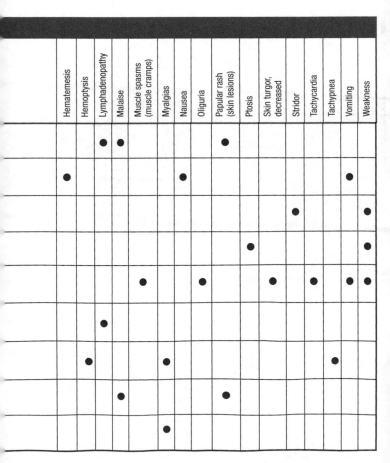

Hematemesis	Hemoptysis	Lymphadenopathy	Malaise	Muscle spasms (muscle cramps)	Myalgias	Nausea	Oliguria	Papular rash (skin lesions)	Ptosis	Skin turgor, decreased	Stridor	Tachycardia	Tachypnea	Vomiting	Weakness
		•	•					•							
•						•								•	
											•				•
									•						•
				•			•			•		•		•	•
		•													
	•				•								•		
			•					•							
					•										

Selected references

Aehlert, B. *ACLS Quick Review Study Guide*, 2nd ed. St. Louis: Mosby-Year Book, Inc., 2002.

American Heart Association. "Guidelines 2000 for Cardio-pulmonary Resuscitation and Emergency Cardiovascular Care," *Circulation* 102 (suppl 8):I1-165, August 2000.

Bickley, L.S., and Szilagyi, P.G. *Bates' Guide to Physical Examination and History Taking*, 8th ed. Philadelphia: Lippincott Williams & Wilkins, 2003.

Braunwald, E., et al., eds. *Harrison's Principles of Internal Medicine*, 15th ed. New York: McGraw-Hill Book Co., 2001.

Buppert, C., "Complying with Patient Privacy Requirements," *The Nurse Practitioner* 27(5):12-32, May 2002.

Dambro, M., ed. *Griffith's 5-Minute Clinical Consult*, 11th ed. Philadelphia: Lippincott Williams & Wilkins, 2003.

Dipiro, J.T., et al., eds. *Pharmacotherapy: A Pathophysiologic Approach*, 5th ed. New York: McGraw-Hill Book Co., 2002.

Fischbach, F. *A Manual of Laboratory and Diagnostic Tests*, 7th ed. Philadelphia: Lippincott Williams & Wilkins, 2004.

Goolsby, M.J. "Migraine Headaches," *Journal of the American Academy of Nurse Practitioners* 15(12):536-38, December 2003.

Goolsby, M.J. *Nurse Practitioner Secrets*. Philadelphia: Hanley & Belfus, 2002.

Habif, T.P., et al. *Skin Diseases Diagnosis and Treatment*.

St. Louis: Mosby-Year Book, Inc., 2001.

McLellan, K.A. "Is Your Practice Ready for HIPAA?" *Patient Care* 37(3):56-68, March 2003.

National Institutes of Health. *The Seventh Report of the Joint National Committee on Prevention, Detection, Evaluation and Treatment of High Blood Pressure.* NIH Publication No. 03-5233, May 2003. Available: *www.nhlbi.nih.gov.*

National Institutes of Health. *Third Report of the National Cholesterol Education Program (NCEP) Expert Panel on Detection, Evaluation, and Treatment of High Blood Cholesterol in Adults (Adult Treatment Panel III).* NIH Publication No. 02-5215, September 2002. Available: *www.nhlbi.nih.gov.*

Nurse's Handbook of Alternative & Complementary Therapies, 2nd ed. Philadelphia: Lippincott Williams & Wilkins, 2003.

Pillitteri, A. *Maternal and Child Health Nursing: Care of the Childbearing & Childrearing Family*, 4th ed. Philadelphia: Lippincott Williams & Wilkins, 2003.

Procedures for Nurse Practitioners. Springhouse, Pa.: Springhouse Corp., 2001.

Professional Guide to Signs and Symptoms, 4th ed. Philadelphia: Lippincott Williams & Wilkins, 2004.

Rapid Assessment: A Flowchart Guide to Evaluating Signs & Symptoms. Philadelphia: Lippincott Williams & Wilkins, 2004.

Index

A

Abdominal aortic aneurysm
  as cause of abdominal pain, 10
  as cause of back pain, 14
Abdominal pain as chief complaint, 10-11
Abrasions, 312. *See also* Corneal abrasion *and* Trauma wounds, open.
Abscess
  incision and drainage of, 333-334
  major, precautionary period for, 328t
  types of, 333
Accelerated idioventricular rhythm, 108-109, 108i
Accelerated junctional rhythm, 101-102, 101i
Acetaminophen overdose, 381-382
Acetylcysteine as antidote, 377t
Acid-base disorders, 46t
Acne vulgaris, 130-132
Acquired immunodeficiency syndrome, 225-231
  opportunistic infections in, 230t
  as sexually transmitted disease, 270-271t
Activated charcoal as antidote, 377t
Acute coronary syndromes, 169-173
Acute respiratory distress syndrome as cause of anxiety, 13
Adenovirus infection, precautionary period for, 327t
Adolescent health guidelines, 415-417
Adrenal insufficiency as cause of excessive weight loss, 40
Adult health guidelines, 418, 418t, 419-420t, 421
Advanced life support for drug overdose, 376

Adverse reactions versus age-related changes, 403, 408-409t
AIDS. *See* Acquired immunodeficiency syndrome.
Airborne precautions, 325, 326t
Alanine aminotransferase, 43
Alcohol toxicity, interventions for, 397t
Aloe-drug interactions, 388t
Alzheimer's disease, 173-175
Aminocaproic acid as antidote, 377t
Amphetamine overdose, 382
Amphetamine toxicity, interventions for, 397-398t
Amyl nitrite as antidote, 377t
Analeptic overdose, 382
Anaphylactic shock as cause of anxiety, 13
Anaphylaxis
  development of, 290
  emergency management of, 289-291
Anesthesia, 334-336
Angina, 169-173
  as cause of anxiety, 12
  as cause of chest pain, 16
  forms of, 169
Angioedema, 162-164
Animal bites, 309-311
Ankle injuries, 366
  grading, 367t
  Ottawa rules for, 368
Ankylosing spondylitis as cause of back pain, 15
Anorexia nervosa as cause of excessive weight loss, 41
Anticholinergic overdose, 382
Anticoagulant overdose, 382-383
Antidotes, 376, 377-381t, 381-387
Anti-HAV test, 57t
Anti-HBc test, 57t

---

i refers to an illustration; t refers to a table.

---

i refers to an illustration; t refers to a table.

---

i refers to an illustration; t refers to a table.

i refers to an illustration; t refers to a table.

---

i refers to an illustration; t refers to a table.

i refers to an illustration; t refers to a table.

---

i refers to an illustration; t refers to a table.

---

i refers to an illustration; t refers to a table.

---

i refers to an illustration; t refers to a table.

i refers to an illustration; t refers to a table.

---

i refers to an illustration; t refers to a table.